The Essentials of Nutrition

by

Gerhard Schmidt, M.D.

D0772186

The Essentials of Nutrition

by

Gerhard Schmidt, M.D.

Bio-Dynamic Literature
P.O. Box 253
Wyoming, Rhode Island 02898

Originally published in 1979 in German with the title *Dynamische Ernährungslehre*, Band II. The English translation by William M. Riggins, Jr. has been authorized by Proteus-Verlag, CH-9000 St. Gallen, Switzerland. The Swiss edition was sponsored by the Consumers' Association for the Promotion of Bio-dynamic Agriculture and Nutritional Hygiene in Switzerland. This American edition is published by Bio-Dynamic Literature, Wyoming, Rhode Island, under the editorship of Heinz Grotzke. Book production: Horace L. Cartter. Editorial Assistance: Anne E. Marshall, Lieselott I. Salva Cartter, Astrid Murre.

ISBN No. 0-938250-22-1

Printed in the United States of America

Table of Contents

Introduction

From Nutritional Insight to Nutritional Practice

Chapter I

Milk

A Universal Foodstuff — 1

Chapter II

Protein

The Indispensible Formative Force of Life — 48

Chapter III

Fat Substances

Stimulators of the Warmth Processes and The Ensoulment of the Organisms — 105

Warmth Production as a Basic Function of the Organism 105

Chapter IV

Carbohydrates (Sugar) as Mediators of Form and Consciousness

The Form and Nature of Carbohydrates — 154

Chapter V

The Mineral World in Nutrition: Spirit Activity in Earthly Matter — 205

Chapter VI

The So-Called Vitamins: The Necessity of Correcting
Our Current Viewpoint

Chapter VII

Nutrition in the East and West: The Hygienic Task
of the Middle — 287

Introduction

From Nutritional Insight to Nutritional Practice

The Essentials of Nutrition is a sequel to *The Dynamics of Nutrition* and has the same purpose as that book. Experience has shown that today we must develop an entirely new conception of the whole question of nutrition and that this is possible only with a view of man and the world which facilitates such a new conception. We find the firm foundation of knowledge for such an enterprise in the modern spiritual science inaugurated by Dr. Rudolf Steiner, which will be our guide in this book as it was in *The Dynamics of Nutrition*. We have already mentioned that Rudolf Steiner himself gave an abundance of suggestions in this field, suggestions which open for us a realistic view of the field of nutrition. We are convinced that today this view is more urgently needed than ever before.

We are glad to see that the interest in questions of nutrition has grown, both in the fields of medicine and natural science as well as with the general public. This is primarily because the quality of our nutrition has become increasingly questionable, the harmful effects more apparent, and nutrition-related diseases far more obvious. Along with the overwhelming spread of improper nutrition is the threatening increase in undernourishment. The authors of the new report of the *Club of Rome* thus write: "Today already 500 million to one billion people . . . are undernourished. And this poses a task of unprecedented scope to the world community." How can this problem be solved, or even approached in a rational way? In *The Dynamics of Nutrition* I gave an answer — negative at first, but thereby capturing our attention even more.

In the introduction, I wrote "that no combination of purely technical, economic and legal measures can bring about a significant improvement." External means by themselves are insufficient to deal with this crisis; we need new insights as well. We must know how such a world-wide crisis could come about in order to develop new possibilities and capacities for overcoming it. To do this, an inventory of the material resources of humanity is by no means enough; the constitution of man's spirit and soul is especially decisive. With respect to nutrition, we must learn to gain real knowledge of the whole field of nutrition, where previously we could safely follow our instincts. But because these instincts are rapidly vanishing or becoming decadent, we have the duty (in no way egotistical) to strive for such new insights and knowledge — that is, to become capable of making sound judgments. This is possible only if we break down the limits of knowledge imposed upon us by a materialistic world-view. Such a path may be taken today, and the signs of the times show all too clearly that it corresponds to an inner necessity. An understanding of man requires an understanding of nature; an understanding of nature provides the basis for the understanding of humanity. This idea, as expressed so concisely by Rudolf Steiner, stands today as a mighty summons to modern humanity to tread such a path of knowledge. And he comes closest to the inner needs and longings of humanity who asks the most questions of nature and himself—including questions about his nutrition. Both man and nature are, however, understandable only with spiritual knowledge.

The material side of things cannot of course be ignored along the path to spiritual insight into nutrition; quite to the contrary, Rudolf Steiner himself pointed out that "materialism has a certain validity." We must "attain to a thinking in material laws," but it is just as valid and necessary to "attain to a spiritual thinking for the spiritual realm." Only in this way can a knowledge of nature begin to become a knowledge of the spirit, and man be comprehended not merely as a material being, but rather as a being who incorporates spirit and soul in his earthly existence. "And thus the lowest material things always lead up to the highest spiritual things." With regard to our theme, this shows that it is precisely an apparently "inferior" or common activity like daily nutrition that requires an especially deep and comprehensive spiritual insight.

On this basis, Rudolf Steiner himself was able to progress from spiritual knowledge to practical life—to nutritional practice —and thus to give many concrete explanations, indications and suggestions, as we have already shown in *The Dynamics of Nutrition.* In the *Essentials of Nutrition,* we hope to take a further step along the path from insight into food to actual nutritional practice. It will become quite clear that one can progress to realistic conclusions about daily nutrition only by means of this type of genuine knowledge, to the extent that it is successful. Cheap recipes and instructions smother one's real inner activity, and they cannot bring about the intended change which is necessary in this field. I am not denying the value of cookbooks and the like, but am convinced that whoever earnestly works through what is here presented will be able to find his own valid nutritional form and develop his daily practice.

The conception of this current volume has developed, to a great extent, from that of *The Dynamics of Nutrition.* A third book will deal with some of the issues that cannot be fully treated in *The Essentials of Nutrition.*

Beginning with *milk*—which makes a natural starting point for our work because of its universal nature in human nutrition— the first point considered is "nutritional factor number one," the *protein question,* since protein forms the basis for our earthly life and appears as the carrier of the vital activity of the formative forces. We are led from there to the *fats* and *oils,* substances which express the forces of the inner intensifications of the soul. Then we progress to the consideration of the *carbohydrates* and their most important manifestations, the *sugar substances.* We thus come to the realm of substances which are capable of serving as the earthly support of the human Ego-organization—a capacity which reaches its highest intensification in the *mineral substances.*

In this way, we can form a picture not only of our nutrition but also of man himself. One sees that man daily renews and builds up his four fold being through his nutrition. With milk, he takes in a primal food which was once his sole source of nutrition and which, even today, reflects this universal character. This is also true in the sense that milk serves the development of all the members of man's being. In contrast, the so-called vitamins appear as a mere offspring of our limited power of intuition. They are not able to give real life, nor are they viable with regards to their definition. It would almost be possible to characterize them as "miscarriages" resulting from our one-sided thinking. Here, too, Rudolf Steiner has shown us a new way of considering these things.

In the last chapter I have added some material which seems especially relevant and important as a result of my teaching in the United States. It is clear that modern man is not merely faced with the task of developing his power of judgment in the face of the frequently one-sidedly materialistic way of looking at nutrition today, but also that he must form a sound judgment about the nutritional tendencies from the Far East which come from ancient traditions. They are often seductive because of their one-sided kernel of truth, and yet they are no longer appropriate to the times and thus can often do more harm than good. Rudolf Steiner quite clearly characterized such eastern practices, usually connected to yoga-culture, as "instruction which is given so lightly today . . . like when children play with fire," while just now "the greatest care in this field" is necessary. In contrast to the theories pressing in from both east and west, our method of consideration — both realistic and modern, born of the spiritual life of the "middle" — will become all the more sharp in its profile. It can give us the certainty that "the spiritual is the basis of everything material" , and thus that "what feeds us in the bread" is really, as a simple grace puts it, united in "life and spirit."

Thus we hope, through *The Essentials of Nutrition,* to make possible for the reader a further step from nutritional understanding to nutritional practice.

Chapter I

Milk

A Universal Foodstuff
Introductory Consideration

There is hardly a better starting point for presenting milk as a universal foodstuff than the description given by Rudolf Steiner on this theme in a lecture for teachers held on January 6, 1922. He states here: "You see, milk and milk products, and most especially mother's milk, work in such a way that their effect is spread throughout the whole person in a uniform manner. All organs are brought into harmony to a certain extent with milk and milk products. All other foods, on the contrary, have the property of influencing predominantly one particular organ-system ... With milk, the whole person comes into consideration; with any other food, a single organ-system."[1]

This result of spiritual-scientific research gives milk a universal position in the entire area of human nutrition. It belongs at the center of human nutrition not only because of its extensive effect on the whole human being, but also because it is of central importance in all stages of human life. Milk is thus not just another food—it represents the basic food which, seen in this light, may serve as a universal creator of energy in all ages and positions in life. It is, thus, indispensible.

It will be our task in what follows to create a picture of milk in such a way that the meaning and justification of this statement emanating from spiritual research are made visible. At the same time, we must remember that Rudolf Steiner spoke here of "milk and milk products" altogether and thus clearly meant the most essential milk products — first of all sour milk and curds, but furthermore the dairy products, cheese and butter. However, we must not forget that mother's milk best embodies milk's universal characteristic.

In discussing this topic, we also hope to take into account the accessible and apparently important results of research in the fields of natural science and medicine. Even in these fields the universal character of milk is supported, as can be seen in the statement of Prof. Halden of Graz who, on the occasion of an "International Milk Day," characterized the consumption of milk as a "white spring of life" for human beings.

The Plant-like Character of Milk

The first thing we would like to point out here is the position of milk in the realm of the creation of the living. As was seen in Chapter 9 of *The Dynamics of Nutrition,* we can look at milk as a product which has a position between that of the animal and plant. "Milk is something which gives only the weakest expression of the animal processes," because the inner soul process — which is most strongly manifest in the production of blood, and thus in all blood-filled organs — "is not allowed to take part" in its formation.[2] Human beings, as well as animals, externalize this inner world of forces in the process of milk production; it is led to the periphery, where it becomes selfless, as opposed to the self-asserting tendencies which dominate in blood. Milk, therefore, comes close to the same kind of process expressed by the green plants, which are devoid of inner life. Because the flowering plants point to something beyond themselves with their flower formations, and because, through the color expressed in their seed and fruit formation, they come into a relationship with the type of force which is internalized as "astrality" in animals and humans — milk comes to have a tremendously close relation to the plants.

This summarizes the above-mentioned material in *The Dynamics of Nutrition* which led to the important assertion that milk and milk products properly belong beside plant foods. A "lacto-vegetarian" diet thus in no way involves reliance on an animal diet — though certain groups of vegetarians, unaware of the true situation, still maintain the contrary; it may certainly be considered as an extended vegetarian diet. Furthermore, as we have already mentioned, milk is more than a vegetarian food; it is a universal food.

2

metamorphosis
female
1st natural ea... nourishment   *blood → milk*

The Milk Formation Process

The actual research of milk began — at least in our culture — towards the end of the last century. Like the rest of nutritional research, it went the way of quantitative analysis, and has not, to this day, become sufficiently free of it. Nonetheless, such brilliant researchers as G.v. Bunge and Abderhalden—and later W. Heupke — could make important statements about the value of milk which are still valid today. We shall have the opportunity to come back to them. First, we shall look at the process of milk formation as such, since a deeper understanding of its universal nutritive value can arise from this consideration.

Such a consideration must take into account the fact that the process of milk formation had to have followed the evolutionary processes of animals and man. We have already mentioned that the production of warm blood is a prerequisite for the production of milk. At the present stage of evolution, milk can be understood as a metamorphosis of — or a new creation from — the blood.

But we must become more specific, as it is well known that, as a rule, only the female organism is capable of milk production. Moreover, within the female organism, this production is accomplished by special organs — the mammary glands.

We have thus obtained a starting point for our considerations: the process of milk formation is a metamorphosis of the process of blood formation. It is bound to a glandular activity within the female organism. Thirdly, we must add: the organization of this milk formation is suited for a new-born animal of the same species. Milk represents the new-born's first natural earthly nourishment.

Let us first consider that milk production is bound to a glandular activity. Glandular activity is widespread in an organism. It is characteristic of the mammary glands that they are located on the surface. From an anatomical point of view, they appear as a complex of modified sweat glands.

As Rudolf Steiner pointed out in the first medical course (1920)[4] and elsewhere, the glands are organs by means of which the etheric finds its way into the physical. This is true, in general, of all glandular activity, as well as for the organs of inner secretion. Thus for each glandular activity we have two things to keep in mind: first, the activity as such — in this case, milk formation;

etheric finds its way into phys thru glands

3

second, the secretion, the milk secretion. In the production of milk, these two processes are closely related.

We may make an observation regarding the related process of sweat formation. A sense process—often quite hidden, many times obvious — always precedes perspiration. Whether it is the impression of warmth which activates the sweat glands, or a soul-impression — perhaps the sight of a fearsome beast — a sense impression always comes first, and is imparted to the glands, thus calling forth their activity. And only then does the outer secretion follow as a third stage. Something else occurs with this externalization. Not only is room made for renewed inner activity, but there is also a separation — a kind of objectification — of the previously interior substance. The externalized substance no longer belongs to the inside; it can now be viewed from without. The inner experience is transformed into something outwardly visible. At the same time, however, this act produces a certain consciousness, a self-experience in relation to the externalized substance. The process of externalization calls forth the inner experience: that art thou.

Rudolf Steiner referred to this phenomenon in a profound way, in connection with the evolution of humanity. He related how, with the descent of man to earth — characterized by the so-called "original sin" or "fall of man" — the cosmically based harmony of the members of man's being was disrupted, and thus imbalances and preponderances arose. "Thus it is with all glandular secretions, with everything in man which is a gland-like secretion process. They all stem from an excessive concentration . . . Otherwise, there would be no secretion . . . The glands would not force anything out, nothing would come out from the glands . . . This excessive concentration brings about what we might call our intuitive feeling of self."[5]

We have already mentioned that the mammary glands are modified sweat glands. If we look at the facts of embryology, we recognize that the milk glands evolve at an early stage, in the fourth week of embryonic development, and thus before the formation of sweat glands. The mammary glands are thus the oldest of the two; they take longer to develop. This fact shows us that we must look at the mammary glands as primary, and the sweat glands as secondary. Furthermore, embryology teaches that these rudimentary mammary glands are formed from the ectoderm, the outer tissue, i.e. from the same genetic structure

4

that produces the entire nerve-sense organism. We may thus say that the mammary glands developed in connection with the nerve-sense system. They are organs which have stopped along the way to becoming nerve-sense organs, just as the entire skin is a lower sense organ.

A phenomenon which is by no means self-explanatory is that the formation of the mammary glands proceeds in a like manner in both male and female organisms, and that the development of these organs is so advanced during the embryonic stage in human beings that (as is well known) they are in both sexes capable of secretion at the time of birth. They then secrete the so-called "witches milk", which contains essentially the same elements as normal mother's milk.

Furthermore, the breasts of both boys and girls develop similarly until, at puberty, they are retarded in the males and undergo a significant further development in the females. Nonetheless, their final development is not reached until pregnancy and childbirth. We shall come back to this.

As the above shows the relatively late differentiation in the formation of the mammary glands, so the early similarity between the two sexes in the functional basis of the mammaries is shown by the so-called "gynecomastia" as well as by the appearance of "witches milk". Alexander von Humbolt describes an impressive experience which he had among the Indians in the South American jungle. He there met a man whose wife had died giving birth. In despair, the widowed father held the crying baby up to his breasts. Stimulated by the child's sucking, the breast began giving milk, and the father fed the child for months, just like a mother.[6]

It has also been described how, among some primitive mammals which may still be found in Australia, the males as well as the females are capable of giving suck to their offspring.

We thus see that the potential for mammary glands is in both sexes. Their development in males stops at puberty, while in females it progresses greatly just at this time, being completed, however, only with motherhood.

During pregnancy, the female organism is profoundly changed. It becomes the bearer of a new organism. It transcends itself, in that it not only remains itself but also becomes the receptacle of a new creation. A bodily separation occurs in the act of

5

birth, but it is just then that milk production in the mammary glands begins. The activity of nursing represents a renunciation of the motherly being in the truest sense of the word.

This aspect can hardly be seen in the milk-production process as such. We shall consider this at first in relation to the process of blood formation.

Blood Formation and Milk Formation as Polarities

Rudolf Steiner pointed to a certain polarity in these processes in the first medical course of 1920, mentioned above. Whereas the process of blood formation "is strongly pushed back to the hidden side of the human organism, the process of milk formation is something which tends more towards the surface." This polarity is worthy of much consideration. It tells us that the female organism is capable of bringing a process to the surface, out of the "inwardness" of the blood. Thus, a centralized occurence is brought into the sphere of the periphery, and an "inwardized" substance is transformed into a substance which can be externalized. This newly-created substance thereby comes into the region of the nerve-sense activity, as can be deduced from the above descriptions.

New light is thus shed on the process of milk formation. In the above-mentioned lecture, Rudolf Steiner also describes how, in the human being, everything peripheral is related to the non-earthly, and everything central is related to the earthly. And he pointed to the possibility "of studying the female gender, when we consider it in its dependence on the cosmic-peripheral forming forces". The male gender, on the other hand, "may be considered in its dependence on the telluric forces of dissolution."[4] In male and female we have before us this polarity of the earth and the cosmos.

In that the female organism externalizes the process of blood formation in the process of milk formation, it makes use of this cosmic impulse, bringing it to the periphery. The intensity with which milk tends toward externalization and blood toward internalization can be seen in the following phenomenon: milk retention — that is, milk which is not externalized — leads to pathological manifestations just as, on the other hand, a significant loss of blood endangers one's health, or even one's life.

The difference in the process of coagulation of milk and blood is of interest here. Whereas blood clots on the surface of the body after a short period of time, milk does not curdle even when cooked but rather only when it comes into contact with rennet or acid. In the coagulation of both, calcium plays an important part, as it expresses its affinity for the earthly. Although with blood, forces promoting coagulation are already elicited upon contact with the surface, this is by no means the case with milk. Without a doubt, there are different forces at work in the coagulation of milk and blood.

The ability of blood to clot is an expression of the forming force of the Ego-organization. This force keeps the human being present in his physical body, whereas with severe bleeding, the higher members of man's being become detached from the body. Rudolf Steiner indicated that the force of coagulation is related to the formative force of the antimony-metal process. "These antimony forces are at work in the clotting of blood. Wherever blood in its continued existence, in its flow, displays a tendency to clot, 'antimonizing' force is there . . ." The antimony forces are especially active in everything "which becomes organizing under the influence of the forces of thought."[4] Thus, in the clotting of blood , Ego forces are at work which act as forces of thought in the upper part of man.[7] This formative Ego-force must constantly work on the blood, from above and from without, in order to protect it from externalization. This is the force of coagulation.

It ought not to work in the same way in milk. The upper forces, which live in the formation of thoughts, must be held back more strongly. It is part of milk's essence that it flows. A thought-force is here expressed which is at work whenever blood tries to avoid coagulation. Rudolf Steiner spoke of the "albuminizing" force, which works from below, creating substance a a protein-forming force. In milk, the formative force active in metabolism rises into man's middle region, as we shall see later. It thus approaches the "antimonizing" force, but may not be affected by it to the same extent that the blood is.

Although the milk and blood processes are, on the one hand, polar opposites, we must nevertheless consider them together, to the extent that blood provides the substantial basis for the formation of milk. It has been known for some time that, in spite of their quite different compositions, milk and blood correspond basically in one respect: milk and blood are isotonic, i.e. the proportions of the dissolved salts in milk are the same as those in the blood. This amazing correspondence in the salt basis has yet another aspect. It is also known that such a remarkable similarity exists between human blood and the salt-content of sea water. Of course, the ocean today has three times as much salt, but this displacement notwithstanding, blood and sea water are isotonic. This fact has, understandably, given rise to a consideration of whether blood is an internalized continuation of the original sea water, which formed the environment of living beings in past conditions of the earth. Thus, George Gray, for example, writes:

> In fact, one can consider the blood as a refined and highly developed portion of sea water, enclosed within the individual organism, which is reminiscent of earlier conditions . . . Thus, every person carries his own ocean within himself . . . Human blood is a remnant of the ocean as it once was when our most ancient ancestors attained an enclosure of sea water.[8]

The conjecture here expressed can be confirmed by the spiritual research of Rudolf Steiner, and thus seen in its proper context.

The Milk Formation Process in the Evolution of Earth and Man

Previous stages of development of the earth and humanity were discussed in *The Dynamics of Nutrition*. We saw how the environment of the beings living then was formed by a living, liquid-gas-like atmosphere (in contrast to the present day solidification), and how these beings could themselves be permeated by the occurrences in the substances outside of them. During the time when the earth was in a transition from the Sun to the Moon stage, the "protein atmosphere" not only formed the stuff of breath and nourishment but also stimulated the sense activity and reproduction of human beings. In fact, this substance was full of living primal forces, and man absorbed these forces and released them, hardly changed, into the environment. The primal life-substance was "the common blood of the whole earth."[9] But we should not imagine this omnipotent substance as similar to the blood of today. The latter is already specialized and internalized in the higher living beings. Rather, this ancient "blood", this "primal protein" is in fact primal milk. Rudolf Steiner explained

8

it as follows in a lecture given on June 30, 1924 in Dornach: "What present day man has from the mother's womb in the present stage of development, this came from air, from the environment, during the previous condition. Then, people had something milk-like during their entire lives. The air today contains oxygen and nitrogen, relatively little carbon and hydrogen, and above all, very little sulfur. They have gone. During this previous condition (Moon condition) it was different; in the environment there was an atmosphere composed not only of oxygen and nitrogen, but also of hydrogen, carbon and sulfur. There was a milk soup all around the Moon, a very thin milk soup which was inhabited."[10] And in the above-mentioned lecture we find the following: "Let us go back to pre-Lemurian times: a condition prevailed where milk was absorbed externally from the environment."[9]

The consideration of the relationship between the processes of blood formation and milk formation led us along the path through isotone to a recognition of the origin of milk in the Moon-condition of the earth. Milk was then cosmic, and it is not for nothing that the old legends speak of an ancient land "where milk and honey flow." It flowed through man as something living. Milk was the cosmic food. Out of this universal substance, man — along with the higher animals — internalized the blood. But the female organism can once again bring forth a creation of milk, out of the blood, in that it externalizes the forces of blood formation at the periphery in the cosmic sphere.

It is thus in accordance with cosmic evolution when man and the higher animals still form and develop the rudiments of the milk-producing organs equally in both genders. During the time of which we write, man was still an hermaphroditic being. Blood formation only came about when man was so far along the way toward internalization and individualization that he was no longer just a cosmic representation of his environment. This development led to the separation of the unified human being into a male and female form. "Let us think of a time when the earth was still united with the Moon . . . Man already had warm blood then, but was not yet divided into two sexes. With the separation of the Moon, we may observe the separation of the sexes."[10]

During the Moon-phase of the earth, primal milk was the cosmic nutrition of man. We may here ask ourselves if there is not, perhaps, at the current stage of development of nature, a kind of memory of this past condition. We should then be directed to the fact that, in the modern plant kingdom, there are a number of families which produce a milky liquid — especially the poppies and the spurges *(Euphorbia)*. This liquid typically flows through all the parts of the plant; the entire being of the plant is filled with milk. Without going into particulars about the significance of this phenomenon, we may say: this milk formation by plants contains an image of that ancient, nonsexual process of milk formation of the Moon period of the earth. The essentially animal-like plant kingdom was then filled with the "milk soup" of the primal life atmosphere. A convincing description of this condition is provided by G. Grohmann in his book *The Plant,* where he describes this milky liquid as "a veiled reminiscence of the animal-plant origin of the plant kingdom."[12]

But then, a new form of nutrition had to come about: "As the Moon left, the previous Moon forces could be concentrated in very special organs in the living beings." These organs are, at first, the lacteal glands of our mammals.

In the remnants of functioning lacteal glands still found today in lower mammals of both genders, we can see a memory of that second condition, when "milk became a universal food."[9] Rudolf Steiner described this as the time of the old shepherd people, represented by Abel, the son of the moon. At this time, milk was the food of mankind. The animals at that time — who, like man, had been forced into a separation into two sexes — were more advanced than humanity in terms of the inwardness brought about by combining the astral body with the physical-etheric bodies. They remained connected to the cosmos, however, in the formation of the lacteal glands and in the ability to produce milk. And man, who took in milk as nourishment, partook of a cosmic-childlike substance in so doing.

Only after further evolution could humanity also develop the mammary glands. Rudolf Steiner indicates in his book, *Cosmic Memory,* that the separation of the two sexes went on into the middle of the Atlantean period. From this, we may suppose that the transition from a universal milk diet, provided by animals, to mother's milk took place quite gradually. It is known that in earlier times, mother's milk was consumed for a longer time: among some primitive peoples today, children are still breast-fed for over a year. The more humanity developed beyond the stage of childhood, the

10

shorter became the time when milk provided exclusive physiological nutrition. Rudolf Steiner recommended to mothers that they nurse their children for five months, if possible.

The Formation of Human Milk Today

We have seen that milk represents a memory of the old Moon condition. When we ask how the formation of mother's milk came about, we must again refer to the above-mentioned unity of nutrition, respiration, sense-activity and reproduction which existed before the division into sexes. As this unity dissolved, the female bodily element remained in a stronger relationship to the cosmic past. The bodily male element on the other hand undergoes a stronger solidification, and the development of earth forces brings a future condition into the present. In the light of this, two of Rudolf Steiner's comments take on a special importance.

In a lecture to the workers at the Goetheanum, Rudolf Steiner said: "This milk liquid . . . is especially necessary for the formation of the brain. The brain in man is actually hardened milk liquid."[13] How can we learn to understand this riddle-like saying? We saw that even in the male embryo the rudiments of lacteal glands are developed, but that their development stops at puberty. Where do the forces go which the male individual does not use for milk production? When we consider that the lacteal glands remain stationary in their development towards the nerve-sense organism, we may assume that these liberated organic forces are used in the male for the further development of the brain. The male brain is not only anatomically heavier than the female, but it also provides a more powerful instrument for the development of logical, abstract thought. The female individual, on the other hand — who in part holds back these forces for milk production — will be less able to develop the forces of intellect. This is especially so during pregnancy. In this light, the saying of Friedrich Schiller about the "milk of the pious way of thinking" gains concreteness.

In another connection, Rudolf Steiner also spoke of female milk formation in an enlightening manner. "The whole mother lives in the mother's milk. We have there something that has merely changed its location within the human organization. Up to the time of birth, it is essentially active in that region which belongs primarily to the metabolic-limb system. After birth, it is

11

active primarily in the region of the rhythmic system. These forces thus move up one step in the organism." And in the lecture quoted above[10] we read, "Even today, the human being still lives in a thin soup before birth. For only after birth does the milk go into the breasts. Before birth it goes to those parts of the female body where the germinal human being is. And that is the peculiar fact, that those processes in the mother's organism which went to the uterus before birth, afterwards go into the breasts."

The forces of milk formation are active in the lower human regions before birth. They nourish the embryo from without, and are to be found in the amniotic fluid and placenta. This is a repetition of the condition in which man absorbed milk from without. This has its image in the fact that the two activities then taking place — which are embodied in the follicular hormone and progesterone — prepare the mammary glands for secreting milk, but the secretion does not take place until after birth. One may justifiably say that these two activities actually hinder the secretion of milk, or restrict the influence of pituitary activity. And it is characteristic that the path to milk formation is free not with the leaving of the fetus, but rather with the expulsion of the placenta. If even part of the placenta remains in the uterus, proper milk production hardly comes about. That is to say, that only when the mother's appendages have ceased their "milk-forming function" — when they are physically eliminated — can the milk formation "move up a level" into the rhythmic region.

Should it move up "yet another level higher", into the head, then "we see all the abnormal symptoms which appear in the mother."[3] The first thing that comes to mind here is the picture of the illness eclampsia and its effects upon the consciousness. The forces of milk production — which in the male organism physiologically "rise into the head" and help to form the brain forces — have a pathological effect on the female organism in such cases as eclampsia.

The Structure of Milk Substance

Having attempted to sketch various aspects of the process of milk formation, we shall now consider the substantial structure of milk from various points of view.

The origin of milk shows us that it is not so much a specialized as a universal substance. This follows both from its origin in

12

human evolution as well as from the present-day production of milk from the element of blood in the female organism. Even today, milk is still basically an image of the primal life substance which filled the atmosphere as "primal protein."

The first thing we notice milk is its white color. Today, this is related to its physical structure. It is not a true solution, but rather an emulsion: in it are suspended microscopic globules of fat. This indicates that milk, as a substance which cannot be crystallized, does not have any purely earthly qualities. Rather, it bears the qualities borne in previous earth epochs.[1] These finest fat globules — 1-6 million per cubic millimeter — have a relation to light known in physics as total reflection and give milk its yellow-white appearance. This is the same phenomenon which gives the moon its color.

These fat globules are encased in a membrane of milk protein (casein), and float in fresh, living milk in a way similar to corpuscles in the blood. But, although the corpuscles gradually sink to the bottom when the blood is outside the body, the fat globules, with a specific weight lower than milk, float to the top as cream. Here, too, blood and milk have developed opposite tendencies. As part of a living organism, however, both share the property of keeping their solid components suspended by the forces of buoyancy.

The fat in milk — composed primarily of olein and palmitin — is the least specific in its organic components. According to the research conducted up to the present, fat, as well as protein and carbohydrates, can be at the basis of the stream of nutrition; that is, it can be included in the metamorphosis of substances. This sheds light on why fat has a middle and mediating position within this group of three important substances. Fat also plays a mediating role in other ways, e.g. with its warmth-bearing property. It is functionally related to the activity of man's central system and thus to the leaf organization of the plant. As the central region in man harmonizes the activities of above and below, so does fat exhibit the same mediating force, which thus most often appears as the result of external forces.

"Fat is the substance in the organism which proves to be least alien when taken into the body from without ... This property of fat comes about because it carries the smallest possible aspect of the nature of the other organism (its etheric forces) into the human organism."[14] Thus, fat can easily be incorporated into the activity of one's own organism. It is there transformed into warmth by the Ego-organization. Rudolf Steiner describes how this warmth appears as formative forces in the fat of human milk. Thus, the mother conveys to the child the forming forces of her own Ego-organization. Fat — which in itself is of a universal nature — thus becomes the carrier of a process of the warmth-ether. This is how the child receives milk. For "the child cannot change anything without life into something of the warmth-etheric nature . . . he must take in milk, which is so close to the human organization, and transform it into warmth-ether. He can then use his forces for the extensive work of growth. This is pre-pared for the child in that a transformation has already taken place in the milk, so that it is easier for him to transform the necessary elements into warmth-ether."[15]

Milk protein and milk sugar behave quite differently. Milk protein (casein) is an extremely specific product of the lacteal gland. It is not to be found anywhere else in the organism. More-over it is specific to the species, i.e. man and each species of mam-mal produce their own casein. Interestingly, this protein is chemi-cally bound to phosphoric acid. This phosphorus proteid is a unique protein combination, and we may assume that, as a car-rier of light, phosphorus brings a special light-ether formative force to milk protein. Casein also proves to be stable under the effects of light and warmth: it does not coagulate even when boiled; it keeps its living structure even under the influence of much warmth. We have already indicated the relation of this "albuminizing force" and the processes of coagulation.

This does not hold for the other proteins in milk — lactal-bumin and lactalglobulin — as we know from the skin which forms on milk when heated. These proteins are more like blood in their sensitivity to external effects, and they give milk properties which are, in a certain sense, similar to those of blood. We shall return to this when considering the formation of colostrum.

The protein forces are the basis of all growth in a living organ-ism. All life, all metabolism, is kindled from protein. Thus, milk protein may be seen as the carrier and transmitter of the forma-tive forces of growth. An important relationship points to this fact, and we may especially thank the physiologist Gustav von Bunge, of Basel, for our understanding of it.

14

The Milk Research of Gustav von Bunge

In 1874, Bunge published his analyses of mother's milk and a number of animal milks. This issue occupied him late into his life. The most important results of his milk research can be found in his *Lehrbuch der Physiologie des Menschen.*[16]

The first analyses which Bunge undertook already showed a highly conspicuous difference in the quantitative composition of mother's milk from that of animals. He straightaway found a fundamental law, which he put as follows: "The more rapidly the suckling grows, the greater is the need for nutrients which further tissue formation, for proteins and for salts. The milk thus has a correspondingly different composition . . . "

This law — later known as "Bunge's Rule" — was first published in his work *Die zunehmende Unfaehigkeit der Frauen, ihre Kinder zu Stillen* (The increasing inability of women to nurse their children). He was thus the first to discover the specific nature of milk, i.e. that each milk contains the optimum nutrients for the corresponding animal species.

This is admittedly a certain limitation of the universality of milk. For a cow's milk is primarily suited for calves, and mother's milk for human infants. But milk still has its universal quality within each respective species. Further, we shall try to show that cow's milk, which may serve as a food for people of all ages, attains a universality in a wholly new sense.

But we first want to mention "Bunge's Rule" and its consequences. The values obtained by Bunge were:

Time for newborn's weight to double (in days)		100 parts by weight of milk contained			
		Protein	Ash	Calcium	Phosphoric Acid
Human	180	1.6	0.2	0.033	0.047
Horse	60	2.0	0.4	0.124	0.131
Cow	47	3.5	0.7	0.160	0.197
Goat	22	3.7	0.8	0.197	0.284
Sheep	15	4.9	0.8	0.245	0.293
Pig	14	5.2	0.8	0.249	0.308
Cat	9.5	7.0	1.0	—	—
Dog	9	7.4	1.3	0.455	0.508
Rabbit	6	10.4	2.5	0.891	0.997

"The expected relationship appears in a surprising way," wrote Bunge about this table. Fast-growing animals have a high concentration of protein and ash in their milk. But of all milks analyzed, human milk has the lowest protein and ash content. The doubling of his weight at birth, which takes place in 180 days, is at the other extreme from that of the rabbit, which needs only six days. Correspondingly, mother's milk contains 1.6g protein and 0.2g ash, as opposed to values of 10.4g and 2.5g respectively for the rabbit.

Because milk is produced in the mammary gland from blood—which has an altogether different composition — Bunge came to the following insight: Nature has given the epithelium in the lacteal glands a wonderful ability: to collect all the solid components in exactly the proportions that the suckling needs from a blood plasma which has a totally different composition." The essential difference between blood and milk again comes into view. The composition of blood is totally oriented toward the needs of the human interior. The formation of milk, however, takes the needs of the suckling — the separated living being — into consideration. We shall see that this is true not only of the minerals and protein, but also, above all, of the sugar. We shall later consider that this relation — apparently — does not hold for iron.

This knowledge was not just theoretical for Bunge. Rather, he came to the following important conclusion: "One cannot replace mother's milk with an artificial formula without harming the infant." He saw in such "artificial nutrition" a sign of degeneration and lack of conscience in many mothers. Since his time, many questionable things have come about in this field. Enterprising businesses have brought new and apparently better nutrient mixtures on the market, as substitutes for breast feeding. They have often done more harm than good, especially when it is claimed that these "artificial milks" are of higher nutritive value than mother's milk.

Spiritual-Scientific Aspects

Rudolf Steiner also left no doubt that mother's milk is the best food for infants. We already mentioned his words: "The whole mother lives in the mother's milk ..." The fact that milk is a totality is thus expressed. This fact is manifest—in the truest sense of the word—in the orientation of milk production toward the infant. A further remark of Rudolf Steiner's is also noteworthy: "A child raised on mother's milk will still be vigorous later, when 65, 66 years old. A child raised on cow's milk will be calcified when 65, 66 years old."[18] This points to the irreplaceable—even by cow's milk—nature of mother's milk. An even more important view of the subject was developed by Steiner in his course on curative education. He there says that the child's soul-spiritual element, which comes into a bodily sheath, must also come into intimate contact with its food. Thus, the food should be so constituted as to facilitate the incarnation of the pre-natal human being in an appropriate way. This is especially the case with mother's milk. For it "is a substance which actually still has an etheric body," i.e. it comes entirely from the mother's formative forces. When taken in by the child, it works "in an organizing way, up to the etheric." And "the inner contact can occur, between what is taken in and what is represented by the astral and Ego-organizations."[3]

This interplay is actually unique and represents an extremely important result of modern spiritual research. It shows that a unique connection comes about between mother and child through breast feeding: a connection between the formative-force body living on in the milk, and the child's soul-spiritual element. Milk, indeed, is the only food which retains its own formative-force organization in this sense. Plant foods have, more or less, only the effect of this organization. We can thus understand why a child raised on mother's milk remains vigorous in old age. We shall consider these relationships again.

Modern Appraisals of Milk

We must now consider the question of the relatively low protein content of mother's milk. We shall also consider it in the chapter on protein. However, it should be noted here that insightful pediatricians have clearly pointed to the irreplaceable nature of mother's milk. Prof. G. Fanconi in his essay on "The Necessity of Breast Feeding" writes: "It is today possible to feed a child right after birth with scientifically developed artificial milks. But even the best artificial milk can never replace breast feeding . . ." Another specialist in this field, F. Vasella, writes, in agreement, that according to "the most recent scientific facts . . . let us conclude that even from a purely scientific point of view, mother's milk is superior to artificial nutrients. Today this is a proven fact."[20] He thus confirms the remark of the medieval scholar, Aldobrandino da Siena, who wrote, in his book on raising children, "what is best is mother's milk." The experienced pediatrician W. zur Linden wrote, in his widely respected book, *Birth and Childhood:* "Breast-feeding a child for four to five months benefits his health for the rest of his life. Even the best milk substitute cannot offer the same protection against disease as mother's milk can."[21]

Thus the life-organization of mother's milk not only leads to health in old age, but also protects a person from sickness and even a premature death. Zur Linden writes: "The mortality rate of the bottle-fed babies is still almost three times as high as that of the breast-fed babies."

One might at first think that these life forces would manifest in a high protein content in the mother's milk. We saw, however, that just the opposite holds true. Not the amount, but the quality, is decisive here. Thus, not only protein, but rather the entire composition of milk must be considered.

The Protein Question with Milk, and the Problem of Acceleration

Bunge already came to the important insight, by means of his milk research, "that the composition of milk is one of the greatest wonders of living nature." He soon discovered a further important fact regarding protein: the protein content of mother's milk is highest during the first days of feeding (during the so-called colostrum), and then gradually diminishes. This corresponds to the at first rapid growth of the infant, who later grows increasingly slower. "The rule which we discovered for the different mammals also applies for the different stages of development of the individual." Bunge concluded from this that a wetnurse can never fully replace the mother's breast, unless she had given birth the same day as the mother. He also maintains that "the mother's organism passes on nothing which the infant cannot utilize."[16] [17]

We are here directed to a number of facts which give us some idea of the wisdom at work between mother and child, and which lead us to ask about their deeper significance. This significance can be found in an intimate relationship with overall human existence, the earthly incarnation of humanity, and the goal of humanity. Thus, these aspects are too close to our subject to be passed by. We thus come to a theme which has proven fruitful not only in the fields of physiology and chemistry, but also in

18

contemporary anthropology. The spiritual-scientific research of Rudolf Steiner can also make an important contribution here, as we shall see.

Let us first consider the anthropological aspect, an important example of which is the research of A. Portmann (Basel), published in his book *Biologische Fragmente einer Lehre vom Menschen.*[22]

Starting with altogether different assumptions, Portmann called man a "physiological premature birth", a "definitely deviant autophagous type." Although apes attain adult proportions earlier on in their embryonic life, and are already "a miniature image of the adult form" at birth, "hereditary factors hold humans back from taking on the bodily proportions of the species as early." Man takes on adult bodily proportions "late after birth." The all-important "holding back" of human development is seen here. Portmann, in his chapter on "The First Year of Life", explains that in this period the human being actually grows more quickly than the ape. But his development is altogether different. In fact, it is only after a year that the human child reaches a level of development "which a genuine mammal of a corresponding species has at the time of birth." Human pregnancy would have to last about a year longer, if we were to attain the same condition at birth which we in fact achieve about one year after birth! We thus repeat in the first year what (physiologically) the anthropoids go through as embryos. Our growth in length seems to correspond to "fetal proportions." The growth into these bodily proportions, during the first year, is, however, determined by the expression of the typical human form of existence: "gaining an upright posture, learning to speak with words, and entering into the sphere . . .of thinking and doing." In coming to these three "important occurrences", the obvious difference between man and animal plays an essential role. "The powerful growth of the [human] cerebral cortex and its paths is related to the weakening of the instinct-organization, the decrease in the number of offspring, and the increasing weakening of sexual drives" on the one hand. On the other hand, it leads to "the development of human intelligence, an upright gait, and the ability to speak." Both are dependent upon the normal development of the brain, which is also the cause of the weight increase in humans during the first year, which is spread out over the entire period of growth

19

among anthropoids. On the other hand, the total growth period of human beings is much longer, and the term "retardation" was coined to express this fact. Whereas the anthropoid apes are in old age after twenty or thirty years, human beings have a life span at least twice as long, in which "an impressive, general characteristic of our type of life — increased individuality" — is expressed, "the expression of the specific nature of the individual."[22]

This awareness comes to expression when we say that an animal "lives" his life, while a person "leads" his life.

Compare this to Bunge's statement: "In human beings, old age — the period of decreasing forces — lasts longer than in any animal. This is perhaps related to the fact that it takes longer to bring up a human being in order to bring about the high level of mental development."[16]

As we have seen, it has long been known that protein is primarily responsible for the growth of the organism and for building up the body. This fact sheds a new light on the low protein content of mother's milk. As the human being grows during the first year, it is not just a matter of building up the body, but also (as we have seen) of taking on the typical human form of existence: an upright posture, speaking and thinking. K. Wetzler, who takes up the ideas of Portmann to a large extent in his short work *Menschliches Leben in der Sicht des Physiologen* (1972) writes:

> If a human child at birth were a genuine mammal, he would have to be . . . similar to the adult, and to have mastery over the rudiments of communication common to the species (speaking in gestures and words.) But this stage — often considered the beginning of being human by biologists and phychologists — is not reached until a year after birth.[23]

The apparent contradiction that man "grows considerably more quickly during the first year than do all anthropoid apes",[23] takes on an new aspect with Portmann:

> The increase in weight in humans up to birth—this much larger size of human babies, compared to anthropoid apes—is meaningful only in light of the following. The difference in weight between the human and ape brains at birth is proportional to that of adults. Moreover, the greater bodily weight of our newborns can only be understood as an approximate adaption to the considerable weight of the brain.[22]

Perhaps one could say that the considerable bodily growth of human beings during their first year can be seen as a sort of

20

adaptation to the brain, a sort of repetition in the entire organism of the intense growth of the embryo brain. But, as the central nervous system is "the most regularly stimulated organ", the brain "is favored by the metabolism." Portmann again emphasizes that the activity of standing upright "is a process primarily directed by the organization of the central nervous system."

The "actual process of becoming human" — corresponding to the time of breast-feeding — thus takes place by means of a clear reduction in protein consumption.

We may consider this conclusion of Bunge's: "The sexual functions [represent] a form of growth beyond the limits of the individual." Thus, protein also serves the development of the sexual functions. In this light, Portmann's statement about the "continuous damping of the sexual drives" becomes unusually interesting: the "tremendous increase in the size of the brain" occurs as the counterpart to the "weakening of the instinct-organization." This polarity may explain the low protein content of mother's milk, which appears to be ideally suited to "actually becoming human." Furthermore, as Bunge discovered, human milk is the lowest in protein because the human being grows the most slowly.[16]

Since then, this problem has taken another turn. This is the problem of acceleration, which Portmann related to nutrition in 1944 (in the above-mentioned book) and which has since been examined from the most varied points of view.

Portmann handles this question of "transformation of maturity" in modern times, maintaining that "twelve-month-old children are today about 1.5 to 2.0 kg heavier, compared to the time around 1890" — just the time when Bunge was pursuing his milk research. "The increased growth in the first year of life is especially strong."[22] He writes, further on: "We must consider, for example, that since the large population increase in the nineteenth century, nutritional conditions in the west have constantly changed. This has meant an increasing share of high-quality protein in the diets of larger segments of the population."[22]

W. Lenz, in his work *Ursachen des gesteigerten Wachstums der heutigen Jugend* (1959), shows that infants "today are, on the average, about 1.5-2.0 kg heavier at the end of their first year than were the infants 50-70 years ago. Moreover, they are about 5 cm taller." He relates this phenomenon to "improved nutrition.

21

especially with protein." We want, finally, to mention Du Pan (Geneva), who has studied this question more specifically. He showed, in his work *Die Ursachen des gesteigerten Wachstums,* that "among the natural foods which improve the size and weight of a well-nourished child", milk stands at the top of the list, and calcium stands above all other minerals.

More pertinent for us is the research of E. Wollny, which relates directly to the "influence of acceleration on the composition of mother's milk."[16]

Wollny confirmed that the time taken for a newborn's weight to double has been reduced from 172 days (1890) to 124 days (1967), i.e. it has accelerated 28%. At the same time, she examined the question of whether the composition of mother's milk has changed in this time, and is thus related to the acceleration.

On the basis of her own extensive research, Wollny concluded that "in the last 70 years the average protein content of mother's milk has increased 0.13g (=12%) and the average ash content 0.03g (=15%)." This is a clear confirmation of Bunge's law. Even more, it shows that the rate of growth today is higher than the protein and ash content would indicate: mother's milk would today have to have 1.37% (instead of 1.2%) protein and 0.256% (instead of 0.23%) ash to correspond to the modern rate of growth. Wollny could show that "there is a surprising correspondence . . . if one gives children the nutrients which, according to Bunge's rule, correspond to the present-day rate of growth." In order to double the weight within 120 days, a protein content of 1.24%, and an ash content of 0.27% in milk is indeed adequate; i.e. it has almost exactly the values which, theoretically, mother's milk today would have! "The fact that it effectively remains behind" is due, according to Wollny, to the fact that "the milk produced corresponds to the level of acceleration of the mother's own generation, and not to that of the child." But this correspondence also adheres to Bunge's law.

Equally important for our theme is Wollny's research into "differences in the rate of growth between artificially and naturally fed infants." She concluded that, today, children who are not breast-fed double in weight more quickly than those who are breast-fed. At the turn of the century, just the opposite was true. At present, bottle babies reach double their weight at birth in only 118.6 days, compared to 136.8 days for breast babies. At the turn of the century — during Bunge's lifetime — the corresponding ratio was 156 to 174.9 days.

Lest one conclude that breast feeding is inferior, however, we should consider the "irreplaceability of the mother's breast" discussed by Bunge.[16] During his own time, Bunge warned of the danger of overfeeding children who are not breast-fed. For "the infant is not satisfied at the right time", whereas breast feeding is an instinctive regulator of the child's intake.

In view of the worldwide discussion of the phenomenon of acceleration, this milk research is again pertinent today, as we have tried to show. Wollny's work shows how this research can be of help. We may thus add the conjecture she presents at the conclusion of her research:

> It is conceivable, for example, that the accelerated and constantly increasing rate of growth of infants must be seen not at all as a physiological phenomenon, but rather as something pathological, or in any case, as something more exogenous and forced on the infant than as an endogenous phenomenon.

E. Ziegler (Winterthur), who has also studied the problem of acceleration (in part from another point of view), expresses his concern as well:

> Today many doctors, psychologists, psychiatrists, educators, social workers, judges, sociologists and politicians are disquieted, and almost no one tends toward seeing the phenomenon as harmless, as was once the case.

He notes, further, that not only before birth, but "also during infancy, acceleration has appeared dramatically, especially during the last decades as more use was made of modern nursing substitutes."[27]

We are here reminded of the "formula" infant food — the product of American research — with 2.5 times more protein and even more salt. The results of this nutrition include "the increase in acceleration with the huge gap between the physical and psychological/mental maturity which so troubles educators."[28]

Portmann certainly speaks in the same sense when he says: "The phenomenon of increasing height — which we do not see optimistically — is for us a crack in a tightly woven whole. Through it, something from the hidden depths looks up, while we look at it with concern, due to our ability to have insight into a complex system."[22]

Portmann alludes here to "the tightly woven whole" of human existence, the earthly development of which has gotten some "cracks". This theme is touched upon in more depth by the spiritual research of Rudolf Steiner. Although only a short discussion of this topic is possible within the framework of this book, we would like to emphasize a number of points which are essential to our "dynamics of nutrition."

Further Spiritual-Scientific Insights

When a person is born, his mode of existence is profoundly changed. Before birth, his developing body was enclosed within the mother's womb, and his nutrition flowed to him. He is then suddenly separated from this enclosure and is on his own, from a physical point of view. He must accommodate himself to the conditions of the earthly world. Mother's milk is the only — and last — thing which comes to him from the sheltered environment he has left. Because "the whole mother" lives in the milk, it is important — indeed indispensible — for the transition from the existence before birth to that after birth. The child receives not only nutrients in the milk, but also the mother's warmth. Since nothing comes between mother and child during breast feeding — i.e. the milk flows directly from one living organism to the other, never coming into the physical environment — we may say that the mother's life-organization, her complex of formative forces, flows to the child in a unique way.

It is here appropriate to look into a certain law discovered by modern spiritual science: that the development of earthly humanity occurs in certain rhythms. At birth, the physical body becomes independent. But its life-organization, the etheric body, does not reach independency until the change of teeth, occurring around seven years later. Until then the "model" received from the mother by the forces of heredity is at work in the child. In addition, the wisdom-filled forces of the pre-earthly world as such are active in the child's organization . At this time, they still act organically, "bound to the processes of growth and nutrition."[29] They work on the "plastic formation of the brain, and the development of the rest of the organization." In this way, they build up the bodily basis for the trinity of abilities typical of humanity: uprightness, speech, and thinking.

These three abilities are the essential difference between man and animals and form the basis for the future development of the three soul forces: thinking, feeling and willing. They are formed during the first three years. One can, indeed, say: man here works upon himself in the most wisdom-filled way — doing so from the unconscious depths of his being which are connected with the cosmic forces.

What has this got to do with milk? Rudolf Steiner here made an important discovery. It was first communicated to the teachers in his lectures on *The Study of Man*[30]. "When we give a child milk, it acts as the only substance — at least in essence — which wakes the sleeping spirit. It is the spirit, which is in all matter, which manifests itself where it should. Milk bears its spirit within itself, and this spirit has the task of awakening the sleeping spirit of the child."

We indeed come to the center of a "dynamics of nutrition" with such an indication. Rudolf Steiner may himself have sensed that he came to a new world of knowlege with such a statement. For he added to the above: "It is not a mere picture, but rather a profound, established, natural-scientific fact, that the Genius of nature — which brings forth the substance 'milk' from the mysterious depths of nature — wakes the human spirit sleeping in the child. Such profoundly mysterious relationships in worldly existence must be grasped. Only then will we understand what wonderful, cosmic laws are really in the world." Such cosmic laws cannot be discovered — or even understood — by our modern scientific way of thinking. On the contrary, this way of thinking leaves us "dreadfully ignorant when we construct theories about material substance, as if this substance were an indifferent contrivance which breaks down into atoms and molecules." In reality, matter is quite different, and that constitutes its dynamic character. Steiner continues, saying that milk is a material which "has the most ardent desire to wake the slumbering human spirit." To speak of "desires" of living substances will appear quite new to modern thought, and could all too easily appear absurd. But a thinking such as we described and developed in *The Dynamics of Nutrition* will have access to this new concept, which we have here as a further element of a "dynamics of nutrition." For "just as we may speak of a 'desire' — i.e. of a force upon which the will is based — with respect to man and animals, we

25

may also speak of desires with respect to matter in general." Steiner here adds a sentence especially relevant to this chapter on the universality of milk: "We have a complete view of milk only when we say: milk, when produced, desires to awaken the child's human spirit."

In this sense, the child is a continuation of "that activity which we allow the Genius of nature to take up, when she feeds the child with her milk and allows the mother to be merely the means by which the child is fed." Thus, "feeding with milk is the first means of education."

What a depth is given to the contributions of Bunge — and of modern anthropological research — by such insights! The above-mentioned problem of acceleration takes on whole new dimensions. We shall return to this later on, in the discussion of nutrition in youth.

First, however, these considerations bring us to a number of further problems.

Milk as the Expression of the Threefold Human Organization

Rudolf Steiner's discussion of this subject contains a further indication concerning the character of milk. We first came across it in this form: milk is related to the human nerve-sense organization, as it is produced at the periphery of the human form. On the other hand, we have seen that milk production takes place in the middle region of man — in the rhythmic organization — and this phenomenon appears to be typically human. Rudolf Steiner says that this process can "rise up a level" in man. It is furthermore significant that the formative forces of milk come from the limb region. This gives milk a third characteristic which Steiner emphasizes in the above-mentioned *Study of Man* where he says that milk "is the only substance in the human and animal kingdoms which has an inner relationship to the limb-being, which in a certain sense is born from the limb-being and which also retains the forces of the limb-being."

This connection of milk to the limb forces gives it the property of awakening the slumbering human spirit. For this connection gives it a sort of will-character. This allows it to take on the role of building a "bridge from the will to the sleeping spirit of the child." Thus, a bridge is built between the time of birth and the point where the educator's activity can be effective. Rudolf Steiner could say, "if milk could not build this bridge, we humans would waste away because of the gap in our development during earliest childhood."[3]

We thus come to a brand-new possibility for assessing milk. It is certainly of the greatest importance, and has never before been recognized and expressed in this form.

In human beings, this will-element in the process of milk formation is, however, raised from the lower limb system to the upper. "In female humans, milk arises in relation to the upper limbs, to the arms." The will-element of milk is thus not eliminated, but rather transformed and humanized. It is raised to the region of the human heart. The will is filled with heart forces.

In the animal this process remains behind in the lower limb region. We thus see another difference between human and animal milk. Mother's milk is, indeed, an expression of the entire, threefold being of man. All forces—the nerve-sense organization the rhythmic system and the metabolic-limb region — are there united in a comprehensive harmony. We again see the indispensable nature of mother's milk in this universality. This cannot hold equally true for animal milk, for animals are unable to form a threefold organization as human beings can do. There is something else here worthy of note. Rudolf Steiner, in his book, *Agriculture,* called attention to the unique nature of the dairy animals.[31]

These dairy animals — primarily cows, but also sheep and goats, as sources of milk for human beings — have been altered by the human art of breeding. Their milk formation process has also been brought into the rhythmic element. "Consider an animal which should be strong in this middle region, where the head organization — the nerve-sense organization — develops more toward respiration, and where the metabolic organization becomes more rhythmic . . . you then have the dairy animals." Thus the wisdom which inspired ancient humanity in breeding animals has brought forth in the dairy animals a form which is oriented toward the model of the threefold human organization. The milk from these animals has thus taken on a character similar to mother's milk, though it can never be the same.

We here see why the milk of domestic animals — in the broadest sense including not only sheep and goats, but also horses and donkeys — can be an appropriate food not only during childhood, but also for the rest of one's life. This insight takes the wind out of the sails of those who argue that these milks are only there for the respective animal and not for human beings. Just the opposite is true: the dairy animals are oriented towards humanity with respect to their milk formation, though not with respect to their meat formation.

This milk takes on the character of the human organization to such an extent that it can have a brand-new function: not only the raising of the species, but also the process of shaping man. This is perhaps one reason why the cow was revered as a holy animal in old India, and its slaughter for human consumption was forbidden.

Dairy animals also produce a product which bears this universal character, though not to the same degree of perfection and uniqueness as human mother's milk. This should be considered with respect to milk products as well: sour milk, curds, cheese and butter.

Rudolf Steiner here emphasized, however, that proper care of this dairy-animal character is necessary, to keep up the quality of the cow's milk. This is a question both of keeping and of feeding the animals.

We mention this important problem only briefly, but we wish to do so emphatically. The free movement of animals—as opposed to their confinement in dismal stalls—stimulates their limb forces and gives them "the chance to relate to the world through sense perception." The feed with enough leaf and herb content stimulates the rhythmic forces of the animal, "and then good, plentiful milk is produced."[31]

We see that the quantity as well as the quality of milk is an important agricultural problem. Without this insight, milk will continuously lose its universal character for humanity. Also, the various manipulations of milk after milking endanger its value.

Milk as a "Biological System"

We should mention a few points before looking at this complex. Modern researchers have rightly emphasized that, in reality, milk "is not an unvarying, uniform, trade article; its composition varies considerably." The composition of milk — as a biological system — is not the result of a chemical synthesis. Rather, it is the fruit of the interplay between the animal and its interior and its environment. We have already pointed to the activity of this inner world in milk production from one point of view. In addition, there are the hereditary factors which influence the process of milk formation among the various breeds. It is, for example, known that the fat content of milk is largely determined by heredity. On the other hand, among the environmental forces not only feeding, but also the forces of the changing seasons, plays a large role. The fat content of cow's milk "clearly varies with the seasons, and is higher in winter than in summer."[32] The fat-free solid components show a similar change: protein and mineral content drop during the summer, while the lactose (milk sugar) content is less clearly affected by the change in seasons. The influence of outside temperature is an especially important factor among the forces of the changing seasons. This warmth factor points to the activity of cosmic forces which is essential to the milk production of animals. Light, as well as warmth, here plays an important role as a cosmic force. Interestingly, the age of the cow is apparently of minimal importance for milk production, according to modern research. The health of the animal is far more important.

Having mentioned the varying fat content of milk, we should return to something previously mentioned: the formation of fat globules with their typical sheaths. This form of milk — an emulsion — has today been especially well-researched through the use of microscopic techniques. It has been revealed that these globules have different diameters. The size of the globules among the different breeds of cattle is affected by heredity. However, their size also varies during the course of lactations. There are 1.5 to 3 billion fat globules per milliliter of cow's milk — an enormous sum. The surface area of milk is correspondingly immense. It has been calculated at approximately 550,000 cm^2 per liter. This property of milk — also characteristic of human milk — is significant for its digestability, for even in the small intestine, fat must be in the smallest droplets in order to be digested. Milk is thus an easily digested food — a fact which Rudolf Steiner also emphasized.

In addition, these globules have a special structure. A fine protein and lecithin sheath surrounds them. It also contains other

29

important substances, such as phosphorus lipids and the metals iron and copper. There are also vitamins A and D there, which are characteristic of milk. One sees that, in fact, these fat globules carry a whole string of important substances. Because the globules are in a state of equilibrium with the plasma (the liquid component of milk) — i.e. they are suspended in it — the forces of buoyancy are also at work in them. They remove milk from the exclusive influence of the earth forces. The spherical form of these innumerable, delicate creations reveals their cosmic character. When milk is left standing, these globules move upwards: a layer of cream is formed. As we shall see later, this property is important for the production of butter.

We would here like to mention a process significant in the dairy industry today: homogenization. Its importance can be seen in the fact that, today, not only milk as such is subjected to it, but also cream, ice cream, condensed milk and some types of soft cheese as well. Homogenization consists of pumping milk through small openings under high pressure, thus breaking the fat globules down into smaller particles. Milk then loses its tendency to form a layer of cream. It is questionable that this alteration of milk's structure by technical means improves it nutritionally. It is more a matter of convenience for the modern dairy industry. It has been argued that homogenization reduces the size of the fat globules in cow's milk to about that of mother's milk, thus making the former similar in digestability to the latter. But it must be kept in mind that this alteration is wrought at a pressure of 300 lbs. and is not similar to the physiological process underlying the production of mother's milk. Milk as a "biological system" is thus profoundly altered.

The Functions of Lactose

Lactose stands out among the component substances especially characteristic of milk. We have pointed out that human milk has the highest sugar content—7%—of all milks. Bunge mentioned this fact but could not see its significance.

The first interesting fact is that lactose is a new creation of the organs of milk production. It is not to be found in the blood nor, indeed, anywhere else but in milk and a few rare exceptions in the plant kingdom. We may assume, then, that this sugar formation
30

is of special value for the infant. Moreover, it is known today that lactose remains longer in the gastro-intestinal tract than any other common sugar. This favors a better utilization of the calcium and phosphorus in milk, which is very important to the infant. Also galactose, which comes from lactose, can be used to produce the cerebrosides, important structural units in the brain and nerves.[32]

These properties point to the special significance of sugar in general, and of lactose in particular. We shall describe, in our chapter on sugar, how sugar is inwardly related to the development of the human personality. The physiology and, even more so, the pathology of sugar metabolism show the close relationship between sugar utilization and human consciousness. A deficiency of sugar in the blood leads to drowsiness, then to sleep or unconsciousness (coma).

We can see that lactose has a special task in light of the function of milk as "the awakener of the child's human spirit."[30] The significance of lactose for consciousness is expressed not only in its crystallization, which shows its earthly structure as opto the cosmic orientation of fat. In addition, the improved utilization of calcium and phosphorus furthers the activity of sugar in the formation of the "personality character," i.e. the formation of the necessary earthliness and the possibility of the development of consciousness as well. It brings people to a "healthy power of judgment in earthly matters." (Rudolf Steiner). This is further seen in the way that lactose stimulates the processes of formation and maturity in the brain and nerves.

In this way, the power of transformation of the growth forces of protein is directed toward the abilities of uprightness, speaking and thinking. The low protein and high lactose content of human milk make clear what is needed for human development. Indeed, man must learn "to stand with both feet on the ground" and still to develop spiritual capacities.

We shall later discuss the significance of lactic acid as a product of the fermentation of lactose. Lactic acid, formed in the organism with the help of bacteria, is hardly less nutritious than lactose. Moreover, it has been used since ancient times in form of sour milk, buttermilk, yogurt, etc. in various ways, in both regular and special diets.

About the Minerals in Milk

The mineral content in milk shows its relation to lactose in its ability to crystallize. We have already mentioned calcium and phosphorus, both of which are plentiful in milk.

Among the minerals in milk, calcium is especially plentiful, and milk is one of the most calcium-rich substances. This should not surprise us, when we consider how much the infant needs the calcium forces and bone-building earthly substance. Calcium makes milk an earthly food to a large extent. The physiological calcium content of mother's milk here plays a role in its proportion to the other substances. If, for example, an infant is given cow's milk too rich in calcium, this can lead to problems in later life. "For example, one can give a child milk from cows whose nutrition comes from an area too rich in calcium. The child can then get too much calcium by drinking the milk of such cows. This may not be apparent at first. . . But the child raised on mother's milk is still fresh when 65, 66 years old. The child raised on cow's milk is calcified at 65 or 66. This shows that milk is a totality. What happens at one time shows its effects much later."[18]

On the other hand, we have already emphasized the high phosphorus content. Both calcium and phosphorus appear in organic compounds and in solution. Phosphorus, as the stimulant of the forces of consciousness, joins company with calcium, the bringer of terrestrial forces.

Equally important is the excretion of magnesium in milk. Magnesium is the carrier and mediator of the light-ether forces, especially in the plant world. It thus plays a central role in chlorophyll. It also works in human beings whenever the directing forces of light are at work in forming the organism — especially in the teeth and muscles. It is essentially a constructive substance. On the one hand, it appears in milk as an excretion of the organism which no longer needs the constructive magnesium force. On the other hand, it is in this way that it comes to the infant.

An obvious contrast to the high magesium content of milk is its low iron content. Much has been said about this phenomenon. It has been argued that the new-born organism brings a store of iron with it and thus does not need any more until this store is used up and it can obtain iron from a different diet. This may be true, but it really does not explain why milk is so low in iron. The indications of Rudolf Steiner, already mentioned, shed light on this phenomenon. He says that milk — in spite of a certain polarity to blood — nevertheless has "a similar formative capacity" to blood. Still, we see "a considerable difference" between these two in the different iron levels. To understand this, we must remember that milk today comes from the blood. But, at the same time, blood is a metamorphosed form of "primal milk."

This metamorphosis resulted in the separation into two sexes. Humanity thereby immersed itself in matter. There came a separation from the cosmic forces, an inwardness, an independence as an earthly being. In falling away from the cosmos, "blood, by its own being, became ill," for every separation from a connection with the cosmos signifies illness. Iron came into the evolution of blood in order to heal it. "The blood must constantly be healed in the organism. In contrast, that is not the case with milk."[4] This shows the creative force of milk. Oriented toward the cosmos, it moves into the periphery with its formative forces. It leaves the iron behind, because it leaves the illness of the blood behind.

Once again, it was Bunge who saw the mineral content of milk (in the form of salts or ash) in relation to the rate of growth of the newborns. It was shown that human milk contains relatively less of these substances than do the animal milks. There is a correspondence between ash content and the rate of growth, as with protein. Moreover, the colostrum has the highest mineral content, and the values later generally decrease.

The following indication should aid in understanding this process, which we shall look at in detail in chapter 5.

It seems significant that a relatively large portion of the minerals are organically bound to the protein in milk. Casein (casein phosphate) in particular exhibits this property, which brings the protein into an active living condition. Its orientation to the forces of growth thus becomes understandable. Phosphorus and calcium are both necessary—in large quantities—for building up the skeleton. Moreover, we must be clear that in man — albeit in a qualitatively more subtle way — all these minerals are put into the service of the consciousness-forming functions. We discussed this in *The Dynamics of Nutrition* (cf. Chapters 8 & 10). In the human organism, the minerals are put at the service of a higher organization which lends man his actual Ego-character.

They thus have a dual function in man. In animals, they remain more strongly bound to the metabolic functions and serve the construction of the soul-organization. Where they have a broad field of activity and can manifest in many ways.

The Curdling of Milk

Curdling may be called a natural process. It comes about from the effect of bacteria on milk left exposed. In this way, part of the lactose is gradually transformed into lactic acid. At the same time, a coagulation of protein takes place under the influence of the lactic acid. This happens with the casein-calcium compound in milk. The calcium frees itself from the casein, and the latter coagulates in a mass. In addition to lactic acid, a number of other acids are produced in small quantities, e.g. formic acid, butyric acid, acetic acid and carbonic acid.

The process here is similar to the digestion which takes place in the human stomach and intestines. Sour milk products are thus rightly considered easy to digest. They therefore play a large role in many special diets. Buttermilk — a by-product of butter production — is especially noteworthy here. It is low in fat, but still contains 3.5% lactose as well as live lactic acid bacteria. Its activity in the large intestine, which pushes back the putrification of protein, was discovered by Metschnikoff. Because of its similar properties, he introduced yogurt — an ancient sour milk product from the east — into curative diets in the west. His belief was that the intestinal poisons — coming from the putrification of proteins — promote arteriosclerosis through the blood. This was interestingly confirmed by Rudolf Steiner.

In a lecture to workers[33] Steiner spoke about the exaggerated consumption of protein then being advocated. "But he [man] does get something from it. For, before leaving, it remains in the intestine, becomes poison, and poisons the whole body! . . . This poisoning often leads to hardening of the arteries."[33]

In this respect, sour milk products are of great importance. We shall later emphasize other dietary aspects of the subject. It should here be mentioned that the nature of lactic acid has recently been more thoroughly researched. It has thus been established that it appears in three different forms. These are at first differentiated by their optical properties under polarized light.

34

In muscles, the dextro rotary L-lactic acid is produced. The bacteria in yogurt usually produce the laevoratary D-lactic acid, and certain intestinal bacteria produce the optically neutral DL-Lactose. All three are physiological products, but they behave differently in the metabolism. In any case, they do not acidify the organism, but are, rather, alkaline. We shall examine this more closely in Chapter 5.

Lecithin has been seen as a valuable component of buttermilk. It contains phosphorus, and is closely related to the nerve metabolism and to the liver functions. Bunge discovered that human milk has the highest lecithin content. He described the effect of this substance with respect to the formation of the brain and nervous system. He found that the brain is the organ richest in lecithin. He writes in his *Physiologie:* "The development of the brain is quite different in different mammals. We would thus expect that the ratio of lecithin to protein in the milk would be higher in animals whose newborns have a relatively heavier brain. In fact, that is the case. The relative weight of the brain is, as follows:

Calves	Cattle	Humans
1:370	1:30	1:7
*1.40%	2.11%	3.05%

*—The lecithin content (in % of protein)

The connection of lecithin metabolism to the liver has since been researched. It was found that the choline from lecithin hinders the depositing of fat on the liver and furthers its function of detoxification.

This leads us to the bridge to the relationship between milk and milk products and to the functions of the liver in general. Not only is milk protein the least problematic for the liver, but there are also other substances in milk which are good for the liver. Cottage cheese has proven to be especially valuable to a liver-cure diet.

Whey and Butter

As important as the sour milk products is whey. It is produced when the protein and fat are largely removed from milk. Sour whey is formed when the whey undergoes a natural fermentation. Sweet whey is produced by adding calf rennet, which comes from the stomach of young calves which have been slaughtered. These wheys—known in ancient Greece—were used for curative purposes even into the nineteenth century in some places. Various things were added to make a tasty combination (e.g. herb whey, apple whey) which was used as a dietary therapy for diseases such as tuberculosis, jaundice, colitis, etc. A saying came from the famous medieval medical school in Salerno: *Indicit que, lavat, penetrat, mundat.* This was expressed in German as follows:

> Von den Molken weiss man dies,
> Dass sie lösen und durchdringen,
> Und recht häufig in dem Leib
> Gute Reinigung vollbringen.
>
> ————
>
> Whey is held, by those who know,
> To loosen up and penetrate;
> It often cleans the body out
> In a way that is truly great.

Whey is today again gaining in respect. It is certainly significant that Rudolf Steiner recommended its use.

We are thus already in the realm of the curative uses of milk, which we shall later consider separately. At this point, these indications are meant primarily to emphasize the universal character of milk. We have seen that milk is a "nerve food" as well as a "metabolism food." Another process brings out the third characteristic of milk, in the making of butter.

Butter-making is an ancient process. As is known, it makes use primarily of the properties of the milk fat: the specific form of the globules. Butter-making was once an art. Today it has become a technique, concerning which comprehensive theories have been made. Essential factors in butter-making are warmth, air, and water, which are shaken in a way which brings the fat globules into a kind of crystalline structure. A complex emulsion results, which makes a mass capable of being spread.

It is here of interest that, in butter, the third characteristic of milk comes forth: its relation to the middle region of man. We shall deal with this in the discussion about fats in general. But we should here mention that Rudolf Steiner ascribed a value to butter in human nutrition. This judgment not only takes the plant-like nature of milk into consideration. It also relates to the appropriateness of milk for human nutrition in general.

36

About the So-Called Vitamins in Milk

Before coming to our final evaluation of milk, we should look at its so-called vitamins. The reader of *The Dynamics of Nutrition* probably noticed how little this show-horse of modern nutritional research was to be found there. In this volume, we wish to consider the vitamins more thoroughly, and have dedicated an entire chapter (VI) to the subject. Here we wish only to mention what is pertinent to our consideration of milk.

Once again, it was Bunge who was among the first to ask if factors other than the known nutrients played a significant role in the human organism. He came to this question through his experiments with milk. In this regard, milk is at the starting point of vitamin research. It therefore seems justified to discuss vitamins here.

Kollath described Bunge's nutritional research as follows: "Bunge concluded: the organism needs something else; it is a task of science to recognize this something else. He thus prepared the way for vitamin research . . ."[34]

At first, the question of what this "something else" was remained open. Bunge's way of thinking leads us to see that he came close to reality. He said, for example: "None of our nutrients are chemical individualities, but rather aggregations." One thus has the impression that Bunge was not searching for new nutritional components along the path of dividing and isolating substances. However, his experiments were given this interpretation.

Rudolf Steiner also knew of these experiments and he often spoke of them. He referred to them, for example, in a lecture where he said: "What does science do today when it wants to research the nutritive force of food? . . . Science analyzes a certain food, and looks to see how many components of one or another so-called chemical substance are in it . . ." He then spoke of the experiments of the "famous physiology professor, Bunge . . . who fed milk to mice." But "the composition of the substance is of no account . . . This is what the gentlemen should have told themselves . . ."[18]

Bunge himself had similar thoughts. In the last year of his life (1920), he wrote to his brother ". . . 'vitamin' is only a name; no one has isolated it. Modern physiological chemistry is in danger of becoming physiological economy. It consists in inventing

37

Latin and Greek names for substances which remain unknown."[35]

In the above-mentioned lecture, Rudolf Steiner said: "The gentlemen said to themselves: well, there must be a new substance in there . . . And the people called this new substance vitamins." He returned to this theme in the same lecture cycle on December 15, 1923. "The pupils of Bunge simply said, well, there is a life substance in milk, and in honey too: it is vitamin." But, Steiner added, "It is just as if one would say 'wasting away comes from emaciation.' Here one says, there is a 'vitamin' in there."[18]

We see clearly here how materialistic thinking again won out. The whole ensuing avalanche of vitamin research took the direction which Steiner predicted.

In contrast, we find a concise statement from him in a medical lecture: "A whole new way of considering things must come about." What way? the reader might ask. In our opinion, a dynamic way.

Wilhelm Pelikan spoke about this clearly in a noteworthy essay. He wrote: "If one removes 'vitamins' from their subtle state and concentrates them in the normal, three-dimensional, coarse state, they lose everything mysterious. Vitamin C becomes a white substance that looks like salt, ascorbic acid, just like all the other acids the chemist has in his laboratory. A vitamin is not

We may say something about the vitamin-complex of milk along these lines.

It should be kept in mind that milk is formed primarily for the infant's nutrition. The processes taking place in it—which precipitate as vitamins—are all meant for the young, growing organism only, even if they have a more general effect as well. And thus the question of the universality of milk again arises.

It is characteristic that vitamins are active in all life processes, in building up the organism, in the metabolism. In the latter —according to one publication—they "are mediators of the processes of building up and breaking down, but do not themselves serve as building material."[37] They thus show their dynamic character, which has to do with activities, not with substance. They "act as catalysts", i.e. they stimulate processes and interplays in the realm of life. They are, indeed, power centers of the world of formative forces.

38

It is no surprise that the two most important vitamin function-chains in milk — vitamins A and D — are connected to the cosmic energies of sunlight in their formation. In order to manifest in the realm of substance, both must be exposed to an adequate amount of sunlight in the human skin.

Vitamin A is formed in milk "in such quantity that it is fully sufficient for the infant and growing child," according to W. Heupke.[38] It is found in the smallest fat globules in milk, which we described above. It is found in these cosmic, round structures, which overcome gravity and reveal their origin in their signature. A deficiency in this process is first manifest as weakness. First comes a decrease in productivity. Finally comes a disease of the human light organ—the eye—called xerophthalmia, which results in an opaque cornea.

The process connected to vitamin D works in a different way. There is also a clear relationship to the light metabolism. The so-called ergosterol, as "provitamin D 3", is found in milk. It is transformed in the skin by sunlight and becomes vitamin D. It furthers and directs the incorporation of calcium and phosphorus into the bone substance. It has thus been called the "anti-rickets vitamin."

The effective vitamin is formed upon contact with light. It is in no way a "building block" in the organism. It is entirely a carrier or stimulator of processes — in this case the calcium process — which are activated by its presence. It is thus clear that the materialization of such a process comes at the end. It represents what Paracelsus called the "end of the way of God." And milk, as the producer of the "provitamin", stimulates man to complete this process which directs the regulation of the calcium metabolism. (cf. Chapter 5)

Such insights make it clear that the addition of synthetic vitamin D to milk works against the true function of this process.

We may assess the vitamin B group — also found in milk — in a similar way. This group works primarily in relation to the nervous organization. Heupke's discovery holds true here, as well: The vitamin B 1 found in the total milk complex "is more effective than synthetic vitamin B 1. Thus, nervous disorders (neuralgia, neuritis etc.) are cured faster, and relapses are more easily prevented, when the patient drinks milk regularly."[38] The situation with lactoflavin — vitamin B 2 — in milk is analogous. It is noteworthy that it is substantially enriched in sour milk, for the bacteria there activate its formation.

We thus come to the realm of the curative effects of milk, which we shall briefly consider later on.

Sheep, Goat and Donkey Milk

Before coming to our concluding discussion, we shall look briefly at other milks used in human nutrition. One example which has recently come to the fore is sheep's milk. Its appropriateness for human beings is seen neither in its high protein content (4.7%) nor in its relatively high fat content (5%), but rather in the quality of the fat. The above-mentioned property of milk fat — the formation of small globules — is especially developed. The globules are smaller than those in cow's milk, and more similar to those in human milk. Sheep's milk is thus praised as easily tolerated and digested, and is therefore of value to stomach and liver patients.

On the other hand, its high orotic acid content has occupied modern research. This is about 350-450 mg/liter, compared to 100 mg/l for cow's milk, 63 mg/l for goat's milk, and much less still for human milk. Modern research has discovered that orotic acid stimulates growth. It also plays a role in the production of certain important substances for the liver metabolism (pyrimidines). Thus orotic acid (or sheep's milk) is used in cases of liver parenchyma disorders, for reconvalescence and in geriatrics.

However, these uses should bring us to consider that this intensive, growth-stimulating property is similar to that of protein (orotic acid contains nitrogen.) It should thus be given the same consideration that we gave to protein earlier on in this chapter. The fact that sheep's milk is clearly higher in protein than human milk also points in this direction. This in no way speaks against the use of sheep's milk and milk products—cheese, yogurt etc. — in special diets. As a remedy, it will prove increasingly valuable. But as a normal food, it should be used sparingly.

In this respect goat's milk is more similar to human milk. It contains less protein than cow's and sheep's milk, but has a higher sugar content (3.7% to 4.6%). Its fat content is similar to that of human milk (4.0%), but it is less rich in vitamins, and its sharp taste is not appealing to everyone. Goat's milk cheese, on the other hand, enjoys widespread popularity. One should keep

40

in mind, however, that in some cases, goat's milk can cause a special type of anemia.

Sheep's and goat's milk play a large role in the nutrition of those peoples who specialize in raising these animals. The original yogurt from Bulgaria is made from sheep's milk and the longevity of these people is today attributed to the above-mentioned properties of sheep's milk.

In recent times, people have been taking special note of mare's and donkey's milk. By the end of the nineteenth century, there were a number of donkey herds which were milked for the children of wealthy parents. Its composition is, in fact, most similar to that of human milk (1.9% protein, 6.6% lactose). But in spite of all similarity — which is doubtless an advantage of this milk — one must remember that all animal milk is different from human milk. For clinical applications, however, mare's milk has its justification and advantages.

Finally, we should mention that even a milk with such an extreme composition as reindeer milk is often consumed by northern peoples (e.g. in Lapland and Siberia). Bunge himself noticed that, with a fat content of 17.1%, reindeer milk represents an extreme. He discovered, however, that the climate plays a large role here. All animals in northern climates have a more or less fat-rich milk. The high point in this respect is attained by dolphin's milk, with 43% fat. The watery environment of this mammal must be kept in mind here.

Final Consideration

We shall now turn to a final consideration of milk and will first look at the use of milk among various peoples.

Without a doubt, milk is one of the most important foods in Europe. This means predominantly cow's milk. A number of countries are even able to export surpluses of milk or milk products.

Milk is also drunk on the other continents. Its use is an ancient cultural element especially in Asia and Africa. Whether reindeer, horses, sheep, goats, camels (in Tibet) yaks or cattle—the most widespread — these animals were everywhere kept and bred. Often, this was done primarily for their milk. Milk was processed, even in early times, as yogurt, Kumys, Kefir (both contain alcohol!), butter and various cheeses. The enormous cattle herds of

41

certain black African tribes have been known of for centuries. The relationship to cows in India is especially interesting.

Milk was there primarily an object of religious veneration. This fact determined the relationship of the ancient Indian toward using cows and milk as food. K. Buhler-Oppenheim, who conducted interesting research in this field, wrote: "The religious use of milk probably originated in pre-historic times."[39] There are many indications of the holiness of the cow in the Indian holy scriptures. The *Atharva-Veda,* for example, says: "The cow is to be revered as the God-world, as the world of the immortals ... " Something is here expressed which we shall continue to look at: milk as the expression of cosmic and earthly forces. Later, in the great Indian epic, *Mahabharata,* the holiness of the cow is expressed in these words: "Whoever kills a cow, or permits a cow to be killed, will burn in hell for as many years as the cow has hairs on its hide." Interestingly, not only the cow itself, but also its five products, are holy: milk, curds, buttermilk, manure and urine. In certain instances, it was indeed required of Brahmins that they live only from these five products. Understandably, a hierarchal priesthood then cared for the animals. This was also true of the holy buffalo herds of old Indian tribes.

The ancient Egyptians evidently also had a religious relationship with milk animals. Similarly, we find indications from the Greek and Roman cultural epoch that milk was used as a sacrificial food, e.g. in the original Dionysius cult. In ancient Italy, Ceres was brought a sacrifice of milk. Also in the large, ancient, African cultures, milk animals enjoyed religious veneration.

Buhler-Oppenheim concludes his enlightening exposition with these words: "Wherever the cow is worshipped as a holy animal, everything related to it is also holy: the milk, the urine, the dung, every hair on its body, even the paths it walks and the tracks it leaves behind."[39] But this is ultimately because the cow is a milk animal, capable of producing a universal foodstuff.

We have encountered this universality in many forms. With respect to the religious nature of milk, described above, the reader is here reminded that, in Chapter 12 of *The Dynamics of Nutrition,* we pointed to Rudolf Steiner's description of milk's character as "primal nutrition." From the cradle of humanity — where it was still a general nutrient, externally absorbed from the environment — onward, it has accompanied man through all stages of develop-

42

ment. This alone justifies its religious veneration.

Milk is literally an echo of the primal food of man. It came from the living formative forces of the world long before it was cast into the world of organisms. The "thin milk soup", as Rudolf Steiner called this primal food, filled ancient Lemuria as a "protein atmosphere," bearing the universal forces which reflected the innocent condition of humanity. This quality is preserved as an echo in milk even today.

The "three phases of milk nutrition" were mentioned in Chapter 13 of *The Dynamics of Nutrition*. They go from the general etheric nutrition, to the condensation into the earthly form of milk, and finally to the "condition where mother's milk is consumed." This points to the wonderful, comprehensive development of a substance which is most intimately connected with human evolution.

In his lectures on "The Development of the Forms of Nutrition" already mentioned, Rudolf Steiner spoke of the "Sons of the moon . . . who raised only animals and fed themselves from their milk." This "moon generation" is represented in the Old Testament by Abel. It is a still child-like stage of human development, in which the Jehovah forces are at work. "If we go back to the most ancient times, there is no other food than milk. It is the food from the living animal, the original food." The Cain people left this stage behind and chose to nourish themselves with grain. At the same time, the transition was made to dead nutrition — a plant diet including roots, and the consumption of slaughtered animals.

Milk, which still remains connected to the process of life, retains this original state within itself. However, it has been transformed according to the development of humanity, and it has increasingly taken on the properties it has at present.

This is also a criterion of its universality: it carries all the phases of human and terrestrial evolution within itself. This can help to explain why milk is able to resist and withstand the attacks made upon it by modern technology — pasteurization, sterilization, homogenization, condensation, etc. Without a doubt, though, milk's value is decreased by these processes.

The development here outlined makes it clear that, in our time, the milk for human beings is primarily mother's milk. In truth, nothing can replace it. Furthermore, during the stage of development after infancy, milk in general serves as a basis of

43

nutrition. We can thus understand what Rudolf Steiner said about milk and honey in his lectures on bees. "One could discover that honey can be significant even for small children. One should put a little honey in the milk: more milk, less honey . . . "[18]

On November 10, 1923, Rudolf Steiner said, "When we are children, we expedite the forming forces from the head by drinking milk."[15] For older people, however, he suggested looking for these forces in honey. "Honey, not milk, is primarily of help to old people."

One might assume from this that Rudolf Steiner did not recommend milk to old people at all, or only in the sense of "a little milk and a lot of honey." But this only applies to the stimulation of the formative forces from the head region.

From the point of view of the universality of milk — which has been our main emphasis — we may come to an altogether different conclusion. Rudolf Steiner presented this view in a lecture on nutrition held on December 17, 1908.[40] He emphasized the fact that in the production of milk "the etheric body comes into consideration." This refers to the living complex of formative forces which belong directly to milk, and which differentiate it from all other foods. "Therefore the consumption of milk in old age is adventageous. It is especially significant for a person because, under the influence of continued milk consumption, he is able to take up special forces into his etheric body which can have a healing influence on his fellow man." This clearly states the significance of milk, for older people, which comes from its etheric force. On the one hand, it works against the aging forces of the astral body. It thereby stimulates of the forces of the nervous system. In this way, milk becomes a medicinal food in old age. On the other hand, a person can himself develop healing forces by consuming milk. "Healers, who heal in a spiritual manner, often see a special preparation for their vocation in such a consumption of milk . . ."

With these indications, we return to our starting point, the universal character of milk. We have seen how milk came from an originally supersensible world of formative forces and filled the entire world at that time. As humanity descended to the earth, milk gradually condensed into an earthly substance. It thereby led mankind into the earthly world, yet continued to bear its vital, cosmic origin within itself. Thus Rudolf Steiner could say: "Everything which comes to the human organism from the consumption

44

of milk prepares it to be a human, earthly creation. It brings it into the conditions of the earth. It makes man into a citizen of the world, but does not hinder him from being a citizen of the entire solar system." The decision to consume milk is to say: "I want to dwell on the earth, to be able to fulfill my mission upon earth, but not to exist solely for the earth."

This is a most appropriate characterization both of milk's uniqueness and of its universality. At the same time, it is clear that milk can be replaced neither by plant nor by animal foods. It is an irreplaceable element of human nutrition. However its true character will be opened to us only when we learn to use the key given to us in the modern spiritual research of Rudolf Steiner.

Earlier times had such a key instinctively. Today, we must learn to use it consciously. We must therefore learn to pay much more attention to the quality of milk, and to the conditions of its production and preservation, than has yet been the case.

References

Milk—

1. Rudolf Steiner, *Die gesunde Entwicklung des Leiblich-Physischen als Grundlage der freien Entwicklung des Seelisch-Geistigen* (GA 303). 1921/22 Fifteenth lecture, 6 January 1922, "Die körperliche Erziehung im Besonderen."
2. Rudolf Steiner, Lecture given 8 January 1909 in Munich, "Ernährungsfragen im Lichte der Geisteswissenschaft."
3. Rudolf Steiner, *Heilpädagogischer Kurs*, Dornach 1979 (GA 317). Reference is here made to the 12th lecture, given in Dornach on 12 July 1924. English translation, *Curative Education*, London, 1972.
4. Rudolf Steiner, *Geisteswissenschaft und Medizin*, Dornach 1920 (GA 312). English translation, *Spiritual Science and Medicine*, London 1975.
5. Rudolf Steiner, *Die Welt der Sinne und die Welt des Geistes*, Dornach 1979 (GA 134). English translation, *The World of the Senses and the World of the Spirit*.
6. J. Schwabe, *Archetyp und Tierkreis*, Basel 1951.
7. G. Schmidt, "Wandlungen in der Anschauung über die Bedeutung der Bakterien," in *Der Beitrag der Geisteswissenschaft zur Erweiterung der Heilkunst*, Vol. III, 1952.
8. George Gray, *Auf Vorposten der Medizin*, Zürich 1944.
9. Rudolf Steiner, Lecture given in Berlin, 4 November 1905, published in *Grundelemente der Esoterik*, Dornach 1976 (GA 93A).

10. Rudolf Steiner, *Heilpädagogischer Kurs*, Dornach 1979 (GA 317). Reference is here made to the fifth lecture, given in Dornach on 30 June 1924. English translation, *Curative Education*, London 1972.
11. Rudolf Steiner, *Aus der Akasha-Forschung, Das Fünfte Evangelium*, Dornach 1975 (GA 148). These lectures were given in 1913/14. English Translation, *The Fifth Gospel*, London 1968.
12. G. Grohmann, *Die Pflanze*, Vol. I and II, 1949/51. English translation, *The Plant*, Rudolf Steiner Press, London, 1974.
13. Rudolf Steiner, *Mensch und Welt. Das Wirken des Geistes in der Natur. Über das Wesen der Bienen*, Dornach 1978 (GA 351). Reference is here made to the seventh lecture, given in Dornach on 31 October 1923.
14. Rudolf Steiner/Ita Wegman, *Grundlegendes für eine Erweiterung der Heilkunst nach geisteswissenschaftlichen Erkenntnissen*, Dornach 1977, first published in 1925. English translation, *Fundamentals of Therapy*, London 1967.
15. Rudolf Steiner, *Der Mensch als Zusammenklang des schaffenden, bildenden und gestaltenden Weltenwortes*, Dornach 1978 (GA 230). The cycle of twelve lectures was given in Dornach in October/November 1923. English translation, *Man as Symphony of the Creative Word*, London, 1970.
16. G. v.Bunge, *Lehrbuch der Physiologie*, Vol. I, ninth lecture, 1905.
17. G. v.Bunge, "Die zunehmende Unfähigkeit der Frauen, ihre Kinder zu stillen," Munich 1900.
18. Rudolf Steiner, *Über das Wesen der Bienen*, Dornach 1923 (Part of GA 351). English translation, *Nine Lectures on Bees*, Spring Valley 1975.
19. G. Fanconi, "Die Notwendigkeit des Stillens," in *Schriftenreihe der schweiz. Vereinigung für Ernährung*, Heft 23a, Bern.
20. F. Vassella, "Über die Ernährung des Säuglings."
21. W. zur Linden, *Geburt und Kindheit*, Frankfurt/M. 1963. English translation, *A Child is Born*, London 1980.
22. A. Portmann, *Biologische Fragmente einer Lehre vom Menschen*, Basel 1969.
23. K. Wetzler, "Menschliches Leben in der Sicht der Physiologen," in *Neue Anthropologie*, Band II, Stuttgart 1972.
24. W. Lenz, "Ursachen des gesteigerten Wachstums der heutigen Jugend", in *Akzeleration und Ernährung*, Darmstadt 1959.
25. R. M. Du Pan, "Die Ursachen des gesteigerten Wachstums."
26. E. Wollny, "Untersuchungen über den Einfluss der Akzeleration auf die Zusammensetzung der Frauenmilch," Dissertation Frankfurt/M. 1967.
27. E. Ziegler, "Wachstumsbeschleunigung und erhöhter Zucker-

konsum," in *Neue Zürcher Zeitung*, No. 239 of 27 May 1970. Also, "Betrachtungen über den säkulären Wandel der Ernährung in der Schweiz," *Schriftenreihe der schweiz. Vereinigung für Ernährung*, Heft 12, Bern 1970.

28. R. Dubos, *Mirage of Health*, Doubleday 1961, J.A.M.A. 182/8.
29. Rudolf Steiner, *Die gesunde Entwicklung des Leiblich-Physischen als Grundlage der freien Entfaltung des Seelisch-Geistigen*, Dornach 1978 (GA 303). Reference is here made to the seventh lecture, given in Dornach on 29 December 1921. English translation, *Lectures to Teachers*, London 1948.
30. Rudolf Steiner, *Allgemeine Menschenkunde als Grundlage der Pädagogik*, Dornach 1980 (GA 293). English translation, *Study of Man*, London 1975.
31. Rudolf Steiner, *Geisteswissenschaftliche Grundlagen zum Gedeihen der Landwirtschaft*, Dornach 1979 (GA 327). English translation, *Agriculture*, London 1977.
32. Jenners/Patton, *Grundzüge der Milchchemie*, Munich 1967.
33. Rudolf Steiner, Lecture given in Dornach on 2 August 1924 to workers. The lecture is published in *Die Schöpfung der Welt und des Menschen. Erdenleben und Sternenwirken*, Dornach 1977 (GA 354).
34. W. Kollath, *Getreide und Mensch*, Bad Homburg 1964.
35. G. Schmidt, *Das geistige Vermächtnis von Gustav v.Bunge*, Zürich, 1973.
36. Wilhelm Pelikan, "Von den Vitaminen" in *Der Sanddorn*, Arlesheim 1964.
37. *Roche Vitamin Kompendium*, Basel 1968.
38. W. Heupke, *Milch, das Schutz — und Heilmittel für Gesunde und Kranke*, Frankfurt.
39. K. Bühler-Oppenheim, *Verbreitung und Nutzung der Milchtiere*, Basel 1948.
40. Rudolf Steiner, Lecture given in Berlin on 17 December 1908, published in *Wo und Wie findet man den Geist*, Dornach 1961 (GA 57).

The publication dates mentioned refer to the latest editions available in German and English.

Chapter II

Protein

The Indispensible Formative Forces of Life

There is no problem in modern nutritional science so hotly contested—and apparently so far from settled—as the question of the significance of protein. The scientific research of this substance began in the middle of the last century and has since been in constant flux; thus it has often produced contradictory and opposing results and views. Such remains the case today. Georg Borgstrom's statement, in his book *Der Hungrige Planet* (*The Hungry Planet*), is especially relevant to protein: He writes: "With the help of the analytic method, we have come, in part, to some good insights. But we are ensnared in the false belief that by assembling the pieces of information in an analytic mosaic, we can come to a true picture of the world. Yet experience and research have shown that a realistic picture can never be had in this way." Unfortunately, however, in spite of this experience, there are hardly any signs that researchers are looking for new methods. Bergstrom acknowledges, in the light of his extensive nutritional research, that "What we need is a fundamentally new concept of research, its tasks and its goals ... A total picture must be created, taking into account the nutritional needs and physiological constitution of man, as well as the social structure."

In *The Dynamics of Nutrition,* I often sought to portray the inadequacy of the analytic method. I tried to show that one must use different methods when researching the living world.

It must be acknowledged that Rudolf Steiner performed a great service in laying a foundation for this in 1886 (at twenty-five years of age!) in his work *A Theory of Knowledge Implicit in*

Goethe's World Conception.[2] In his autobiography[3] he wrote, "I want to show how one must go about gaining knowledge in order to penetrate into the phenomena of life in the consideration of Goethe's organics." Although "the ideal of the non-organic sciences is to work the totality of all phenomena into a unified system . . . the ideal of organic science must be to find — as perfect as possible — in the species and its manifestations, what we see evolving in the individual beings." This holds especially true for protein, for it represents a prototype of life.

Such viewpoints can lead to understanding "that for a realistic evaluation of the facts, the gross material substances and their direct effects do not stand in the foreground. The world presents itself to the unprejudiced observation of the process of knowledge as an organization springing forth from spiritual forces. Thus, the basic insight is opened into substances as the carriers of the expression and effect of the non-substantial." These words of Herbert Witzenmann are from his work *Ueber die Erkenntnisgrundlagen der Biologisch - Dynamischen Wirtschaftsweise.*[4] They relate to a passage from one of Rudolf Steiner's few special nutrition lectures:[5] *"Behind everything material is spirit. Thus, behind all the matter we take in through our nutrition, there is also spirit . . . By means of nourishing ourselves with this or that, we enter into a relation with something spiritual, with a substrate which is behind the material . . ."* This means, however, that "in the consumption and entire digestion of food in the human organism, not only a material, but also, at the same time, a spiritual process" takes place.

An exact knowledge of these processes can come only from a realistic view of human nutrition. It is therefore no surprise that the spiritual-scientific indications about nutritional hygiene are in no way merely theoretical but also bring about highly practical results. They shed a significant light on today's pressing questions in this field. They are, doubtless, even able to fructify modern research.

General Characteristics of Protein

In order to be able to point to such concrete results within the framework of our presentation, we shall here turn to a topic especially important and widely discussed today: the *question of protein.* We must, of course, limit ourselves to an outline of this difficult and broad-reaching subject, but this should still allow for the consideration of some essential aspects of the problem. One can clearly see the relevance of what Rudolf Steiner said in another lecture on nutrition. "Protein is something which is usually falsely evaluated when one does not look at it from a spiritual-scientific point of view."[6]

To characterize the problem quite clearly, let us begin with the statement of a modern nutritional researcher, Professor H. Aebi of Bern. He calls protein the "number one nutritional factor."[7] This means that "protein is not only the most important, but also the most valuable nutritional component." The name "protein" points to this. The researchers of the nineteenth century chose this name — based on the Greek word "proteios," the first or most important — for this *forming substance* (as Justus von Liebig called it.).

On the other hand, the German word for protein, *Eiweiss* (literally "egg white") points to a fact discovered by William Harvey. He wrote *"Omne vivum ex ovo"* — everything living comes from the egg — showing that protein is the "bearer of life" (Aebi). This is the most important role of protein and brings up two further points. Protein serves reproduction as well as regeneration in the living world. Furthermore, because life is manifest in an infinite number of ways in the organism, protein is also a substance, which, according to Rudolf Steiner, "can be transformed by its formative forces in the most manifold way."[8] Therefore "every living being" must build up protein "according to its own blueprint" (Aebi); i.e. every organism has its own specific protein. Human beings, however, are able to build up an individual protein, even a specific protein for each organ. This capacity makes each person a "physiological individuality" according to the American, Williams, and others. Nonetheless, in Steiner's words, protein must also "have the ability to give up the form which nature gave its material components, when called upon to take a form for the sake of the organism." Aebi describes this situation as follows: "The deeper significance of digestion is this: to remove the foreign character of the ingested protein . . . and to construct it according to the appropriate blueprint."

The following statement from K. Lang's *Biochemie der Ernährung*[9] is also significant for our theme. He writes: "The older authors wrote that entire proteins — or large pieces of

50

them—are absorbed from the intestines. This has been shown to be false. Research has been done using methods beyond any objection. Even with the most sensitive experimental arrangements, no peptides or proteins were found in the mesentery blood or the blood in the portal vein. Using immunobiological methods, it was determined that tiny amounts of entire molecules of protein can be absorbed. These amounts are so small, however, that they cannot be detected with the most sensitive method of immunoelectrophoresis today. Even in newborns, immunoelectrophoresis showed no entire mother's or cow's milk proteins which pass through the intestinal membrane..."

Somewhat further on, he writes: "Human beings absorb only immeasurably small traces of entire protein. This absorption is nonetheless important, as it brings about the allergic reactions that many people have to certain foods."

We thus see how a person guards against every foreign protein in order to maintain his "physiological individuality," which is also immunological individuality. This is done from the first day of life.

This brings us to a second important fact relevant to nutrition. Protein, as the bearer of life and as "building material", is constantly subjected to renewal in the organism. For, ultimately, life is the present, the moment. Protein therefore cannot be stored or conserved like fats or carbohydrates. It is constantly changing, coming and going. It is always subjected to an intense process of renewal, *pantarei* as the Greek sage Heraclitus called it. "Everything flows" is a significant characterization of protein. In the words of modern spiritual research: "Protein is always on the point either of being taken into the activity of the etheric body (i.e. into the organization of formative forces) or of falling away from it."[8] This leads to the constant building up and breaking down of protein in the organism, to the necessity of its being renewed daily through nutrition, and of being excreted every day.

Moreover, modern research has shown that this process of renewal "occurs at a widely differing rate, according to the type of protein and the organ."[7] Here are a few examples which help us to characterize protein. The protein in the ganglia in the brain is renewed, on the average, every nine hours. The so-called half-life of enzymes is likewise only a few hours. In contrast, the liver takes about ten days for its protein to be renewed, while the mus-

51

cles take 150 days, and the interstitial tissue about 160 days. Thus, the most varying rhythms of building up and breaking down protein hold sway in the organism. Its healthy functioning requires that it execute this process in every moment at the right time, at the right place and in the right way. We thus come to the activity of the "body of formative forces", as Rudolf Steiner often described it, especially as it is expressed in the protein activity. There is, however, a polarity here which is also known to modern protein researchers. It is the separation of protein into "globular protein" and scleroprotein. The latter appears primarily as "frame material", e.g. as collagen in tendons and cartilage, as the so-called connective tissue. The globular proteins appear primarily as the components of egg cells, of blood and of enzymes. The scleroproteins last a relatively long time, the globular proteins, a short time.

We thus have a functional polarity which is of importance to the human organism. Our whole protein organism is divided into two parts. One has more to do with reproduction, and also with the forces of inflammation. The other is related to hardening and the sclerotic forces, which also have a strong formative tendency. The forces of reproduction are here held back.

We should pay attention to this polarity when trying to understand the effect of protein in human beings. This is the functional polarity which is expressed in the metabolic organism which is set against the activity of the nerve-sense organization. We should here like to mention the description given by Rudolf Steiner in the lectures *Spiritual Science and Medicine* (1920).[10] In the first lectures, our attention is directed to these "formative forces", which are reproductive and regenerative in the metabolism — in the "lower" organism — but which are also especially strong in the embryo and in the lower animal kingdom. Rudolf Steiner called them "forming forces" *(Plastische kräfte),* which reminds us of Liebig's "formative matter" *(Plastizierungsstoffe).* In human beings, however, these "forming forces" are partially "lifted out of the organs," — e.g. in the nerve and sense cells — and then appear as soul-spiritual forces. "Whenever I think or feel, I think or feel with the same forces which exercise a formative activity in the lower animals or in the plant world."[10] They also work similarly in the human metabolic and reproductive processes.

52

Protein thus comes into the "upper" man under the influence of forces which push back this "plasticity." They are transformed into the ability of the soul to think and feel. The protein itself is transformed in its character and structure. It becomes scleroprotein, appropriate for the building up of form and frame. As such, its rate of renewal is decreased.

An important statement by Rudolf Steiner, in a lecture entitled "Heilweise und Ernaehrung im Lichte der Geisteswissenschaft" (October 22, 1906),[11] makes the basic character of protein clearer. Among other things, we read there: "The greatest imaginable care must be taken, that neither too little nor too much protein is taken into the body. Just the right amount absolutely must be found." We are here confronted with the question still discussed today: How much protein does a person need? The answer here given by Rudolf Steiner is purely qualitative. He speaks of the polarity between the upper and lower human being. "When the lower is not in harmony with the upper, this gives rise to trouble." For the proteins in the digestion correspond to the production of mental pictures (*Vorstellungen*) in the thought activity. If we burden the metabolic sphere with consumption of too much protein, the higher activities, "which make for effective thinking", will correspondingly suffer. A person is then "overpowered by his ideational activity, from which he should become free." This means that this thought activity becomes too strongly bound by this corporeality. "Therefore, the consumption of protein should be kept within certain limits."

With this description by Rudolf Steiner, we come to the center of the protein problem. We see clearly that there are definite limits to the need for protein in human beings. This is related to its nature and purpose. As the bearer of life, it is indispensible. Nonetheless, it must not hinder the other pole of the human being, that of consciousness. There must be a proper balance between the two poles. Otherwise, one activity would overpower the other. Therefore, "just the right amount absolutely must be found."

Taking this fact as a start, we may proceed further into the question of protein. It will prove to be a key to many as yet unanswered questions and can shed light on many important results of modern protein research.

Indeed, the research into protein in the last decades has opened new perspectives in the fields of bio-chemistry and phys-

53

iology. As a result, some central questions have been revived, questions concerning the riddle of life, the problem of evolution and the existence of man and nature.

An eloquent witness for this is a passage from the introduction to a modern American work, *Structure and Function of Protein* by Dickerson and Geis:[12]

> If you asked a chemist a hundred years ago about the difference between living and dead matter, he would probably have referred to the "life force", *vis vitalis* or some special property of living matter. Today, the difference would be made according to the complex, ordered and differentiated reactions. In principle, the chemistry of living cells is no different than that of dead matter. It is only more intricate, refined and therefore stimulating, just as a pocket watch is more interesting than a sling shot, and a computer is more interesting than a pocket watch.

We shall later deal with this important statement more specifically. It is presented here as an indication of the direction of modern protein research, and of the conclusions reached through the methods of this research.

Historical Aspects of Protein Research

The first considerations of protein did not raise such a question. At this early point, one could not imagine anything but the living. The view at this time led much more to questions of metabolism, digestion and assimilation.

Hippocrates, in the *Corpus Hippocraticum,* developed the view that there is a basic substance in all foods which is taken into the human body by means of a double cooking process. The necessary heat — the *calor innatus* — originates in the heart. The cooking *(pepsis)* of the nutrients takes place in the stomach, where the fluid "chyle" is formed. In the second step, the spleen with its black bile steps in, transforming the nutrient fluid into blood. When the latter coagulates, it forms the inner organs, as well as the other bodily fluids.

This view of the important role of warmth in the digestion of food was taken up centuries later, first by Paracelsus and then by van Helmont. They are looked upon today as the originators of the "chemical digestion theory." But it is significant for both that they considered the *Archaeus* to be the actual *director digestionis,* the ruling force of digestion.

Here we have a conception which summarizes the last remnants of an originally instinctive insight into the essence of the

54

living. The human being, as a being of warmth — of fluids living in a fourfold stream — was not yet seen as the interplay of physical and chemical forces, such as are found in lifeless nature. One saw, rather, an inner process, at once living, ensouled, and permeated with spirit. One experienced the reality of the "etheric body" in the vitality of the fluid movements. The warmth streaming from the heart was experienced as *pneuma,* as spirit. This view, which Hippocrates drew from consciousness of the etheric, was only a shadow by the time of Paracelsus and van Helmont. Finally, in the seventeenth and eighteenth centuries when the so-called "dynamic school" appeared, the idea of a "life force" was invented, for it was believed that such a theory was necessary. It is to this abstract theory that the American authors refer in the quotation above.

Rudolf Steiner described this development in a lecture cycle, *Der Entstehungsmoment der Naturwissenschaft in der Weltgeschichte,*[13] given in 1922-23. He came to the following significant conclusion: "What modern physiology or anatomy says about man — that is not man." It is a mechanical understanding of man which, in changed form, is once more applied to living human beings. The same holds for chemistry. "And thus, the natural-scientific concepts arose which are applicable to nature, and their great triumph was celebrated. But they are of no use in taking in the being of man." The comparison of the human interior to a computer is merely a continuation of the thinking exhibited in the eighteenth century by La Mettrie in his *L'Homme Machine.* It is a mechanistic view of man. This thinking is, in truth, not modern, but, at most, has become "more complex and refined."

We in no way wish to call the enormous achievements of modern biochemistry into question. Yet we must show that this path—in spite of its great discoveries—has lead to a dead end with regard to a realistic knowledge of the human being. This fact is clearly reflected in protein research.

From a purely medical-historical point of view, it is interesting that the word "albumin" is to be found as early as Pliny (23-79 A.D.). He used it as a special name for egg white, *albumin ovi.* The concept of "protein", in contrast, was first used in this form by Jean Paul at the beginning of the nineteenth century. In his work *Zur Geschichte der Eiweissforschung,*[14] H. Schadewaldt relates that the words "albuminosa" (protein), "saccharina" (carbohydrate) and "oleosa" (fat), were used by the English doctor William Prout in 1834.

Soon afterwards, the first amino acid—as a product of the decay of protein—was discovered: glycine. In 1846, J. von Liebig analyzed a further compound, which he called tyrosine. The name "amino acid" itself comes from Berzelius, who introduced it in 1848 to describe the products of the division of protein.

With these discoveries, an era of protein research was opened, applying itself ceaselessly to this remarkable substance. In discovering more and more such products of division, it sought to comprehend the riddle of this carrier of the life process. In 1900, sixteen amino acids were already known. Thus, of these twenty products of the destruction of protein, most were then accessible to research. In the twentieth century, a molecular biology of protein was developed on the basis of this research. The resulting picture appeared as follows to the above-mentioned American researchers:

> If we imagine the living organism as a factory, these small molecules are the nuts, bolts, and cogs which keep the factory going ... The steel beams are the chemically resistant basic substance: bones, teeth and chitin in insects. Lipoids—fats, oils and their derivatives—are the plaster for the factory walls. The design for everything produced in the factory — including the blueprint of the factory itself — is stored in the nucleic acids, DNA and RNA. But the proteins are, in many respects, the most remarkable compounds in a living organism.[12]

The Incomplete Image of Man and Its Correction

This image of man — as consequential and persuasive as it might appear in the area of protein research — is a clear sign of what Rudolf Steiner recognized a half century ago: its uselessness for understanding the being of man. It is most significant that today American researchers are appearing who have begun to speak in a whole new way. An example is John C. Eccles, a neurophysiologist at the State University of New York. In his book[15] *Wahrheit und Wirklichkeit* he writes:

> We know that human beings are not just active units, because we can look into ourselves and recognize our own conscious individuality. Therefore, I warn against philosophies which explain man exclusively as a reacting being and which lead to a caricature of man as a computer, a cybernetic or robot human. For many people, these philosophies provide satisfactory ex-

planations of man, when seen from without. But they fail horribly when they are applied to the human beings being considered. These words are quite clear, and they pass a stern judgment on the proudest triumphs of modern research.

Let us not overlook the fact that this thinking nearly compels one to the conclusion: "A few DNA play a teleonomic (i.e. endowed with purpose) role. A few RNA form the most important part of the mechanism which translates the genetic code ... However, there are also specific proteins in this mechanism which bring about an interplay between proteins and nucleic acids at almost every step." Thus wrote Jaques Monod in his book *Zufall und Notwendigkeit.* (1970).[16] Further on, he writes: "The organism is a machine which builds itself up ... Our knowledge of the developmental mechanism is less than inadequate. Nonetheless, we may already say that the building up takes place by means of microscopic molecular interplays, and that the molecules involved are essentially, if not entirely, proteins."

Protein is here ascribed a central significance in the construction and functions of the organism. This concept is used as an alleged proof of the mechanical nature of the latter. We see clearly where research into the nature of protein — a substance which least of all follows mechanical laws — has led. The deeper reason for this is to be found in the fact that a research method valid only for grasping the inorganic world fails when confronted with a carrier of life.

We here turn anew to Rudolf Steiner's basic book, *The Theory of Knowledge Implicit in Goethe's World Conception*[2], which was followed by his *Philosophy of Spiritual Activity*[17], a book resulting from "spriritual observation based on the natural scientific method." In this fundamental — and, even today, scarcely discovered — book, Steiner shows that human thinking is neither based on, nor a continuation of, the bodily organization. Rather, it develops by pushing back this organization. Thus, our individual human abilities are not developed from the human blastoderm (in which modern protein research discovered DNA), but rather in opposition to it. The "interplay" spoken of by Monod is actually a resistance, against which "our own conscious individuality" (Eccles) is activated.

In his book *Vererbung und Wiederverkoerperung des Geistes*,[18] Herbert Witzenmann takes on the task of "testing the methodological pillars" of Rudolf Steiner's modern spiritual

57

research with respect to present-day scientific enterprise. He writes the following:

> The soul-spiritual abilities of man are expressed in a three-fold way in his living body. First, they find the instrument for doing things in a specially constituted body, organized for them from birth. These accomplishments show them to be expressions of the human being which are not determined from outside. Secondly, they can modify themselves, either remarkably or slightly. This happens in that they push back the bodily organization either almost by habit, or progressively more consciously. They thus give a new form to the body in the form of its pliancy. Thirdly and finally, they can develop a certain predisposition in this bodily organization. This predisposition demands a new possibility of expression, which this body cannot offer.

Human Life and Death Processes

At this point, we may return to our comments at the begining of this chapter. We remember that protein was characterized as a "bearer of life." And we made clear that human protein activity is arranged in a polarity, expressed by the metabolic and the nerve-sense poles. It was further mentioned that, in the upper pole, this plastic protein activity is pushed back to make room for something higher: the thought forces.

This was of central concern to Rudolf Steiner and is discussed in his *Philosophy of Spiritual Activity*. We here meet it again. In the ninth chapter of this work, Steiner begins with the assertion that the "organization plays no part in the essence of thinking" (this refers to the inherited organization.) He then explains "how peculiar the relationship is between the human organization and thinking. The former has no effect on the essence of thinking. Rather, it pulls back when the activity appears. It gives up its own organization, and makes a free space: and in this free space, thinking appears. The essence of what works in thinking is two-fold. First, it pushes back the activity of the human organization. Second, it puts itself in this place. Even the first, the pushing back of the bodily organization, is a result of thought activity."

Later on, in his book *The Riddles of the Soul*[19] (mentioned in *The Dynamics of Nutrition*), Steiner points to Fortlage, a researcher forgotten today, who published his book *Acht physiologische Vortraege* in 1869. Fortlage writes:

> We call ourselves living beings, and thus ascribe to ourselves a property which we have in common with plants and animals. In so doing, we understand that the living condition is something

which never leaves us, and continues through both waking and sleeping. This is the vegetative life of the nutrition in our organism, an unconscious life, a life of sleep. The brain is an exception here, in that this nutritive life, this sleep life is there overcome during the periods of waking by the life of consumption. In these pauses, the brain is given up to an overwhelming consumption. It comes into a condition which, if extended to the other organs, would lead to a total weakness in the body, or to death . . . Consciousness is a small, partial death. Death is a large and total consciousness, an awakening of the entire being in its innermost depths.

In spite of comprehensive brain research in this century, this problem apparently has either not been paid enough attention or has had few results, a fact certainly related, among other things, to the tremendous complexity of the human brain and its function. This may be an indication that its activity is totally different from that of a typical metabolic organ. A. Hopf (quoted by Marfeld)[20] writes about the complexity of the brain's structure: "Of all the organs of the body, the brain exhibits the most complicated structure. The liver, for example, has a similar mass — about one and a half kilograms — and exhibits a uniform tissue structure throughout the entire organ. In contrast, the microscopic structure of the brain changes within a few millimeters, or even fractions of a millimeter." This tremendously high level of differentiation corresponds to a similar functional differentiation. Eccles writes: "It is impossible to imagine the complexity of the reproduction of the neuron chains, where every neuron is linked to hundreds of others, and where the transmission of many impulses within a few milliseconds is necessary in order to discharge a neuron."

Moreover, Hopf relates that, for this process, "very little energy is needed; it is about the same as in a 25 watt lightbulb." It is amazing that "the human brain has about 15 billion nerve cells, which may be looked at as the functional element." It is true of these neurons that "in general, a neuron does not divide itself. We live and die with the same neurons, with the exception of those which gradually disappear in old age," or are destroyed by illness etc. A constant death process is here to be found. It is a genuine pushing back of growth and reproduction, as they correspond to the function of protein. On the other hand there are about ten times as many glia cells in the brain. These glia can reproduce by

59

division. "These approximately 100 billion glia cells are significant for the metabolism of the brain."

We thus see that, within the actual nerve-organization of the brain, we are, indeed, "given up to an overwhelming consumption," to a partial death. Rudolf Steiner and Ita Wegman characterize this pushing back or laming of the life forces in their book *The Fundamentals of Therapy*,[8] where they write: "It is of the greatest importance that we know that the usual thought forces in man are sublimated forces of form and growth ... Even the emergence of thinking within the etheric body does not come from a continuation of the etheric being, but rather from its destruction. Conscious thought does not take place in processes of formation and growth, but rather in those of unforming, of withering and dying away ..."

This brings us back to the question of the amount of protein we should consume each day, and to the answer given by spiritual research: "Therefore the intake of protein substances should remain within certain limits."

Questions of Protein Digestion

Let us begin by turning to the complex of questions which arises from the constant renewal of protein. As a result of this renewal, it is necessary to take in protein daily. Modern research has tried to determine a measure for this by calculating the nitrogen balance in the human organism. However, the result of this research is not satisfactory — not least of all because of the artificial conditions of such research. Nonetheless, the assertion has been made that when an adult is given no protein, but an otherwise sufficient diet, he "burns" about thirty grams per day of bodily protein. This, however, is a crude starting point for the proper amount of protein. It was clearly seen, even at first, that qualitative considerations were also important with regard to this amount. It was noticed that the relation of protein to carbohydrates played an important role.

From the first, there was no disagreement with the fact that all protein from nutrition must be broken down in the digestion in order to be of use in building up one's own bodily protein. In this way the amino acids were discovered as the products of the breaking down of the various proteins. It was noticed that the amino acid spectrum was different, according to the protein from

60

which it came. At this point, however, an error crept into the interpretation of these findings, in that the amino acids were called the "building blocks of protein." In truth, just the opposite is so: they are products of break-down, products of decay.

Every protein which loses the living connection to its organism is thereby subject to physical and chemical forces. These ultimately strive to decompose it into the organic forces of nitrogen, carbon, oxygen and sulfur. In contrast, protein which has remained part of the living organism "repels this tendency, and fits itself into the formative forces of the etheric body."[8] In fact, this breaking down occurs in human digestion. Its purpose is to rid the protein taken in of its alien nature, to rid it of the "after-effects of the processes of the living being from which it was taken."[8] Grain protein should continue the after-effects of the life-force of the grain plants in the human interior just as little as chicken protein should bring in the life-sphere of the chicken. In addition, though, the chicken has ensouled its living protein organism, and this also creates an "alien activity" in the human being. We here touch upon the further problem of the difference between plant and animal protein.

This elimination of alien activity is a special activity of the human organism. It becomes visible in the destructive activity of ferments, pepsin, trypsine etc. The products of the decay of protein — the amino acids — appear. In the cell metabolism, the above-mentioned chemical elements appear: "Protein becomes lifeless upon contact with trypsine."[8] The force which is active in an enzyme—itself a protein body—is of a higher order than the mere life force of the organism. It is the same force which alone is capable of building up a new protein — specific to the body and based on the pattern of the individual — out of the ruins, the substance which has become dead and physical. It must, therefore, be a force possessed of "Ego-character." In fact, Rudolf Steiner spoke of a human "Ego-organization," i.e. a spiritual element also active in the body. "Everything that comes into the realm of the Ego-organization dies . . . This deadening effect is exercised upon protein where trypsine—a product of the pancreas—is active in the digestive organization."[4]

It becomes clear, at this point, where the limits of animal experiments with regard to protein lie. An animal, even though it may produce trypsine, cannot activate the same quality of forces. This is because the animal has a soul-organism, but no Ego-organization. Animal protein thus cannot be compared with human protein in this respect.

One is subject to such errors when one tries to determine the "biological valence of protein" by experimenting with rats. There, the "effect on growth and the maintenance of health"[2] of the rats is determined by factors different from those involving man. In the animal, the forces of growth, regeneration and reproduction in protein do, in fact, largely hold sway. But the human being must push these forces back in developing his spiritual forces, his Ego-consciousness. It may thus be true that "it is much easier to measure the biological valence of a nutritional protein in experimenting with animals than with human beings, even regarding the largest expenditures using the nitrogen balance. The rate of growth of young rats with different foods is followed."[7] The proper yard-stick, however, will be found only when one keeps in mind that, ultimately, "every person must seek his own personal optimum."[7] For this result, animal experiments offer little help. The criteria mentioned — which will be examined in the following paragraphs — will be of much more help.

Contradictions in Modern Protein Research

We would here like to further our considerations. It is noticeable that Rudolf Steiner does not speak of amino acids. As we saw, most of these fission products had been discovered at the turn of the century. Yet we don't find a word about them in the "protein chapter" of *The Fundamentals of Therapy*.[8] The following statement sheds an important light on this problem: "Protein which has been removed from the organism to which it belongs tends to become a compound substance which joins the inorganic forces of hydrogen, oxygen, nitrogen and carbon." The amino acids — as intermediate products of the decomposition of protein — are just such products which have been removed from the life stream of the organism, or synthesized outside of it. The fact that, using amino acid mixtures, a protein synthesis of the organism can be stimulated, does not speak against this. As we showed in *The Dynamics of Nutrition,* the human organism is capable of creating its own protein from the simple chemical elements by taking them into the formative forces of its etheric body.

62

Nonetheless, there is here again a clear, noteworthy polarity between the brain and the metabolic organs, such as the blood, liver and muscles. An insufficient protein synthesis is quickly expressed in muscular atrophy, in a loss of muscle. But a protein deficiency is important for the brain only if it appears before birth, or in the first years of life, when the brain is still being formed. Moreover, "a later protein deficiency is of little consequence for the central nervous system."[9]

It is, without a doubt, of great and far-reaching importance that modern protein research has succeeded in bringing about such a comprehensive knowledge of the amino acids. The work by Dickerson and Geis[12] is an eloquent testimony to this fact, although the authors' comparison of the living organism to a factory leads one to doubt whether, fundamentally, the right path has been taken toward comprehending the essence of protein. They are certainly correct when they say: "Proteins are, in many respects, the most remarkable connections of a living organism." But they base this assertion on the idea that proteins "are at the same time building materials and machines at the molecular level." Such a statement makes clear how little this method of research is capable of solving the problem of protein, in spite of how obvious or even convincing such thoughts might appear to natural-scientific thinking today. This inadequacy is not expressed when the authors say, for example: "According to the conception (or should one say 'dogma') of that time, proteins are synthesized as linear polymers ..."

The whole artfully created structure, then, possibly rests upon a new dogma, one which includes a view of all matter as built up and directed by atoms and electrons. Consequently, it has been calculated that "the universe has a mass of 2×10^{55} grams. This is equivalent to about 500 billion galaxies, each with about 20 billion solar masses." The molecular structure of protein, on the other hand, allows for 20^{61} or 5×10^{79} possible (protein) combinations. "... This number is about equivalent to six times the number of atoms in the universe." The conclusion: "With such variety, the versatile application of proteins is easily understood." Using this calculation — which lies beyond the human power of imagination — not only all of "evolution," but also the origin of man is "explained." This explanation then reads: "If the structure of protein were determined by pure chance, one would almost have to

63

believe in miracles." There had to have been "at some point a winner" in the "game box" . . . "Thus, in the end, a considerable evolutionary gain came about, namely humanity," as "only one of the very many possible, but by no means necessary, structures of the biosphere."[22]

Monod had already expressed an idea central to this kind of thinking: "According to the modern theory, evolution is by no means a property of the living being. For its source is in the imperfections of the preservation mechanism . . . which represents its only advantage. One must thus say that the only source of disruption which would slowly destroy a lifeless — i.e. a replicative — system, stands, in living nature, at the beginning of evolution . . ."

Such an assertion is tremendously significant, for it actually means: "Evolution is therefore not construction. It is not the development of expressive archetypes by means of a developmental process which creates expression and unity. Rather, it is the destruction of the momentum of a mechanism which otherwise has as its purpose self-repetition, that is, the return of the same."[18]

W. Heitler expresses his opinion in his work *Zum Verstaendnis des physikalischen Weltbildes*.[23] He writes: "An electron is not a 'tiny ball' as it was earlier imagined" or even as it is still pictured today through the use of x-ray deflection experiments on crystals and the use of electronic microscopy. "It is not a question of tangible matter. Rather, it is one of spiritual structures whose human expression is found in mathematics."

The question remains open: what is meant by "spiritual structures?" What does this mean concretely? If this represents a further step in the above-mentioned direction, it could lead to the knowledge spoken of by H. Witzenmann. "It is never even considered that the relation of cause and effect could, in Monod's conception, be just the opposite — that the physical constitution and function could be the expression of something soul-spiritual."[18] Even Dickerson and Geis show no sign of such a transition. Their description of the history of a protein as "molecular evolution" uses the concept of "evolutionary clocks" which is, however, called "possibly misleading."[12] "For it appears to suggest an internal mechanism which simply runs on its own and is like a kind of screenplay which all evolution must follow. This is, of course, nonsense. The speed of evolution and the changes in the protein sequences change from one period to the next, ac-

64

cording to how the forces of natural selection working on the species affect them." We see that the protein researchers in no way arrive at uniform results, but rather at greatly different ones. Yet in their thinking they are all under the spell of dogma from which they still cannot easily free themselves.

Rudolf Steiner's observation, mentioned above, is here reconfirmed: "Protein is something which is usually falsely evaluated when one does not look at it from a spiritual-scientific point of view."

Formative Processes of Protein

Rudolf Steiner, in his time, saw with surprising clarity the inadequacy of "molecular physics" and "molecular atomic chemistry." He spoke about it to the doctors as follows: "This atomic chemistry — it so to speak looks into that into which one cannot look, into the inside of the bodily constitutions. It invents all sorts of pretty notions about atoms and molecules . . ." But, in plants, "those are not the forces connected with atoms and molecules. They are, rather, the forces which work from beyond the earth, and which work into the earthly substances."[10]

This leads us concretely into the question of plant, animal, and human protein. They are identical from a molecular point of view, because this way of viewing them yields no true differences. One has come through this research to the construction of a phylogenetic tree of living beings. Differentiations are made, but the result is: "From the point of view of yeast — if indeed it has one, for this is a genuine, if anthropocentric differentiation — a moth, a bullfrog and a man are equally distant from one another. Notice, too, how backward our means of understanding living nature are. The differences between different mushrooms are greater than those between insects and vertebrates." One is justified in calling such a view a "consequence of this atomistic way of thinking about the structure of protein."

An organic view leads to a totally different result. I will here continue the remarks I made in Chapter 9 of *The Dynamics of Nutrition*. There I said that the ensouling of the animal is not a continuation of the life forces of the plant. This is replaced in the animal and human organism by an inner light which ensouls and inwardizes. It constructs the nervous system as the instrument of a soul-life.

65

There are four or five basic substances at work in the creation of protein: carbon, nitrogen, oxygen, hydrogen and usually sulfur. In reality, they are not the bearers of a molecular structure, but rather are active as the physical carriers of a specific spiritual force. For "that is what is peculiar about everything we have on the earth: the spiritual must always have physical carriers."[24] The chemical elements found in protein are carriers of the following forces: "Carbon is the carrier of all formation processes in nature," it is "the great sculptor." Oxygen carries the life influences into the earthly world. Nitrogen, on the other hand, becomes the carrier of sensations, of soul forces, of the astral body. Hydrogen is the lightest element and is related to warmth. In it, protein has a substance "which is as closely as possible related to the physical and yet is also as closely as possbible related to the spiritual." Sulfur, finally, is "the carrier of the spiritual" the "bearer of light" similar to phosphorus.[24]

Plant, Animal and Human Protein

The cosmic forces of formation are united in protein, but they take hold in plants at a different point than in animals and human beings. In the latter, they are inwardized and therefore organically active. The plant, on the other hand, receives the protein-forming forces from the periphery. The green terrestrial plants take carbon from the air, in the form of gaseous carbon dioxide. This process of assimilation is the basis of all life on earth. It is stimulated and sustained by the light and warmth forces of the sun. We thus see that the most important building material of protein — carbon — comes to the plant from outside, through the help of cosmic forces.

Nitrogen, as well, comes from the periphery. However — aside from its function in the legumes, to which we shall return — it takes a detour through the earth. Hydrogen, finally, is present everywhere.

Thus, the plant constructs its protein by using the formative forces of the periphery. Animals and human beings inwardize these forces, thereby connecting onto the hereditary stream and constructing protein from the inwardized universe. Rudolf Steiner presents this mystery of human protein formation in his first medical course. He describes four organs — the liver, kidneys, lungs and heart — as structure-forming centers of force. These

66

organs form the "stable" protein-formation centers in the organism, an inner world-system which gives the impulse for protein formation.

In this respect, animal protein is always a polar opposite to plant protein. The latter comes directly from the activity of the cosmic periphery. In animals and human beings, the periphery is turned into the interior. Other, higher types of forces — which we call forces of soul and spirit — are thereby able to work. In taking in plant protein, one is dealing with an altogether different quality. One thus confronts a world of forces which has remained free from internalizing forces, free from soul forces at any level. This is an essential characteristic of plant nutrition which is hardly realized today. It is one of the secrets of protein.

The Protein Secret of the Ephesian Mysteries

The "secret" which is completely forgotten today was an important concept in the past, an essential element of the great ancient cultures. Rudolf Steiner repeatedly revealed that this protein secret belonged to the teachings of the ancient mysteries and was especially cultivated in the Mystery of Ephesus.

Ephesus was a mystery center in Asia Minor, the bridge between the orient and occident. The old oriental wisdom there joined the Hellenistic spirit, and Artemis was revered as the highest divinity. The pictures of her which remain depict her as a goddess "everywhere abounding with life," i.e. with an abundance of breasts. The Ephesian pupil at the climax of this mystery would contemplate her statue. He was then led to the primal forces of life, and to the primal condition of the world and humanity. In this condition, there existed a living protein atmosphere as the world ether, as the womb of the future creation. Rudolf Steiner described it with the following words: "Such spiritual vision into the earth's primal condition arose in the pupils at Ephesus, when they identified with the image of the god. They learned to understand how the present earthly atmosphere was once totally different. Rather, what was present in the place of the atmosphere now existing in the earthly environment was extraordinarily fine, liquid, volatile protein — protein substance."[22] This was during the early Lemurian time, a period in earth evolution long before the Atlantean epoch. It occurred in a region which, as we have seen, was the cradle of many cultivated plants — sugar-cane, the

67

first grains and the early fruits. This was in the region presently between Indonesia and Australia.

This primal-life atmosphere was also the first formative force, which we have recognized as "primal milk." The original nutrition flowed from this primal milk to a humanity still in its pliant state.

In ancient times, the future creatures of nature lived in this atmosphere in an undifferentiated way. Only gradually were the earliest plant forms moulded out of this primal-life atmosphere. Their condition was that of coagulated protein. The present-day sea algae form the last image of this earthly plant creation. In his lectures about the form of the mysteries,[26] Rudolf Steiner described the great processes of creation, how they expressed themselves in "greening and fading," gradually resulting in the creation of plant and then animal life resembling forms still living in the oceans today. From the interplay of etheric forces "the plants — at first in a volatile, fluid form — developed at the earth's periphery by assimilating the atmospheric substance . . . In addition to the silicic acid [of the first plant formations] there was embedded in this albumin atmosphere finely dispersed calcium. Again, under the influence of protein coagulation, the animals arose from this calcium substance.[20]

The human kingdom was unified with the kingdoms of nature in this primal protein atmosphere. Later came the separations: the release of the plant world and the separation of the animal world. Thus, the pupil in Ephesus experienced "the plant world as a part of himself. One felt an intimate love of the earth, because the earth had taken in this piece of humanity — the plants — and allowed them to take root . . ." This "piece of humanity" corresponded to its own realm of life. Another part of the human being, which already bore higher forces — soul forces — appeared in the animal creation. Man "felt as if he had pushed the animal kingdom away from himself in order to become human without the burden of the animals, who thereby were stunted in their development."[25] The animal world took on the principle of the inner life of protein, which has its prototype in the ensouled human being. There thus followed the original polarity between plant and animal protein of which we have spoken.

This primal experience of the plant and animal kingdoms was impressed upon the ancient pupil of the mysteries. We can

68

thus understand why these pupils were required to nourish themselves from plants and to avoid meat as well as such plants as legumes, which represent a certain transition from the plant to the animal kingdom. One also understands why, even today, people often have feelings about plants and animals which may lead to vegetarianism for ethical reasons.

We shall consider the modern scientific evaluation of plant protein in detail later on. Such scientific evaluation has concluded that plant protein is completely sufficient, if the vegetarian foods are "judiciously combined."[27]

Further Results of Modern Protein Research

We here want to express the immense and profound difference between such an organic world-view and one based on molecules. The latter appears in modern bio-chemistry. Man can understand the organic world-view because he is himself a part of it. With the structural-analytic view, the person remains outside: he is expelled. We may here remember the evolutionary analysis to which the molecular world view leads. The opposition between these two views should thus be clear.

We do not want to undervalue the results of this type of research, in our attempt to characterize its one-sidedness.

For example, the following result of this research is interesting. One works "in the apparently confusing multitude of life processes with a few basic but similar principles of the chemical construction of molecules," for "the chemical reactions which serve to keep up the life of all organisms show an amazing similarity." Hemoglobin — found in all mammals — is an example of this. Likewise, "we find the same means of constructing complex and compound connections in the animal and plant kingdoms, as well as in the micro-organisms."[28]

Without a doubt, it was a significant step forward when Darwin, Haeckel and others brought the concept of evolution into natural science. "Macro-evolution" has since been described in various ways. Today, however, a new research method — based on "micro-evolution" — has been formed. Lund writes about it: "Until now, one primarily considered evolution anatomic — morphologically." But "morphological differences are necessarily the result of differences on a molecular basis." One thus concluded "that one can look at nucleic acids and proteins as living documents of evolutionary history . . . The research and interpretation of molecularly based evolution — of micro-evolution — is the task and goal of chemical paleogenetics." With such research, one does, indeed, arrive at the assumption of a "primal protein." But this evolves in a purely mechanical way, according to the principal of selection, which "randomly determines changes or mutations." We again meet with the way of thinking which considers only certain physical-chemical processes. It does not even pose the question: "What are these structures the carriers of?" or "What different forces are perhaps revealed through similar or identical structures?" And the human being is to be found even less in the "micro-evolution" than in the "macro-evolution." The passage at the end of Lund's work is symptomatic of this type of research. "The evolution which led to these primal proteins remains — at least for now — hidden. We have known only the result, and not the process of this evolution."

There is another characteristic symptom of this way of thinking. It deals with the proof that "the number of all possible protein molecules is practically unlimited." Assuming "that a protein molecule is comprised of a total of 100 amino acids, and that only ten of the twenty possible amino acids are used, there are already 10^{100} possible protein molecules. That is about as many molecules as are needed to fill the entire universe with protein . . . These 10^{100} molecules correspond to a mass of 2×10^{28}g. The earth's mass is about 6×10^{27}. Thus, the earth's mass is about half an order of magnitude smaller than the mass corresponding to these 10^{100} molecules. Consider, too, that there is a total of twenty different amino acids, and that protein often includes not only 100, but sometimes also 300 to 600 amino acids. It is thus clear that nature uses only a small number of the possibilities at its disposal. There are no limits to the formation of specifically constructed protein molecules."

Such a mathematical calculation is very appealing to the abstract thinking of today. One finds such a proof "elegant." But we must ask: What has it got to do with reality? Does it give an indication how protein behaves, how it comes into being and dies in constant creation? Does it point to the ability of protein to be formed by an individuality and to lend an unlimited power of transformation to the formative force which it fills? We may see from such considerations that "we can, indeed, form an infinite

70

number of words with the twenty-six letters of our alphabet. Goethe's *Faust* and Dante's *Divine Comedy* can be created with them. But we would never conclude that such works of art arose in this completely abstract manner. They arose, rather, from the creative ideas and thoughts of those artists who used the alphabet as an instrument to bring about their unique creations. Perhaps even a computer can analyze the work afterwards. But that has nothing to do with the conscious ability and activity of the creative spirit. The cosmic book of infinitely varied protein formations, similarly, arose and arises from the creative power of the cosmic formative force."

The Polarity: Germ Protein - Body Protein

We may now make it clear that protein—when it comes into the sphere of the earthly forming forces — primarily serves reproduction. It becomes propagation protein. No living being can appear on the earth without the activity of germinal protein. We showed at the beginning of this chapter that protein is the bearer of life. All growth and regeneration are connected with protein. We can thus see the primal function of protein in reproduction. All growth and regeneration, then, can be seen as a shadow or weakened form of reproduction. We may just as well say, however, that in growth and regeneration part of the protein's formative force is transformed—it is freed from the function of reproduction. However, it remains in the organism as a higher function, expressed in nutrition and respiration. Here we see the inner relatedness of the processes of reproduction and nutrition, and also of sense-perception. The phenomenon of "pushing back," which we examined earlier, again comes into consideration. Modern protein research speaks of "spheroglobin" and "scleroglobin,"[7] thus characterizing this gradation which can become a polarity. Rudolf Steiner differentiated germinal and body protein in this manner. He also explained what really happens to the germinal protein at the moment of fertilization.

To modern researchers, protein appears as a very complicated substance. It is, indeed, complex, when grasped with the means developed by bio-chemical research. If one studies a book like Hugo Fasold's *Die Struktur der Proteine,*[29] one has the impression that the tremendous complexity of the different proteins can be fathomed by using these methods. Nonetheless, all this research,

71

using chromatography, electrophoresis, x-rays, etc. is nothing but a kind of *post mortem*. One may be amazed by what the protein "corpse" reveals, but such methods have increasingly removed us from the life of protein, and thus from its real essence. The structural diagrams which fill these books are an eloquent testimony to this fact. Although this direction in research is only a few decades old, it is interesting that in 1923 Rudolf Steiner had already characterized its tendencies and purposes in the following way: "Today, one thinks: protein . . . that is surely a complicated, compound substance. Thus, one already has the ideal of a compound — as thought of by an atomist — in protein. One must depict the atoms and molecules there in a complicated way." In reality, however, living protein is quite different. "In reality, the protein of the mother animal is not assembled in a complicated form. Rather, it becomes completely corrupt and chaotic" when set forth in the reproductive processes. The remaining body protein, which serves growth and regeneration, remains "more or less ordered." But " a protein upon which reproduction is based is inwardly completely shaken into chaos and disarray. The matter is completely led back to chaos, and no longer has any structure."[30]

When this chaos comes about, the protein is led back to its original sphere of formative forces — to its true "primal form." It is then no longer subjected to earthly forces and therefore not accessible to research methods based on earthly laws. It is removed from the central forces of the earth, thus coming into the sphere of influence of the peripheral forces. This means that, in its true, determining moment, "every single piece of protein is an image of the entire universe."

A Practical Consideration

As a practical consideration, we add the following comments. This reproduction protein must be kept in view in evaluating the quality of nutritive protein. In lower forms of life — e.g. bacteria, yeast, etc. which are used today as protein sources — the reproductive component is unusually high. Consider, for example, caviar (which comes from fish eggs) or even chicken eggs. This reproductive protein appears in a much different way in the plant seeds, e.g. in grains, beans, peas, lentils, or the various nuts. We must here differentiate between plant and animal protein, thus coming to the appropriate criteria which have already been mentioned.

72

The reproductive protein of animals manifests an altogether different cosmic sphere than does that of the plants. Animal protein is from the start permeated by the forces of inwardization, or is open to the peripheral forces which make this inwardization possible. The chicken egg, however, has a special position, as it is excreted by the mother-being from its own organism. A similar process accompanies this "gesture" of excretion from within, as we saw in the formation and excretion of milk. It is a renunciation of the soul forces and a restoration in the realm of the life forces.

The Most Realistic Protein Picture

Structure formation — frame formation — is also a property of protein. It comes essentially from the carbon found in all protein. We have already described carbon as the form component, as a sculptor. "Carbon is the bearer of all formative processes in nature" and is, as such, especially related to the earth forces. One only touches upon reality when making structural analysis. In contrast, hydrogen is at work at the other pole, as it "actually dissolves everything." For "it bears everything which is at all formed, all enlivened astrality, back into the expanses of the cosmos. This is done in such a way that it can again be taken up from the cosmos."[24] Protein is enlivened by oxygen, and nitrogen acts as the "bearer of sensation." Sulfur, or phosphorous — which is often connected to protein (hydrogen itself has an essential similarity to phosphorous) — "in protein is the mediator between the spirit spread out over the earth, between the forming force of the spirit and the physical realm."

Such a picture of protein, which comes from modern spiritual research, in no way denies natural-scientific research. But it is nonetheless necessary for coming to a realistic view of protein. Rudolf Steiner's claim — that the essence of this substance cannot be understood without spiritual research — here becomes apparent. We can now see the full meaning of what he said in this respect: "This is what is peculiar about everything here on the earth: the spiritual must always have physical vehicles. The materialists only look at the physical vehicles, and forget the spiritual . . ."[24]

In these processes, we encounter a protein working together with calcium and silicon. This cooperation can here reveal to us its spiritual nature. "It is so, that in earlier epochs of earth evolution, the only substance deposited was carbon. Only later, for

73

example, did calcium come into use for man, to create a more solid basis . . ."[24] Together with carbon and protein, calcium gives man "the earthly forming force." We here see the combination of calcium and protein, active in the formation of the bones. But there is also the pathological degeneration of protein in amyloidosis, where calcium is used in the process leading to arteriosclerosis. In contrast to these typical animal configurations, the formation of plants is at first furthered by silica in combination with carbon which brings forth the "cosmic forming force" in plants. Ultimately, however, both calcium and protein, and silica and carbon, can be found as the formative basis in the plant, animal and human kingdoms. They act as the forces of form on the earthly and cosmic sides.

We see how protein works together with minerals and thus has a certain direction in its effects. Protein works differently with the various metals, such as iron. The most striking combination of protein and iron is in hemoglobin, which gives blood its red color.

Protein and Minerals: The Protein-Iron Process

Let us look at this relationship. It has long been known that living protein enters into significant compounds with certain minerals. Among the latter are the metals iron and magnesium. In the green plant, it is primarily magnesium that enters into such a protein-metal compound and appears as chlorophyll. On the other hand, in human beings and higher animals, iron and protein come together in hemoglobin. Both substances influence the character of the respective organism, and both are necessary for its life. Moreover, it is significant that "all nutritional proteins — even those in the body (living proteins) — soon become ineffective without minerals."[31] Without these minerals, the protein appears in a lifeless condition only.

What binds proteins and minerals so inseparably? How can we learn to understand this "life association"? We shall discuss some aspects of this connection, especially as it concerns iron, an important metal for human beings.

Iron is most obvious and most concentrated in blood. But it would be false to assume that its important role is restricted to the blood. On the contrary, iron is found as a trace element in all bodily cells. It is omnipresent in the entire human organism.

74

However, it never appears as free iron but is always combined with protein. In every organ, in every cell, a protein-iron component can be found.

Let us first consider the blood, where we find the hemoglobin of the red corpuscles as a protein-iron compound. These structures go through a long maturation period of many forms. They then enter the blood stream and become the carriers of oxygen. This period of maturation takes place primarily in the bone marrow. There, the erythrocyte takes in iron, and thus becomes a functioning blood corpuscle. However, at the same time it loses its cell nucleus. This means that it is no longer capable of growth and reproduction. Basically, it has already grown old. In other words, the pure life forces of the protein have been pushed back by the forming forces — now bereft of life — of the iron. In this condition it circulates in the blood. However, it only lives for about one hundred and twenty days before being destroyed in the liver and spleen. If it moves rhythmically in the blood stream through the organism, then its formation and destruction in conjunction with the iron metabolism also fall into a rhythm. Every morning, during a phase of assimilation, the liver cells take in iron from the "blood moulting." This makes room for the reverse process: the "secretion" phase in the evening. Correspondingly, there is more iron in the blood serum during the morning hours than in the evening. Moreover, modern bio-chemistry ascertains that "above all, cosmic, and other external stimuli are received and passed on in this way."[32] This rhythm is none other than the one to which Rudolf Steiner often drew attention: the rhythm of twenty-four hours. During this period, a person takes 25,920 breaths, which correspond to the number of years needed by the sun to pass through the entire zodiac. "Here you have, in the course of a single day, a rhythm which is expressed, in the world, on a larger scale."[10] Iron combines with and separates from protein according to cosmic laws. Thereby, it goes through a process of death and resurrection every day. And the director, the impulse behind this event, is the human Ego itself. This twenty-four hour rhythm represents the human "Ego rhythm," to the extent that the human Ego connects itself to, or frees itself from, the living body in the daily rhythm of sleeping and waking. The high iron content of the blood serum in the morning represents the dominance of the consciousness-awakening iron-impulse. In contrast, the protein life forces — which tend toward sleep — win the upper hand in the evening.

In his *Occult Physiology*,[33] Rudolf Steiner described this "dull life process." It represents the iron process which extends from the blood, liver and spleen into the metabolic organism. To the extent that it becomes unusable, this iron is excreted with the gall into the intestine. There, it sets itself in opposition to the flowing nutrients—especially the fats and proteins—in order to overcome their alien nature. This process is actually a healing of the invironmental influences which bring sickness. For if the flow of nutrients were not overcome—if the natural effect of the food were not removed — the food's own nature would have a harmful effect within the human body. That would actually be a process of illness.

We may here see something of the task performed by iron, in the human being, with respect to protein. A constant healing process occurs within the blood by means of the rhythmic exposure of iron to the cosmos. As Rudolf Steiner explained in a lecture to doctors, blood is "always ill . . . simply because of the human constitution." It must "constantly be healed by iron."[10] The protein forces have also been drawn into the "fall of man" by "original sin." But, with respect to the personality forces, the rhythmic infusion of iron brings about cleansing and purification. The "selfless" metal forces from the iron — exposed to the cosmos — develop a healing force.

This confrontation between iron and protein occurs not only in the blood but also in the rest of the human organism. We said earlier that every cell in the body contains iron and that the latter is always combined with protein. Rudolf Steiner spoke, in this connection, of a "radiating iron effect" which branches out into all limbs. A "congesting action" is set against this by protein, which acts to "impede the radiation."[10] A balance must always be found between these two polarities. "This battle is constantly present in the organism." If this "interplay between iron and protein" does not balance "the beam of the scales," illness results. Furthermore, it is clear that this question of balance is, to a large extent, a problem of nutrition — a question of the intake of iron and protein.

The daily loss of iron has been calculated at 1-2.5 mg. A normal diet contains 10-20 mg. iron. However, it is a question of how much of this the organism can take up and use. This is largely dependent on both the condition of the organism and the quality of the nutrition. It should here be remembered that the iron in our food is typically combined with protein. It is not a question of the iron alone, but rather of the total plant-formation process. It is noteworthy that, according to recently published research results, the iron content in experimental plants fertilized bio-dynamically was 77% higher than in those chemically fertilized"[34] A. Fleisch determined something equally important: wholegrain bread contains seven times as much iron as white bread.[35]

Following is a short list of iron-rich plant foods, demonstrating that they are able to meet the need in human beings for iron.

Leek bulb	41.0 mg.% Fe
Millet	9.0 mg.% Fe
Wheat sprouts	8.1 mg.% Fe
Spinach	6.6 mg.% Fe
Dried peaches	6.5 mg.% Fe
Carrots	3.5 mg.% Fe
Dried apricots	4.5 mg.% Fe
Crisp-bread	4.7 mg.% Fe
Wholegrain bread	3.5 mg.% Fe
Hazelnuts	5.0 mg.% Fe

(taken from various tables)

Let us further examine the process of plant formation. We ultimately come to the question: from what sources do the plants and the land produce iron? We are often referred to the weathering of stone, which allows the plants to absorb the freed iron. Rudolf Steiner, for example, mentions the wild strawberry. Its roots branch out quite far, and have "a great power" to draw in "traces of iron from afar."[36] Wild strawberries are thus an important food in special diets for stimulating the blood process.

The plant also receives its iron from another direction: directly from the cosmos itself. Today, it is reported that the earth is constantly in a state of exchange with the cosmos. From the so-called solar wind, the earth receives "no less than 1.6 metric tons of matter per second." Regarding meteoric iron, we are told that "evidently, large quantities of cosmic material — as a fine rain of

77

metal — constantly reach" the earth.[37] This cosmic substance contains iron, nickel and cobalt. The amount reaching the earth in a year has been calculated at five million metric tons.

Rudolf Steiner also spoke quiet concretely about this "meteor rain," e.g. regarding how it falls on the earth as a result of the dissolution of comets. "It goes into the air... into the water... into the roots of plants" and from there "into that which we lay on our tables."[38] We can thus understand how iron comes from the cosmic realm in two ways: as, meteoric rain into the plant world, and through the daily rhythmic process of the production and destruction of our red blood corpuscles. For "a process takes place in every corpuscle when the iron compound shoots into it. This process in man is — on a small, minute scale — the same as that which occurs when a bright, radiating meteor rushes down through the air."[39] This activity is especially intensive during the season of Michaelmas. Human beings take in this cosmic iron directly by way of "cosmic nutrition." This provides, then, a third source of iron.

And what about protein, the other pole? It originally also came, as "pro-tein," from cosmic forces. We can still see this process repeated as "the first step" in the formation of every plant, in the production of chlorophyll by means of sunlight. Along with magnesium, chlorophyll also contains iron, though the latter does not occupy a central position. Thus, with plant foods, we take in forces "which bring a person into a kind of cosmic connection with the entire planetary system." However, animal protein — especially reproductive protein — is at first also a product of cosmic forces in its construction." But it is so indirectly, as animal protein "would never come into being if the earth were not here."[40]

We thus see that the quality of plant protein is different from that of animal protein. As mentioned above, the iron-protein compound likewise has a different quality. Seen from this perspective, nutrition with protein and iron from plants takes on another significance. In the above-mentioned "iron plants," the plant itself produces a manifold balance between these two poles. These plants thus serve man as the best stimulation for his own inner activity.

The Significance of Plant Proteins

We have looked at the specific constitution of plants with regard to iron. We would now like to turn to the general question of

78

the significance of plant protein and its evaluation by modern nutritional research.

The question of whether or not a pure plant diet (i.e. a strict vegetarian diet) is sufficient has long been argued. Often, this matter is not approached with enough objectivity. Many arguments for the inferiority of plant protein have been made, based on analytic protein research. However, the experimental methods have often been one-sided, so that one could not expect any objective results. Nonetheless, we might listen to the important American nutritional researcher, B. Mark Heystead, who came to the following conclusion in 1951: "The condemnation of plant protein as inferior comes largely from the fact that the research was based only on refined grain protein."[41] In contrast, as late as 1971 the biochemist Aebi still clung to the notion of "the rather incomplete plant proteins" which should be "increased in value" by animal protein.[7]

Recently, H.D. Cremer—whom we have already cited—raised some essential points, in his book *Die Bedeutung des pflanzlichen Eiweisses*,[27] which strive toward an objective evaluation. He makes a basic assertion about "vegetarinism," saying "that with the appropriate selection or mixture of plant protein, the amino acid requirement can be met." This statement is in complete contrast to Aebi's, yet it comes much closer to the truth. Thus, "a satisfactory diet can be composed from plant foods alone." Such statements contradict the dogma of the inferiority of plant foods. However, we shall see that these assertions are sometimes based on problematic assumptions, which decrease their value.

Cremer's study was based primarily on the results of research done in America. He came to the interesting conclusion that "the serum cholesterol levels in vegetarians are significantly lower than those in meat and fish eaters." A vegetarian diet therefore has a preventative as well as a curative effect, especially with regard to heart attacks. Of course this is related to another factor which other authors have described: the effect of the roughage or crude fiber in plant foods, which also leads to a reduction of pathologically high serum cholesterol levels. Apparently there are a number of factors at work here. Cremer sees the appearance of heart and blood vessel diseases as "the clear result of a chronic deficiency in the consumption of fibers and roughage." Finally,

79

the pectines — as they are found in our fruits — also reduce the cholesterol level of the blood.

We must place a question mark before some of Cremer's further statements, however. For example, he speaks of the so-called TVP (textured vegetable protein) products which are made from soy beans and are 50% protein. Cremer says about them: "The vegetarian has a pure plant food here, which nonetheless affords him the pleasure others have in eating meat." In fact, the manufacturers strive to make this product as "meat-like" as possible. And, they add, it is "almost as nutritious as meat."

There is, here, an obvious conceptual confusion. Cremer's confession that these products have not been successful speaks primarily for—rather than against—the good taste of vegetarians. This food is as similar as possible to meat. In addition, its extremely high protein content comes from a legume — plants which we have previously characterized as having an animal-like metabolism. If vegetarians were to prefer such a food, it would speak quite badly for their so-called vegetarianism.

Cremer mentions other products, manufactured in the USA, whose development is even more dubious. Here the protein itself (again from soya) is so manipulated that it can be spun into fibers. A transparent liquid comes from the soy protein, "with the properties of a mass of plastic and the appearance of liquid honey." It is pressed through small nozzles and bathed in a coagulating solution. The result is "innumerable fibers which can be processed into meat-like structures." The fibers are colorless, odorless and tasteless. They are processed into any number of "foods" with the addition of flavors, vitamins and minerals. They keep well, and are easily prepared, being pre-cooked. They are also relatively inexpensive, high in protein, and derived from plants. Furthermore, we are told that "they can be made to accomodate any eating habits and any religious or dietary rules and they can be modified to suit the tastes of the people in any part of the world."[27]

We cite from this work so extensively because it is important that the reader be able to form his own clear judgment about nutrition. Considering what we have discussed earlier, there should be no doubt but that we have here a very serious error in the field of nutrition. We can only see it as the expression of the way of thinking which predominates today.

In the search for new sources of protein — especially for those regions where there is real hunger — the use of yeast and bacteria protein has been considered. We have already shown that such protein — based on the reproductive forces of lower organisms — is inadequate for modern humanity. Cremer speaks of "the difficulties in determining its harmlessness with regard to health." These should be taken into account and ought not to be underestimated.

Finally, we may consider the frequent recommendation that *algae* be used in human nutrition. We here again find the argument that these lower plants are exceptionally rich in protein — up to 50%. Algae were used in prehistoric times as food both in the far east, and in the far west, among the Aztecs. Even today, algae products play a significant role in the diet of the average Japanese person. These facts have led to the establishment of research projects dealing with the breeding of various species of algae for human consumption. One is attracted to the idea of finding substances which, in addition to their high protein content, are also rich in vitamins and minerals. But one important fact is not considered: we are here dealing with a very old plant formation. As we saw, it originated in the distant past of the earth. At that time, human beings were still far from their later, and present, organization. The forces in these plants in no way correspond to the level of development humanity has since attained. Even though these algae from ancient times are still used as food in the present, a person should see — by means of his modern consciousness — that an algae-based diet is no longer appropriate. Algae correspond to a level of development which today leads to decadence, not to progress. This statement is meant in the light of something we have often emphasized: a person's nutrition works not only on his corporeal nature, but also upon his consciousness. It is precisely from this point of view that we must understand why the consumption of algae should not be revived. The protein appropriate to our culture comes more from the green plants rooted in the earth. This leads us primarily to grain protein. We shall see how it can be complemented with fruit and milk protein to form a valuable protein nutrition. The brilliant intuition of M. Bircher-Benner in this field led to his creating "Bircher-Muesli," which combines these three components in a manner which has proved to be successful.

The protein from grain and fruit—combined with crude fibers

81

and pectin—provides the amount of resistance to the human organization which is appropriate for arousing one's own forces of nutrition. In this way, a person is called upon to activate his inner digestive forces in the manner necessary for maintaining his life processes. A person's food thus becomes so "stimulating" that the inner play of forces of actual nutrition is carried over into the entire organism. We here come to the activity of substances which, in recent times, have been the subject of increasing research. These are the *enzymes*, which we shall consider in the next section.

The Essence and Activity of Enzymes

We previously spoke of trypsin, and of how it serves to get rid of the alien character of protein in the small intestine. We have thus already referred to one enzyme in the organism. The study of enzymes goes back to the last century (e.g. in the case of trypsin). Since the 1920's, when the importance of their significance for metabolism was recognized, enzymes have been increasingly studied by bio-chemists, although knowledge of them was at first rather modest. In this context it is especially interesting that Rudolf Steiner mentioned and characterized them in various ways. However, he approached their essence only in a certain way, as we shall see.

Let us first ask what present-day research says on the subject. All researchers agree that, chemically, these substances are protein bodies. This is an essential point, as it shows that they belong to the substances in the realm of living formative forces. In fact, they have proven to be carriers of exceptional forces which inhere in the smallest amount of matter. A few decades ago, one could believe that human beings had only a couple of dozen enzymes. Today, one knows—or believes he knows—that even the cell of a single bacterium contains thousands of them. Their number in human beings is today reckoned to be in the millions.

The distribution of enzymes in the realm of the organic is manifold—one can say that, without enzymes, no metabolic activity would take place. However, it is amazing that they appear in all levels of life according to an identical or similar blue-print, at least in regard to their chemical constitution.

82

Modern research describes enzymes as follows: "Living cells . . . use active catalysts in order to accelerate, by a magnitude of ten to a hundred thousand, reactions which occur extremely slowly under normal conditions. The cells have a unique catalyst ready for this purpose for every small metabolic step. These catalysts are called enzymes." In other words, if we combine two elements of fat—e.g. glycerine and fatty acids—after even a few days, no fat will be formed. But as soon as these substances come together in a living cell or organ they will rapidly react chemically with each other. Enzymes are the substances which cause this reaction.

Of course, various conditions accompany their activity. The environment must have a certain acidic or alkaline level — i.e. a specific pH — and the organism must be at a certain temperature. In other words, the chemistry and warmth of the liquid play an essential role. There is another fact: the enzyme itself is not chemically altered but remains unchanged after the reaction, and is ready in the next moment to again be active.

The word "catalyst," coined by the chemist W. Ostwald, simply means "accelerator." It thus does not say much. In spite of enormously extensive research in this field, including the work of J. Monad, many unsolved riddles still remain.

We said that enzymes are protein bodies. However, they are often supplemented with metals such as copper, zinc, etc. Nonetheless, the protein is always the specific carrier of activity.

As early as 1894, Emil Fischer put forth the thesis that enzymes are related to the objects of their activity as a key is related to a lock. It is believed that modern x-ray structural analysis confirms this interpretation. Dickerson and Geiss write: "In fact, there are two separate problems in the activity of enzymes: on the one hand, their great specificity or selectivity, and on the other hand, the actual reaction mechanism of the catalytic process."[12]

As research into these relations began, something occurred which is both enlightening and typical of such situations. "Although he had a cold, Alexander Fleming was working in his laboratory in 1922. On impulse, he put a few drops of his nasal mucus into a bacterial culture to see what would happen. To his surprise, he discovered a few days later that something in the mucus killed the bacteria. This substance was the enzyme lysozyme. Since then, it has been discovered in most bodily secretions, as well as in

83

large quantities in egg whites." This lysozyme, which kills many bacteria by dissolving their cell walls, has since been studied especially intensively with regard to its structure.

This work gave rise to the question of how enzymes could not only accelerate metabolic processes but also direct them. It was concluded that certain hydrogen bridges serve as the points of attack for the enzymes. The concept "steady state" was at the same time applied. One thus sees that the previous conceptions of the activity brought about by these substances were not sufficient. For example, one had to assume that the products in metabolism "are not closed, but rather open systems. Initial reagents are constantly fed into them, and products are constantly removed."[29] In other words: the essential thing in metabolism is the movement, the constant accelerations, changes of speed "whereby equilibrium is never attained," but rather the concentrations are in constant flux. Hydrogen — the element which, according to Steiner, "wants to dissolve everything" and which is least of all bound to earthly conditions—appears to play an important role here. Steiner gave an entire lecture to the workers at the Goetheanum on the "being of hydrogen."[42] He there showed how hydrogen, which is found everywhere in the world, is especially active "where there is reproduction." Hydrogen stands in opposition to everything dying and decaying. It constantly "lifts that which makes life from that which is decaying. When hydrogen develops itself in light...it is there a vivifying force." It is essentially related to phosphorus, the bearer of light. It is "really amazing, when one looks out into the world, and sees how, by means of 'enlightened' hydrogen, new being arises from the old, which would otherwise die away." Working with another substance — soda, sodium carbonate — it constantly inflames new life and reproduction processes.

Modern spiritual science here approaches the question of enzymes — posed by bio-chemistry — from an entirely different viewpoint.

Hydrogen processes are at work where seeds are formed as carriers of reproductive forces. They are also in the seminal fluid of human beings. The creative formative forces from beyond the earth play a decisive role, here, in making substance chaotic.

In this way, we may be able to track the activity of the enzymes, for they control the actual metabolism (the changing of

84

matter) and are thus constantly dissolving and creating anew. We again find that natural science is able to pose the question but is unable to provide an answer. For example, Mohler asks such questions. Regarding the purposeful attachment of enzymes to their metabolic substrate, he writes: "How does the enzyme 'know' that it should attach to this — and not to any other — substrate? Did it learn this, or did it have this knowledge from the beginning, when it was formed?"[21] To divert this question to a consideration of the hereditary forces alone does not answer it; it only diverts the question into a dead end. One will approach reality only when one allows for the extension of the methods of knowledge inaugurated by spiritual science. But is it not true that in earlier times an instinctive power of spiritual perception was still cultivated, and that one then had a much deeper and more valid view of this question than we do today? Then, one did not speak of enzymes, protein, etc. as we do today. But one understood the secret of creation and clothed it in a pictorial language. The letters of this language were veiled in the ancient mysteries and extended as far as the medieval alchemy of Paracelsus and Jacob Boehme.

In his book on medicine,[8] Rudolf Steiner wrote about the actual metabolic activity — the unceasing construction and destruction of substances, as caused by enzymes. These significant words may serve to lead our way in this field. "The point is not that the organism excretes substances into the outside, but rather that it undertakes the functions which lead to these excretions. In the carrying out of these activities, there is something which the organism needs for its continued existence. This function is just as necessary as those which take matter into the organism, or deposit matter there." The enzymes show us clearly that the essence of a substance does not lie in its material vehicle, but rather in what it does—in its activities. Should a substance become inactive, it would mean illness for the organism.

A discovery of modern bio-chemistry is here important. Among the substances accompanying enzymes are not only metals but also what are today called "vitamins." Therefore, such research went in a direction that caused the concept of vitamins to be revised. A clear expression of this can be found, for example, in the Hoffman-La Roche *Vitamin Compendium* mentioned above.[43] We read there that "vitamins are active agents, necessary for life." These active agents "are mediators of the processes of construction and destruction, though they do not themselves serve as building material." The question is thus raised: are vitamins enzymes? do they have an enzyme character? In the above-mentioned book, we read: "Vitamins fulfill catalytic functions. Their intervention makes possible the construction and destruction of the primary nutrients and thereby directs the metabolism." Is that not the same characterization which we made of enzymes? In any event, it is clear that in researching these substances and their activities we have begun to free ourselves from old concepts. We have crossed a threshold into a region in which the activity of substances calls for new criteria of judgment.

The True Nature of Enzymes

It is certainly of interest that Rudolf Steiner repeatedly spoke of the activity of enzymes. We have mentioned that he spoke about the working of trypsin, among others. A few statements in the book *Fundamentals of Therapy*[8] may shed particular light on our subject.

The ninth chapter of that book is devoted to the role of protein in the human body. We there find a description of the digestive path of protein, from the pepsin activity in the stomach to the trypsin functions. The influence of the latter is characterized as one of the human Ego-organization. For "everything which comes into the region of the Ego-organization dies," as does protein, when it comes under the influence of trypsin. "Upon contact with trypsin, protein becomes lifeless" for a moment. It can then be taken up into the individual's life-organization. Mohler's question is here clearly answered. We also see that the same trypsin which is found in animals comes under the direction of the Ego-organization in man. Thus, the same chemical substance can be subject to different, higher influences.

Rudolf Steiner addressed this problem in one of his lectures to workers.[44] He spoke of the three-fold salivation of food by ptyalin, pepsin and trypsin. The Ego is also at work in the sphere of ptyalin activity — in this case, on sugar. But "in the sphere of pepsin activity, the astral body drowns out the Ego-organization." Only under the influence of trypsin does the Ego-organization reappear. However, there are other points to be considered

86

here. This three-fold activity awakens at the same time a perceptive activity among the inner organs: "That which comes from the swallowed food is now perceived, tasted and felt by the liver, and thought by the kidneys."

We here come to the sphere of the interplay between inner and outer digestion, outlined in Chapter Three of *The Dynamics of Nutrition*. It is again clear that the views and concepts of academic medicine prove especially inadequate in regard to protein. Rudolf Steiner said that, with the words "'pepsin,' 'trypsin' etc.," modern science "unfortunately gave these things such abominable names," names which are altogether inadequate.[44] Protein activity leads us into a process which cannot be grasped with fixed concepts. If the word "dynamic" applies anywhere, then it is here. We spoke earlier of the protein atmosphere which filled the environment as the sphere of life and formative force during the distant past of man and earth. This protein atmosphere actually lives on in the inner "liquid man," the "protein man" which penetrates the entire human form. The tissue fluid, the "inner ocean," is today beginning to be discovered. There is a constant, unconscious perceptive activity there, even in the enzymes which are always perceiving. Looking at it in this way, we shall have to judge the purpose of protein differently. We thus come to a central description given by Rudolf Steiner in his second medical course. In the sixth lecture, he poses the question: "What is the task in the human organism of the protein taken in as food?" For what does the human organism need protein? To answer this question, we must again refer to the polarity between the upper and lower man, between the nerve-sense pole and the metabolism. Without this, we cannot come to a realistic view of human nature. In this regard, we see how the coarse material intake of nutrients has its center in the metabolism, in the digestive organism. The latter, however, is refined higher up in respiration and finally undergoes another metamorphosis toward the sense organism. "Sense perception is nothing but a refined process of respiration." Three organs represent such functional metamorphosis: the liver as the central metabolic organ, the lung as an organ of respiration, and the brain. We see at the same time that all three are metabolic organs, all three are organs of respiration, and all three are sense organs — but at different stages of metamorphosis.

The Actual Function of Protein in Human Beings

The possibility of answering the question of the actual function of protein in human beings is thus opened. We at first find protein in the liver processes, in the metabolism. Yet we shall at the same time have to consider the other metamorphosis — the transformation in the higher organ functions — as well. The activity of breathing takes place in an interplay with the outer world. Its counter-image, its counter-process, is found in an occurrence which we cannot directly follow with physical means. Rudolf Steiner described it as follows. "In breathing outwards, it (the organ) develops inwardly another activity — the polar opposite of breathing, the activity of freeing the spirit, of freeing the soul."[45]

We here again come to the important sphere of the actual activity of man. The organs which he forms all fall under the mastery of his soul-spiritual forces. The metabolic organs primarily serve the metabolism and transform the formative forces. They thus transform the formative forces, active at first in the life organization, into something soul-spiritual. The activity of our soul and spirit then appears as liberated, transformed formative forces.

This applies especially to protein, which we have seen as the direct carrier of these life forces — these formative forces. Therefore, we can only begin here to grasp the actual purpose of protein in the human organization. In the building up of protein — in every formation of protein — two activities are developed: one inward and one outward. "Only when we know this can we really become clear about the role played by nutrition." Only then can we grasp how the processes of nutrition and digestion everywhere in the human being pass over into breathing and are "spiritualized." The "plastic" protein force in the metabolism constantly transforms itself into something higher. It stimulates this metamorphosis, provided that the right quantity and quality are found. In *Fundamentals of Therapy,* Rudolf Steiner writes: "The spirit is not developed in the human being on the basis of constructive material activity, but rather on the destructive activity of the processes of 'unformation.'"[8] But the forces of the higher organization must be able to master this process. Otherwise, sickness appears — sickness as the result of false, excessive protein consumption. This is why it is so important to grasp this occurrence

88

in its reality. It begins in the metabolism, in the inner digestion, in the interplay of protein with the liquid organism, with the tissue fluid. This "action of the living play of forces in the tissue fluids maintains life."[45] And life is constantly stimulated by protein — kindled anew — so that the metamorphosis into breathing and "spirit liberation" can be made. At this point, we come to a basic statement by Rudolf Steiner: (Whenever you combine foods in such a way that they stimulate this activity in the tissue fluid, you thereby maintain life.") The central question of the purpose of protein in the human organism is thus answered.

Everything we have said about protein quality and the amount of protein consumption comes together in this presentation. Everything having to do with the evaluation of protein — the measuring rod we must lay beside protein — also has its point of reference here. And it is understandable that without this "measuring rod" all efforts regarding this question will remain more or less imperfect — or even, until now, misguided. Indeed, many researchers are today quite aware of this.

For example Mohler, in his book *Sense and Nonsense in Nutrition*[21] (*Sinn und Unsinn unserer Ernahrung*), clearly emphasizes that the biological indices for the evaluation of protein are unsatisfactory. He writes: "The correspondence between chemical and biological results, and among the biological results themselves, leaves much unanswered."[21] Nothing is changed simply by looking for new examples like the chicken egg—a strong reproductive protein — or bacteria protein, which is also one-sidedly determined by its capacities for reproduction and growth. On the other hand, this search for new examples led to the assessment that milk protein "in its totality is an ideally composed foodstuff," although milk's amino acid spectrum presents only one aspect of its ideal nature.

It is already clear that, in general, a person should moderate his consumption of protein. He thus takes his consciousness-forming organization into account. This organization — to the extent that it is based on the brain — is also physiologically independent of protein as a carrier of energy.

This knowledge, gained from modern protein research, is extraordinarily important. It indicates that protein in fact plays a role in "construction material" metabolism, and appears in the nerve-sense organism in destructive processes. "Protein substance decomposes in the nerve tissue. In an egg germ, it is built up again. But in this nerve tissue, it simply decomposes." In just this way the nerves can become the most material organs. They develop no life of their own, but rather serve as the mediators of perceptions which make use of these nerves either from the inside or from the outside. This termination of the protein processes in the nerve-sense sphere is related to their being limited to the "building material" exchange. They go beyond this limit only when they are forced to act as "energy carriers" due to a person's over-consumption of protein. But this already represents a degeneration of protein — an alienation from its essence.

Here a fact learned from modern physiology is significant: the brain fulfills its need for energy "solely from glucose, and has no alternative."[7] This means that the forces of consciousness-formation do not need protein to become substantial. Rather, they need another substance, namely sugar. Rudolf Steiner said this quite precisely over half a century ago: "In general, one can say that the consumption of sugar typically raises a person's personality-character." It lends him "a kind of innocent ego-hood." These are properties which are related to consciousness-formation. A more precise indication can be found in *The Fundamentals of Therapy:* "Glucose is a substance which can work in the sphere of the Ego-organization. It corresponds to the taste for sweets, which has its existence in the Ego-organization."[8] Protein, in contrast, is active in the sphere of the life-organization, as we have shown. Of course, this is individualized in each person.

The Contested Question of Protein Requirement

The old assumption — that a person needs one gram of protein per day for every kilogram of bodily weight (i.e. 70 g. on the average) — has today been largely abandoned. For, as we mentioned, experiments with human beings point to a considerably smaller amount: about 30 g. per day. H. Aebi, correspondingly, writes: "The minimum daily requirement for protein is 0.5 g/kg bodily weight." But, according to his own argument, we must doubt him when he continues by saying that "the optimum protein consumption, accordingly, is 60-80g. per day"[7] "Optimum protein consumption" is ultimately a qualitative term, and its quantitative equivalent can only be obtained by considering all relevant factors.

90

The strong effect of protein consumption on reproductive processes has today been clearly demonstrated. For example, K. Lang writes in *Biochemie und Ernährung:* "A protein deficiency has serious consequences." In animal experiments, a diet completely devoid of protein led "to a practically complete sterility because of the reabsorption of the embryos." Protein deficiency led to an increase in still-births. And these animal experiments have been confirmed among human beings. On the other hand, apparently no one has observed the effect of an over-consumption of protein on the reproductive forces. Rudolf Steiner, though, spoke quite clearly about this. "By eating too much protein substance, one calls forth the dominance of the reproductive forces. The control of the sexual passions is thereby made very difficult."[11]

Modern spiritual science offers further help in our search for the appropriate amount of protein, but even this help must be considered in the light of pathological factors. On the basis of such considerations, Rudolf Steiner concluded that a healthy adult person actually does not need more than 20-30 grams of protein per day. He once even said, "It is actually impossible for a person to eat too little protein."[46]

How are we to judge such statements — especially in light of the fact that the daily consumption of protein in the so-called industrial nations often exceeds 100 grams per person?

Bircher-Benner called for a "nutritional economy" with the following words: "Every excess of nutrients and calories — and especially every excess of protein — works not to the advantage, but to the disadvantage of a person's health."[47] Rudolf Steiner dealt with this question in a similar way. His conclusions, as we shall see, have today been largely confirmed by modern medical research.

In a lecture given on January 23, 1924,[46] Dr. Steiner warned especially against feeding children too much protein. For "we today see the children who were fed too much protein in the 1870's and 80's. Today they go around with calcified arteries, or have already died from arteriosclerosis." Somewhat later, on July 31, 1924, he spoke on the same theme. "Many people get arteriosclerosis too soon . . . because they are fed too much protein." This extremely important statement has since been confirmed in an impressive way. For example, in 1957 an American publication included the statement that "the intake of protein plays an important role in the development of arteriosclerosis. This is especially true of the intake of animal protein."[48] An important result of research has recently been disclosed: the body deposits excess protein in the inner peripheral layer of the capillary vessels. Thus a "degenerate mucus membrane protein, insoluable in water" is formed. It also furthers an increase in the cholesterol level of the blood: "Here, too, the over-consumption of protein is at fault . . . Thus arteriosclerosis comes about."[48] Finally, we again turn to the research of P. Schwarz. He wrote, in the *Deutsche Aertzeblatt,* that the depositing and gradually destructive effect of amyloid (a waxy, fatty protein mixture) is "the most important cause — and perhaps the determining factor — of decline in old age" and especially of arteriosclerosis. It is again emphasized that, regarding amyloid, we are dealing solely with the degenerate, break-down products of protein. They are heavily enriched with amino acids primarily from animal protein.[49]

Interestingly, the origin of this amyloid is traced back to the formation of "pathological fine fibrous scleroprotein." This is the protein which, under normal conditions, we already classified as belonging to the group which causes hardening of the formative forces. It is apparently just as important that, in animal experiments, such amyloid was easily produced when poisons were introduced. Rudolf Steiner already described how excess protein remains in the intestines, and then "poisons the entire body. This poisoning often gives rise to arteriosclerosis."[48] Indeed, at the eighth European Rheumatologists' Congress in Helsinki, in 1975, B.M. Ansell reported on twenty-eight children with "bi-optically determined amyloidosis."[50] It thus appears that the hardening forces resulting from feeding children too much protein lead to such pathological protein degeneration even in childhood.

Pathological Effects of Protein

The danger of poisoning is present every time protein is consumed, for it is in the nature of protein that it creates putrefaction products in the intestines. The life-force organization of man must constantly fight against this process. "It is so in the human body, that the etheric body is the fighter and victor over putrefaction."[46] This fight is today made extremely difficult by the "lots of protein" mentality.

There is still much to be said in this respect. For example, there is the frightful increase in gout, which entails deposits of uric acid in various places thoughout the body. Again, Rudolf Steiner provides an exact spiritual-scientific description. "This organ (the kidney) is then overburdened with uric acid which is not overcome by the Ego-organization." In this way "focal points come about, where sub-human (animalistic) processes are pushed into the human organism. It is then a case of gout."[8] A recent report claims that this disease has increased eighteen-fold in West Germany during the post-war period.

Equally important is the relation of the over-consumption of protein to the difficult problem of accelerated growth. We spoke of this acceleration earlier, in the chapter on milk. Last year, the *British Medical Journal* reported on the overfed infants in Great Britain. "Instead of 20 g of protein per day, as recommended by the Ministry of Health, the children received, on the average, 33 g. Such excessive protein consumption leads to accelerated growth, and a shorter life-expectancy."[51]

Finally, we here mention the last of the pathological degenerations of protein metabolism. It is the protein metabolism of cancerous growths. In this cell-growth, protein decay is accelerated and toxic degenerative processes take hold. The afflicted organ can no longer be controlled by the Ego-organization in its processes of building up and breaking down. The forces of cell-formation and dissolution become independent. They fall away from the direction of the organizing, forming forces of the organism and become uncontrolled. Embryonic forces of growth and reproduction are activated at an inappropriate time. The resulting toxic protein products threaten to overwhelm the entire metabolism. The liver — whose function is to detoxify such putrefaction processes — is overburdened. It fails increasingly, so that most cancer patients — according to the cancer researcher Zabel — "do not die from their tumors, but rather from protein poisoning."[52]

The Alternatives to Animal Protein: Fruit, Grain and Milk Protein

In the face of this development, which we are right in the middle of, one question becomes ever more urgent: how can we find a way out of such a fatal situation? We might expect that here, too, spiritual research can point out new directions, requiring a further clarification of protein quality.

We have seen that the methods common today for determining protein quality give us a few starting points in weighing this problem. On the whole, however, they are inadequate because they are unable to adequately grasp the nature of protein and the nature of man.

The archetype of protein — as we have already shown — is characterized by its plasticity, its formative and transformative abilities. It is by nature half liquid, colloidal. This means that it joins in with the earthly crystallization forces, which are opposed to the heaviness of earth formation. Therefore, it is especially related to plant formation as such, which also represents an interplay of earthly and cosmic forces. "The plants raise up earthly material from the earth effects." For "in making the transition to life, matter must pull away from the outwardly radiating (physical) forces, and join itself with the forces raying in (etheric)."[8] In this respect, plant protein is archetypal and is thus of special importance for human nutrition. With it, we consume the protein formative forces, as such.

The following question is raised: is this the case with every plant protein, or are there also special qualities of protein within the plant world? The latter is, indeed, the case. It is here that we find new starting points for evaluating protein quality with spiritual-scientific methods.

There is a region in the plant form which opens itself to the forces of reproduction. It is localized at the upper pole, in blossom, fruit and seed structure. The plant here communicates most strongly with the cosmic peripheral forces, which are expressed in light and warmth. At the same time, the plant here is most withdrawn from the gravitational forces of the earth. We may thus suppose that in this region the protein formation of the plant most intensively approaches its archetypal image. Thus, fruit protein is indeed of special significance in human nutrition. "To build up the organs of nutrition, a person needs protein in his diet. One needs the protein in plants, and preferably as the plant contains it in the flower and in the fruit of itself."[46] Therefore, the "protein from the fruit of plants" — e.g. apples, plums, oranges — is especially valuable.

But—one might object—there is quantitatively so little protein there, often little more than one percent! Nonetheless, this protein is qualitatively very valuable, for the reason outlined above. Quantitatively, it furthers a limited intake of protein. It stimulates the dynamic of the human metabolism primarily by means of its dynamic forces. For example, it helps regulate the construction and destruction of proteins, detoxification, and the removal of deposits. We might also mention the well-known effectiveness of raw fruit juice therapies.

In a broad sense, Rudolf Steiner also included the "grain fruits" — and thus grain protein — in this type of protein source. However, further differentiations are to be made here. The protein in a whole grain is in such a proportion to the other nutrients that there can be no question of an over-consumption of protein. Moreover, modern research shows that the carbohydrates, which dominate in grain, have a "protein-saving" effect. Recently, some attention has been paid to the question of quality-raising combinations of different plant proteins. These combinations include those of plant and milk protein.

We thus come to the third important protein source we wish to discuss: milk protein. Quantitatively, it is in a well-balanced composition with regard to carbohydrates and fats. Its form can be characterized as a sort of polar opposite to that of fruit protein. The fruits open themselves to the cosmic peripheral forces in their formation. Thus, in their coloration and scent, they approach the super-earthly forces which Rudolf Steiner called "astral forces." Milk does just the opposite in its formation and in its flowing out toward the periphery of the organism. It leaves behind the sphere of internalizing forces and thus takes on a sort of plant character, the character of flowers and fruits.

This triad of fruit, grain and milk protein, and their sensible combination, stands out as the basis of a rational protein nutrition. These proteins can fully satisfy the requirements of a qualitatively and quantitatively appropriate protein nutrition. Of course this holds true only if an important condition is met: the production and processing of the products must fully take into account the protein character of these foods.

Our considerations also point to the fact that animal protein must receive a different qualitative evaluation, for the animals internalize the forces which the plant meets outside itself. In this

95

way, sensitive substance comes about. Thus, the cosmic influence upon animal protein is indirect. Animal protein is therefore essentially different from plant protein in its effect on the human being. With animal foods, a person takes in something "in which the astral forces were already developed," the internalization and ensoulment of the peripheral forces. Thus, "a person must first overcome what the animal's astral body has brought about." In fact, this process is expressed by the nervous system, which serves as the instrument for the development of the forces of soul. "Whenever a person takes protein from the plant world instead of from the animal world . . . he develops forces within himself which make his nervous system more healthy and fresh."[15] For the plant has not laid claim to these forces for itself. And the animal, in producing milk, again externalizes these forces.

The spiritual research of Rudolf Steiner thus leads, step by step, to the elements of a new understanding of protein. This understanding will form the basis of a truly rational nutritional hygiene.

The Protein Habits of the Modern Consumer Society

We do not want to end our discussion without looking at another problem which plays a large role in the modern approach to the protein question. The suggestions of spiritual research here outlined may bring it substantial illumination and correction.

Many contemporary presentations repeatedly emphasize that "in a reasonable nutrition, a greater quantity of protein should be consumed."[53] Protein should account for 20-25% of one's daily caloric intake — i.e. its consumption should be raised to 100 g or more. As we already noted, this amount of protein corresponds to a great extent to the habits of the modern consumer society. How is it justified scientifically?

It is supported by—among other things—the stimulating effect of simple sugars on the appetite. Refined sugar, common today, has a stimulating effect on the insulin formation of the pancreas. This, in conjuction with an overconsumption of fat, leads to overeating and overweight. It has thus been recommended that people drastically reduce their consumption of carbohydrates while greatly raising their protein quota. One is to avoid grain products for the most part, thus allowing one "to begin breakfast with ham, cheese and/or eggs and to eat as much meat and fish as one wants during the course of the day."[53] The consumption of milk is to be "limited to one quarter liter daily," and honey is "banished from the diet."

These highly official suggestions come from the *Deutsche Klinik für Diagnostik* in Wiesbaden. From even these brief indications, one can see what massive errors they are based on. They assume an attitude which is unrealistic from a purely quantitative point of view. Thus, they lead to a neglect — even a degradation — of the real significance of grain and milk foods. In addition to this, they contradict knowledge of modern nutritional physiology itself.

We here return to the work of H. Aebi.[7] We shall look more closely at a further characteristic of protein: its so-called specific dynamic effect. In the breaking down of food substances in the living organism, there is a basic difference between protein and fats and carbohydrates, even with respect to energy. In breaking down amino acids, nitrogen must be freed and eliminated in the form of urea. This means that it is necessary that "a relatively high amount of energy must be used, in the form of an investment." This situation brings about the known fact that "upon taking in protein, an increase in the total energy expenditure can be observed. This increase is clear, lasts for a few hours, and can be followed by measuring the increased heat given off. In principle, this specific dynamic effect of protein can only mean that energy obtained from protein is extraordinarily expensive . . ."[7]

Much is hidden behind this, at first, abstract statement. The warming effect of concentrated protein from animals is well known. It explains why, especially in winter and in the polar climates, people prefer animal protein. But we must ask about the quality of warmth upon which these increased metabolic processes are based. The so-called specific motor effect of protein can be of help here. This effect is expressed in a "general disharmony of the organism in the sense of an increase in all preparatory reactions." Subjectively, it is expressed as a "stimulating effect." We have already mentioned what is thereby "stimulated": the "stimulating" forces from the metabolism, or as Rudolf

97

Steiner put it, the forces rising up from the abdomen which "create an excess of those forces which correspond in the lower bodily activity to what forms ideas in the upper activity."[11] In other words, "One eats meat especially when the body loves meat. For thus does one satisfy one's lust."[13] These plain words of Rudolf Steiner go to the heart of the matter. Fleusch's views on this subject are quite different, though equally significant. "The stimulating properties of protein — especially animal protein — lead to their over-estimation and over-consumption. This cannot be justified by nutritional physiology, because it leads to 'extravagant combustion'."[54] It is today known that this stimulating effect comes from uric acid, which is also produced when protein is broken down. It thus effects a "constant incitement of the ergotropic nervous system" — i.e. a stimulation of the sympathetic nerve, with its increased production of physical activity and its reflection in the mood of soul.

With high protein consumption as a "source of energy," there is at the same time an increased storage of carbohydrates and fats in the organism. This is because their possibilities for action have been blocked and they must lie fallow. The result is the present tendency towards over-nutrition and over-weight, as well as the idea that one should drastically reduce the consumption of carbohydrates. When this happens, only protein—with its stimulating effect—remains dominant. One can then begin breakfast with ham and eggs, and the essential carbohydrate-sugar effects, previously alluded to, are lost completely when the refined products are over-consumed.

On the other hand, a true quality nutrition will in any event be limited with regard to carbohydrates and will be "protein-saving." Then the actual quality protein — from fruit, grain and milk — can come into its own. Then, too, protein will retain its true purpose as a building material. Its degeneration into an "energy source" will not be forced upon it, and the results alluded to will be avoided. Thereby, Fleusch's "extravagant combustion" will not come about. It is not limited to an "energy component" and a stimulatory effect. Rather, it also brings on profound pathological processes in the organism, as we have mentioned.

This is not all. The effect of this type of protein over-consumption also extends into the socio-economic region, where it has amazing consequences.

98

Economic Aspects

The fact that animal protein is extremely expensive has often been mentioned. A rule of thumb is that 7 kg. of grain are needed to produce 1 kg. of beef or pork. It has been reckoned that "in transforming grain into animal products . . .about 6/7 of the calories in grain are lost for human nutrition."[55] In the American magazine *Newsweek,* an article entitled "Running Out of Food?" contained an interesting conclusion. "If Americans would reduce their consumption of meat by ten percent, enough grain would be saved to feed sixty million people." Professor R. Durmont put it even more bluntly. "Last year we — the rich of this earth — fed 395 billion tons of grain to animals for meat. The amount of grain is sufficient to sustain two billion Asians or Africans for a year."[57]

conscience

These statements are significant from many viewpoints. First, they show how "irrational" it is to produce animal protein from plant products. We must here ask: how is it that an animal needs about seven times as much food as it produces in body weight? As a result of our previous discussion, we can assume that this fact is related to the transformation of living substance into sensitive substance, to the construction of the nervous system. The resulting substance, however, is by no means seven times as valuable — neither calorically nor according to any qualitative criteria. On the contrary, one must speak of a real devaluation, or at least revaluation, when we consider the concerns mentioned above. Moreover, from a socio-economic point of view, the irrational production of animal protein can be clearly seen. In an important table, Aebi shows how (in Switzerland) animal products are about seven times as expensive as grain products. "This comparison shows quite distinctly that meeting one's caloric needs with protein is a luxury, not only metabolically, but economically as well."[7] And we must also consider the fact, that in feeding such enormous amounts of grain to meat animals, one of the most valuable proteins for human nutrition is lost.

This economic aspect of protein has recently been approached in a remarkable way. H.D. Cremer called the transformation of nutrients from plant feed into animal products a "losing business." For "the level of efficiency of this transformation is about 10-15%. There would be a sixfold gain with respect to calories and — most importantly — protein, if the appropriate products

99

were consumed directly by people and the detour through stomachs of animals were avoided."[27]

This "loss of transformation" is, interestingly, especially distinct with regard to the consumption of fish, where it can be as high as 90%. Such a reckoning is not applicable to our discussion, however, since fish are consumers of phytoplankton, a substance which is not significant in human nutrition.

Summary Statements on the Protein Problem

In reality, the difference between plant and animal protein is qualitative. We have seen that animal protein "especially binds man to the earth" and makes him unfree with regard to the body-free will forces. Milk protein provides earthly forces but does not alienate man from his super-sensible nature. And plant protein—like all plant nutrients—connects man to the entire cosmos. "The lightness of the organism which is obtained from plant foods" can be experienced by anyone. It is, in fact, a "real relief" on the path of spiritual development.

Cosmic forces are formatively active in animal as well as in plant protein, but they work only indirectly in the formation of animal protein, i.e. they take a detour over the earth. Animal beings manifest a process of increasing emancipation from the cosmos. They thus internalize another type of force which allows them to develop their own life of soul. Protein is everywhere the basis of life, but it is transformed into an endless number of types until, finally, it can be the bearer of an individual spirit in the human being.

We have been able to deal with only a few aspects of the protein problem in our discussion, for the breadth of this problem is unlimited and its depth is inexhaustible. Nonetheless, we hope we have provided something essential, by way of a "dynamics of nutrition," from a consideration of the totality of this subject. We hope that this may show the way toward an understanding which can lead into daily, practical life.

Drawing a conclusion from all these facts, we come to five essential points:
1) The increased consumption of protein, preferred and recommended today, has more and more been shown to produce or facilitate critical diseases.

100

2) The unrestrained consumption of protein — at least of animal protein — brings forth an increasingly distinct animalization and brutalization of humanity.
3) With regard to the world economy, the high level of protein consumption is an irresponsible luxury for a small minority of the world's population.
4) This presents a considerable social problem, an enormous source of danger for the entire world-situation today.
5) People are hindered from coming to the real facts of the protein question, which is of the greatest significance for the continued existence of human culture.

The impulses from the modern spiritual research of Rudolf Steiner can help us in treading the path toward a solution of this worldwide problem. Here again, there are five essential points to consider:

1) Insight into the right amount of protein will grow out of insight into its character, which furthers life, growth and reproduction. It is the polar opposite of the consciousness-forming forces in human beings.
2) The right amount is about 20-30 g of protein per day. Of course, the individual's situation and age must be considered.
3) The three most valuable proteins come from fruit, grain, and milk. Such a protein nutrition, however, requires that they be in harmony with the appropriate qualitative criteria of the other nutrients and that they be sensibly combined.
4) The protein factor in nutrition is thus also a problem of hygienic, social and economic significance for the whole world.
5) At the same time, appropriate methods for the production and preservation of high quality are needed, both in agriculture and in processing.

If these guidelines are followed, the significance of protein as the "number one nutritional factor"[7] will become increasingly evident.

References

Protein—

1. Georg Borgstroem, *Der hungrige Planet*, Munich 1967.
2. Rudolf Steiner, *Grundlinien einer Erkenntnistheorie der Goetheschen Weltanschauung*, Dornach 1979 (GA 2). English translation, *A Theory of Knowledge based on Goethe's World Conception*, New York 1968.

3. Rudolf Steiner, *Mein Lebensgang*, Dornach 1982 (GA 28). English translation, *The Course of My Life*, New York 1970.
4. H. Witzenmann, *Über die Erkenntnisgrundlagen der biologisch-dynamischen Wirtschaftsweise*, Geneva 1975.
5. Rudolf Steiner, Lecture given in Berlin on 17 December 1908 under the title "Ernährungsfragen im Lichte der Geisteswissenschaft," published in *Wo und Wie findet man den Geist?*, Dornach 1961 (GA 57).
6. Rudolf Steiner, Lecture given in Dornach on 31 July 1924 under the title "Über das Verhältnis der Nahrungsmittel zum Menschen — Rohkost und Vegetarismus", published in *Die Schöpfung der Welt und des Menschen. Erdenleben und Sternenwirken*, Dornach 1977 (GA 354).
7. H. Aebi, "Eiweiss, Ernährungsfaktor Nummer Eins" in *Schriftenreihe der schweiz. Vereinigung für Ernährung*, Heft 17, Bern 1971.
8. Rudolf Steiner/Ita Wegman, *Grundlegendes für eine Erweiterung der Heilkunst nach geisteswissenschaftlichen Erkenntnissen*, Dornach 1977, first published 1925 (GA 27). English translation, *Fundamentals of Therapy*, London 1967.
9. K. Lang, *Biochemie der Ernährung*, Darmstadt 1974.
10. Rudolf Steiner, *Geisteswissenschaft und Medizin*, Dornach 1976 (GA 312). English translation, *Spiritual Science and Medicine*, London 1975.
11. Rudolf Steiner, Lecture given in Berlin on 22 October 1906 under the title "Ernährungsfragen und Heilmethoden," published in *Ursprungsimpulse der Geisteswissenschaft*, Dornach 1974 (GA 96).
12. Dickerson/Geis, *The Structure and Action of Proteins*.
13. Rudolf Steiner, *Der Entstehungsmoment der Naturwissenschaft in der Weltgeschichte und ihre seitherige Entwicklung*, Dornach 1977 (GA 326). English translation, *Natural Science in the History of the World*, typed only.
14. H. Schadewaldt, *Zur Geschichte der Eiweissforschung*, Munich 1964.
15. J.C. Eccles, *Facing Reality*, Springer Verlag 1970.
16. Jacques Monod, *Zufall und Notwendigkeit*, 1971.
17. Rudolf Steiner, *Die Philosophie der Freiheit*, Dornach 1978 (GA 4). English translation, *The Philosophy of Freedom*, London 1970.
18. H. Witzenmann, *Vererbung und Wiederverkörperung des Geistes*, Geneva 1974.
19. Rudolf Steiner, *Von Seelenrätseln*, Dornach 1976 (GA 21). English translation, *The Case for Anthroposophy*, London 1970.
20. A.F. Marfeld, *Kybernetik des Gehirns*, Berlin 1970.
21. H. Mohler, *Sinn und Unsinn unserer Ernährung*, 1972.

22. M. Eigen/R. Winkler, *Das Spiel* 1975.
23. W. Heitler, *Zum Verständnis des physikalischen Weltbildes*, 1975.
24. Rudolf Steiner, *Geisteswissenschaftliche Grundlagen zum Gedeihen der Landwirtschaft*, Dornach 1979 (GA 327). English translation, *Agriculture*, London 1977.
25. Rudolf Steiner, Lecture given in Dornach on 26 December 1923 under the title "Das ägyptisch-chaldäische Zeitalter. Gilgamesch und Eabani," published in *Die Weltgeschichte in anthroposophischer Beleuchtung und als Grundlage der Erkenntnis des Menschengeistes*, Dornach 1980 (GA 233).
26. Rudolf Steiner, *Mysteriengestaltungen*, Dornach 1974 (GA 232). English translation, *Mystery Knowledge and Mystery Centers*, London 1973.
27. H.D. Cremer, "Die Bedeutung des pflanzlichen Eiweisses für die menschliche Ernährung" in *Ernährungs-Umschau*, 3/76, Frankfurt/M.
28. Horst Lund, *Evolution und Struktur der Proteine*, 1968.
29. Hugo Fasold, *Die Struktur der Proteine*, Weinheim 1972.
30. Rudolf Steiner, Lecture given in Dornach on 30 December 1923 under the title "Das Verlorengehen des Wissens um den Zusammenhang des Menschen mit der Welt in der Neuzeit," published in *Die Weltgeschichte in anthroposophischer Beleuchtung und als Grundlage der Erkenntnis des Menschengeistes*, Dornach 1980 (GA 233).
31. Edwin A. Schmid, *Sinnvolle Ernährung — Gesundes Leben*, Zürich 1953.
32. K.H. Schäfer, *Eisenstoffwechsel*, Stuttgart 1959.
33. Rudolf Steiner, *Eine okkulte Physiologie*, Dornach 1978 (GA 128). English translation, *An Occult Physiology*, London 1951.
34. W. Schuphan, "Ertrag und Nahrungsqualität pflanzlicher Erzeugnisse," in *Ernährungs-Umschau,* Frankfurt/M. 1974.
35. A. Fleisch, *Ernähren wir uns richtig?*, Stuttgart 1961.
36. Rudolf Steiner, Lecture given in Dornach on 9 September 1924 under the title "Von den Planeteneinflüssen auf Tiere, Pflanzen und Gesteine," published in *Die Schöpfung der Welt und des Menschen. Erdenleben und Sternenwirken*, Dornach 1977 (GA 354).
37. F.L. Boschke, *Die Schöpfung ist noch nicht zu Ende*, Düsseldorf 1962.
38. Rudolf Steiner, Lecture given in Dornach, 20 September 1924 under the title "Was will Anthroposophie? - Vom Biela-Kometen," published in GA 354 (sec above).
39. Rudolf Steiner, Lecture given in Dornach, 5 October 1923 under the title "Die Michael Imagination," published in *Das Miterleben des Jahreslaufes in vier kosmischen Imaginationen*,

Dornach 1980 (GA 229). English translation, *The Four Seasons and the Archangels*, London 1968.

40. Rudolf Steiner, *Welche Bedeutung hat die okkulte Entwicklung des Menschen für seine Hüllen — Physischer Leib, Ätherleib, Astralleib — und sein Selbst?*, Dornach 1976 (GA 145). English translation, *The Effects of Spiritual Development*, London 1978 .

41. Mark B. Heysted, in *Magazine of the American Dietetic Assoc.*, March 1951.

42. Rudolf Steiner, Lecture given in Dornach, 20 October 1923 under the title "Über die Wesenheit des Wasserstoffs," published in *Mensch und Welt. Das Wirken des Geistes in der Natur. Über das Wesen der Bienen*, Dornach 1978 (GA 351). English translation available only of last nine lectures under the title *Nine Lectures on Bees* , Spring Valley 1975. Above lecture is not included.

43. Hoffman-La Roche, *Vitamin-Kompendium*, Basel 1970.

44. Rudolf Steiner, Lecture given in Dornach 16 September 1922 under the title "Der Ernährungsvorgang, physisch-materiell und geistig-seelisch betrachtet," published in *Die Erkenntnis des Menschenwesens nach Leib, Seele und Geist. Über frühe Erdenzustände*, Dornach 1976 (GA 347).

45. Rudolf Steiner, *Geisteswissenschaftliche Gesichtspunkte zur Therapie*, Dornach 1963 (GA 313).

46. Rudolf Steiner, Lecture given in Dornach 23 January 1924 under the title "Von der Ernährung," published in *Natur und Mensch in geisteswissenschaftlicher Betrachtung*, Dornach 1967 (GA 352).

47. R. Bircher, "Zur Eiweissfrage,"in *Diaita*, 1972.

48. R. Bircher, *Wendepunkt*, 10/1974.

49. P. Schwarz, *Deutsches Ärzteblatt*, 1970.

50. B.M. Ansell, *Wendepunkt*, 4/1976.

51. *British Medical Journal*, 1973.

52. W. Zabel, *Die interne Krebstherapie*, Bad Homburg.

53. B. Knick, "Wie sollen wir uns ernähren?" in *Universitas*, 7/1974.

54. A. Fleisch, *Ernährungsprobleme in Mangelzeiten*, Basel 1947.

55. O. Matzke, "Die Welternährungslage heute und morgen," in *Neue Züricher Zeitung*, 7 July 1974.

56. *Newsweek*, 11 November 1974.

57. *Weltwoche*, 6 November 1974, Zürich.

The publication dates mentioned refer to the latest editions available in German and English.

Chapter III

Fat Substances: Stimulators of the Warmth Processes and Ensoulment of the Organism

Warmth Production as a Basic Function of the Organism

Among the substances necessary in our daily nutrition, fats occupy an important position. We saw protein as the "building material" of the organism. Analagously, the primary function of fats is the development of warmth. In this respect, man cannot do without them. They also play an important role in the plant and animal kingdoms. Looked at from the point of view of analytic chemistry, they are 90% hydrogen and carbon. The proportion of these warmth substances in fat is substantially higher than in carbohydrates, where they make up only 46%. In terms of physics, the oxidation of fat releases about 9.3 kcal, as opposed to carbohydrates or protein, which release about 4.1 kcal. Thus, right from the beginning of our consideration, we are led to the "warmth-man." "This comes from the fact," wrote Rudolf Steiner, "that fat plays its special role in the production of internal warmth." This also holds true for the so-called fat deposits. This is the cushion of fat, a source of warmth which can be mobilized at any time, a depository. However, it is by no means a passive depository but rather an active member of the metabolism. Moreover, fat is combined with the process of warmth regulation in the organism and there exercises an equally irreplacable activity. Finally, the fatty tissues serve as supports and cushions in the organism. We shall see that this is an absolutely essential function. All these activities are closely connected to one another. In reality, they form a unity in their multiplicity.

105

The frame which encompasses all these activities of fat in a human being is his "warmth-organism." It is an organization as complete in itself as the fluid or air-organism. In fact, fat brings "nothing into the human organism except its ability to develop warmth."[1]

Fat Formation Processes in the Plant Kingdom

We have already mentioned that all living organisms on the earth are capable of producing fat substances. Nonetheless, plants occupy a special position here. This is clear from the fact that they do not possess an actual warmth-organism. On the other hand, only in the plants do we find original fat production. Human beings, as well as animals, need to be stimulated by way of the plants in order to come to their own fat production.

The formation of fat or oil takes place in various ways in plants. This means that the resulting fat displays varying qualities. We need mention only olive oil, wheat-germ oil and sunflower or linseed oil to refer to a row of formations which are used in human nutrition. There are clear differences here. Some oils are concentrated in the germ; others penetrate the whole seed or even take hold of the entire fruit.

It is nonetheless false to think that the actual process of oil formation takes place in these organs — e.g. in the embryo of the wheat kernel or the seed of the sunflower. We must, rather, look for its place of origin in the green leaves of the plant.

We can become conscious of the fact that the leaves of the plant are the organs which open themselves to the forces of warmth and light — the forces which radiate in from the expanses of the cosmos. We then come closer to understanding the process of oil formation. In fact, the production of oil substances — the actual fat synthesis — takes place primarily in the leaf region as long as these cosmic forces radiate onto the earth from the periphery. At night, when this stream ceases, the substances formed in the leaves go into the above-mentioned regions — i.e. primarily into the germ, seed or fruit, and occasionally into the roots. Of course, oils or fine, fat-like substances can be found in the entire plant organism. It is no mere coincidence, however, that oils are concentrated in various organs of the plant where they create a protective sheath of warmth. More than that, they form an entrance-way for a higher kind of force which is related to the blossom and fruit.

In the leaf region, the plant opens the largest possible surface to the cosmic forces of warmth and light. The greatest dynamism of fat formation is found here. Where the oil is stored — in the seed and fruit structures—the plant approaches the forces of internalization.

Fat Formation in Animals and Human Beings

The step toward internalization can first be completed in the animal kingdom. Thus, fat takes on a new function there. It becomes the mediator of soul forces. In this regard, warm-blooded animals are different from cold-blooded ones. Among the latter, various animals fall into a kind of "cold rigidity" as their use of energy or warmth sinks to almost zero. The behavior of salmon is especially amazing here. The fully grown and well-fed—one might almost say fattened — fish swim from the ocean to their spawning ground (up to 2,000 km away) in the mountain waters without taking in any food. In so doing, they use up their fat deposits, i.e. they convert fat into energy and warmth.

Migratory birds behave in a similar way. They also over-feed themselves and store a kind of "flight fat" which they consume during their long journey. Their weight increases about 50% before migration. Interestingly, the light conditions also play a role in this phase of their lives.

Real hibernators, like the woodchuck or marmot, develop a huge appetite before the beginning of the cold season. Their fat cushion not only protects them from the winter cold but also makes possible a greatly reduced metabolism and the development of warmth during their hibernation. These few examples give us some idea of the central role played by fat in the human organism.

In the plant kingdom, fat places itself in the service of the life forces streaming in from the cosmos and is primarily an expression of these cosmic forces. In the animal kingdom, fat becomes a carrier of soul functions. In human beings the formative forces of fat bring their warmth potency to the highest organizational form, the Ego-organization. In a healthy organism, the animal [astral] forces will only produce or take in as much fat as can be carried over into warmth processes by the Ego-organization."[1]

Man has this in common with the warm-blooded animals: he not only generates warmth, but he must also keep it at a certain level. He must regulate his warmth. Therefore, he must process external warmth and cold in such a way that they are transformed into his own warmth.

We spoke in detail of these relations in the chapter "Temperature in Nutrition" in *The Dynamics of Nutrition* and will continue to do so here. We have seen that the human being is a warmth being: i.e. he lives in his own individual warmth and expresses his individuality through it. Warmth is here a mediator between the living world and the soul-spiritual aspects of man. "Warmth both outwardly surrounds physical bodies and resides within the human organism. And insofar as the warmth itself is orginated in man, the soul — that which is soul-spiritual — takes hold in his warmth-organism."[2]

Fat is the important, substantial basis for this "warmth-man." It is thus important that we follow this substance in its formation, distribution and chemical nature in the organism. The first thing we notice is that the body forms special fat cells. They are set up during embryonic development and are brought to an individual number during the first years of life. It appears that the number of fat cells, once determined, hardly changes during a person's life. However, the amount of fat in them can, indeed, change.

Although the main mass of an infant's body fat is first accumulated during the last months of the mother's pregnancy, the infant at delivery has about the same proportion of fat as an adult. This is about 10-16% of the body weight. The difference between men and women is here significant. At fifty years of age, a man's body is about 20% fat by weight, whereas a woman's is about 30%. On the average, fat accounts for 1/5 to 1/4 of a man's body weight.[3] It should be mentioned here, though, that hereditary and constitutional differences can be a large factor. In the case of actual fat addiction, the fat tissue can be filled up to 100% with fat — something which otherwise does not occur. Moreover, a hypertrophy of the fat cells, and even the new formation of such cells, can take place.

We mention hereditary and constitutional differences in this regard to make it clear that one type of person has more fat cells than another. With their cells filled to the same extent, one can

108

appear thin, the other fat. These differences are also extended to the soul. Everyone knows that large fat deposits convey different soul qualities of warmth than do smaller ones. People who are cold in the soul are, as a rule, gaunt. The rounder types are generally also warmer in the soul. The typology of Kretschmer, as well as modern behavioral research, offers many interesting insights here, although the relationships so described must be differentiated from the degenerate pathological conditions related to fat addiction which we shall deal with later.

Further Characteristics of Fats

Before going into a greater differentiation of the human fat organism, we must examine a few more properties and characteristics of fats.

The first property is that they are not water-soluble. They have no "salt character", and are thus unlike carbohydrates, for example. In this regard, they are similar to proteins and stand opposite the salts (e.g. table salt) which dissolve straightaway in the mouth. Thus, fats do not directly take part in the typical earthly substantiality.

This property is shown not only in their chemical characteristics, but also in the physical property already mentioned: they form themselves into fine droplets, a phenomenon emphasized in our characterization of milk fat (see chapter 1). This is certainly an indication of the cosmic character of fats. We might also say that fats are related more to the inwardly radiating (etheric) forces than to the outwardly radiating (physical) forces. The fat droplets in the fat tissue and blood both show this globular form as well.

This state of being in an emulsion plays a special role in the absorption of fats. Much modern research has been done in this area.

If we follow the present-day division, we come to two groups of substances which are characterized as fats (lipids). The so-called neutral fats are the more important and it is to them that we refer when speaking here of fats or oils. Seen chemically, they contain fatty acids and glycerin. Their typical representatives are called triglycerides.

The other group is related to these fats with regard to their solubility as well as with regard to certain other characteristics;

it contains substances such as lecithin and cholesterol, as mentioned in *The Dynamics of Nutrition.* It also includes other substances characteristic of the construction of the brain and nerves, such as kephalin, sphingomylin, etc. In this chapter we will deal with the actual lipids, sometimes called lipoids: the fats or oils.

Fat Digestion

What happens when a person takes in one of these fats with his food? It is striking that nothing happens to it in the mouth and that even in the stomach the fat is not substantially altered. According to present-day knowledge, the fat is separated from the protein components with which it is usually combined. But the main digestion of fat begins in the duodenum. We could also say that man relates to fats in an altogether friendly manner; he allows them to enter, unchanged, into his small intestine. This stands in contrast to carbohydrates and proteins, as we can see from our small overview:

Mouth: Carbohydrate digestion
Stomach: Protein and Carbohydrate digestion
Small Intestine: Fat and Protein and Carbohydrate digestion

Bile acid and cholesterol stream into the small intestine from the gall bladder. Both are necessary for emulsification and hydrolysis (i.e. the transition to water-solubility). Pancreas lipase, a typical enzyme, is secreted by the pancreas and enters the same part of the small intestine where, at the same time, it breaks down fat into fatty acids and glycerine. The intestinal lipase, active in the intestinal fluid, also takes part in these processes.

Spiritual-scientific research has thrown new light on these processes and can be significant in helping us to understand them. In the chapter on fat in *The Fundamentals of Therapy,* Rudolf Steiner writes: "Fat is the substance in the organism which, when taken in from the outside, shows itself least of all as an alien substance."[1] The amazing fact is that "it carries over the least possible of the nature [i.e. the etheric forces etc.] of the foreign organism into the human organism." This relation of fats to the human organism is primarily connected to their warmth-nature, which we have mentioned by way of introduction. Of course, we must consider whether we are dealing with plant or

110

animal fat. The chemical structure of fats also plays an important role. The situation of milk fat is especially important, as we have mentioned. (see chapter 1).

Let us first consider what physiological research has examined with regard to these processes, especially with regard to the absorption of fat. According to the latest research, the broken-down fats enter the intestinal membrane either as so-called chylomicrons (with a diameter of 5 microns), or as "microchylons" (with a diameter of .5 microns) or even possibly in a "microemulsion", with a diameter of .05 microns. But the authors of this research add that "in spite of the most modern methods and equipment . . . this problem . . . cannot yet be considered as fully solved."[3] Equally open is the question of the intake and transportation of these tiny particles in the intestinal membrane. However, it is agreed that the primary transport vehicle for absorbed fat is not the blood but the intestinal lymph. About 75% of the fat in a meal is taken in from the cells of the intestinal membrane by the lymph capillaries. What actually happens at this point — the extent to which the measurable fat in the lymph already belongs to the body — can hardly be examined with natural-scientific methods. Even after the lymph lipoids — after flowing into the pectoral lymphatic duct — come into the blood in the left subclavian vein, "it can never be determined with certainty how high the endogenous or exogenous portion is."[3]

On the whole, then, we see how physiological research, in spite of its high level of technical development, must to a large extent admit that it has come only to a piecemeal understanding of this problem.

A Spiritual-Scientific Aspect

It is characteristic of fats that they find their way to the human interior primarily by way of the lymph, rather than by way of the blood. Here there is a problem which we wish briefly to touch upon. Lymph is a bodily fluid which is at a lower level than blood. It is more similar to the general tissue fluid — a carrier of the life forces as such — than to the highly specialized blood which actively carries the forces of individuality. Similarly, fats are, at first, more the carriers of general warmth-forces at the service of the individual warmth-processes.

111

Regarding the orgin of fats, Rudolf Steiner pointed to a clear difference between plant and animal fat. Plant fat — like all natural substances — must in fact be completely broken down and then built up again anew. "Plant fat does not go beyond the intestine; it is destroyed in the intestine. However, the fat contained in meat crosses over into the human being . . . When people eat animal fat . . . it is not completely destroyed." This means an "easing in nutrition." But whoever brings forth the forces to nourish himself from plant fat will thereby gain more inner forces.[4]

Saturated and Unsaturated Fatty Acids

In another respect, modern research has discovered important differences among the fatty acids. They can either be saturated or unsaturated. The saturated fatty acids have an especially intensive connection to carbon, are chemically neutral, and show a tendency toward rigidity and fixation (e.g. grease and bacon fat). The unsaturated fatty acids have a strong connection to warmth in that they have parts which can be saturated with hydrogen. Most plant oils belong in this category. They are liquid at room temperature. The melting points of fats also come into consideration here. The unsaturated fatty acid most common in nature is oleic acid, found in olive oil. Linoleic acid has various unsaturated fatty acids. It appears in many plant oils and is described as "polyunsaturated."

This division, however, requires a further description which will allow us to find a concrete relationship to the human being. Let us begin with the plant oils.

Let us first consider the well-known fact that the organization of plants varies greatly, according to what part of the world they are found in. This fact plays an extremely important role in connection with the quality of the oils. In contrast to the animal kingdom, among plants the oil formation is stronger the warmer the climate is. We could say that the tropical plants produce the most oils, with regard both to quantity and to the intensity of the formative process. They are the most productive plants, because the sun forces work most strongly on them in the tropics. The intensity of oil formation decreases in the Mediterranean region and continues to decrease as we proceed northwards (or towards the poles). This is a further criterion for considering the process

112

of oil formation. For example, linseed oil — which comes more from the north — will be correspondingly different from an oil produced in the tropics. The olive, which grows in the Mediterranean climate, occupies a middle position. Its oil-formation process represents something quite special. In this way, the olive indicates that it forms a middle point between the terrestrial poles and the tropical vegetative region.

Olive

We may now turn our attention to something not immediately obvious but nonetheless accessible to observation. The forces of light and warmth which stream to the earth from the periphery exhibit different — or even opposite — effects, according to whether they come down in the tropical region or more toward the poles.

Anyone who spends some time in the tropics can notice that the daily rhythm predominates. The days are of equal length, and at the equator there are no seasons. Just the opposite occurs at the poles: there, day holds sway for half the year and night for the other half. The situation there is the complete reverse of that at the equator. Thus, the activity of the cosmic forces which stimulate oil production occurs differently. There is something else which may be observed. In the equatorial areas, the cosmic forces of warmth and light are absorbed at once, something that can quite typically be experienced in this warmth area. One can also say that, in the equatorial region, warmth becomes earthly. The more we go northwards, the more splendid do the warmth and light phenomena become. In the polar regions, warmth and light are not taken in by the earth but are radiated back. The earth acts as a reflector. It radiates back into the atmosphere. In his lectures to doctors, Rudolf Steiner described this phenomenon as resulting in something which gives oil formation another quality. Although this perception should not be handled schematically, it does express itself in a certain tendency which plays an important role in evaluating oils. This is especially important with regard to nutritional oils — although it also applies to the fatty oils used therapeutically on the skin — and refers to the character of the so-called unsaturated oleic acid. Every fatty oil has a specific oleic acid spectrum. The closer we come to the warm equatorial regions, where the forces of warmth and light become terrestrial, the more saturated oleic acid is formed by the oil-producing plants. It is an advantage of the oil-producing plants which grow more in the north that they can form more unsaturated oleic acid. It can thus be seen that a certain polarity is manifest, as expressed in the property of being saturated or polyunsaturated.

We find a similar polarity in the human being. Summer holds sway in the metabolism, and winter rules in the nerve-sense system. Spring and autumn alternate in the rhythmic organism and harmonize both poles. We might ask if the polarity between saturated and unsaturated fat is also found in man. There are important research results in this regard today. A person weighing 70 kg has about 7 kg of fat, of which 4.7 kg are unsaturated and 2.3 kg saturated. The saturated fatty acids are found primarily in the nerve-sense organization — in the human "winter sphere" — and the unsaturated fats predominate in the metabolic organism.

Fat Deposits and Organ Fat

We must make a further differentiation, for fat appears in human beings both as so-called fat deposits and as organ fat. The fat deposits primarily take on the general tasks of fat, i.e. they serve as warmth reserves and as warmth regulators. The organ fat, on the other hand, has a more intimate relation to the function of the organ to which it belongs, e.g. the kidneys, the liver, the brain, etc.

Let us first consider the so-called fat deposits, which appear as a subcutaneous fat tissue at the periphery of the organism, as well as in the abdomen and peritoneum. A significant discovery has been made here, namely that this fat is not a deposit but "an organ of prominent importance."[3] It is a highly active metabolic organ which constantly exchanges its substance. There is an interesting differentiation here, too. "The closer to the skin, the more unsaturated fatty acids and the lower the melting point. The more deeply in the organism, the higher the melting point and the smaller the amount of unsaturated fatty acids."[3] The fat more on the periphery is thus the more active; but, in reality, it is still connected to the fat tissue which belongs to the metabolic organism. The fat in the cheeks, on the other hand, is high in saturated fats. There, in the nerve-sense pole, those fat structures predominate which bring out the more plastic, formative components. We can observe quite clearly that this particular fat is at the service of the forces of soul and spiritual expression, in

114

that it is an essential element of the form of the personal countenance.

The fact that the human organism necessarily contains both types of fatty acid — unsaturated and saturated — appears to be of great importance for the practical side of fat consumption. We shall return to this later on.

It should first be mentioned that Rudolf Steiner clearly indicated the form-producing, "padding" function of fat. In a lecture to workers, he designated this "filling out" of the body as an integrating function of fat. Modern research has also become aware of this function. Among other things, the structure and function of the foot-sole fat — and its significance for human standing and walking — has been studied. The fat droplets swimming in the cells of the elastic tissue can be shifted, and they conform to every change of position or pressure. They form an important prerequisite for the elastic gait of humans — for the ability of the lower limbs to lift, carry and move. At the same time, this turgor of the fat cells gives the entire skin its beautiful form — that is, once again, the possibility of expressing the soul and spirit. Such facts also yield new possibilities in the field of cosmetics.

We should not forget that these fat deposits also take part in the other tasks of fat: the production and regulation of warmth.

As we already mentioned, the so-called organ fat should not be seen as being functionally all too different from the deposit fat. Let us first look at the liver, one of the most important organs of lipoid metabolism, which contains a high proportion of fat. This fat is subject to constant change. It is thus understandable that, with respect to its fatty tissue, the liver can degenerate quite easily. Then, the so-called fatty liver — a disease quite frequent today — appears.

On the other hand, the fat in the brain and nerve tissue also plays an important role. Every nerve is surrounded by a fine, fat-like "myelin sheath" which not only protects and isolates but also has a functional relation to the nerve. Let us again recall the phospholipoids of the brain: lecithin, cerebroside and cholesterol. The lipoid composition of the white and grey matter is different. In the white matter — called by Rudolf Steiner the actual "thinking substance" — there is four times more free cholesterol than in the grey matter, which serves more the metabolism and nutrition of the brain. Stanley put forth this remarkable thesis on the basis

115

of such research: "There are direct connections between the lipoid metabolism in the brain and the nervous and mental activity of the person in question."[3] We have already mentioned this problem, and the light shed on it by Rudolf Steiner, in the discussion of phosphorus in *The Dynamics of Nutrition*.

It has today been discovered that the fat around the kidneys, as well as the fat stored in the heart's pericardium, plays a direct role in the metabolism of the respective organ.

These few examples show how fat plays an extraordinarily dynamic role in the organism. On the one hand, it goes toward the plastic-form-active side; on the other hand, it lives primarily in the metabolic functions. In any case, our picture of fat activity in the human organism must be radically transformed. Only with such knowledge can the problem of fat nutrition and the important problem of obesity be discussed in a way that leads right into daily practice.

On the Problem of Fat Consumption

The modern recommendations regarding fat consumption are, understandably, based upon the methods and results of research recognized by present-day nutritional science. They thus contain all the limitations which we have previously mentioned. To the extent that they bring out phenomena which are valid in themselves, these recommendations can be significant for our discussion here — but only if they meet the methodical criteria which we must put forth.

Recently, important research involving fat arrived at conceptions which presuppose a "dynamic of the biological system". This dynamic is based, on the one hand, on the "plasticity" and on the other hand, on the "elasticity" of a living organism.[7] Equally interesting are the observations regarding fat which reveal a person in a special psychological situation. We spoke of this by way of introduction and shall return to it. We here want to mention an important statement by G. Debry, made at the above-mentioned symposium in Zürich: "In fact, physiology can only help to understand the mechanism of the balance of energy . . ." Nonetheless we must keep Eldholm's statement in mind: "The human being is not a rat."[7] There are symptoms here which show the limited possibilities of natural-scientific research regarding warmth. In reality, warmth can never be grasped from a physical, chemical or physiological standpoint alone. It is always also of a soul and spiritual nature. Every one-sided consideration of the fat problem must flounder on this point.

We mentioned at the beginning of our consideration that nutritional fat "brings nothing into the human organism except its ability to develop warmth."[1] Something further, in this regard, is of great significance. This warmth is found in all the members of a person's organization: his physical organism, his vital activity, and his soul-being. But ultimately, this warmth is always an expression of the person's individuality, which extends its feelers into the warming-through of his corporeal nature. To the extent that fat "plays its special role in the production of inner warmth", this warmth is "that in which the Ego-organization primarily lives in the physical organism."[1] Natural warmth — whether from a living or a lifeless source — never proceeds directly into the human being. Rather, it stimulates the person — and especially the highest member of his being — to produce his own warmth. Human warmth is thus always individual. It necessarily engenders illness when it cannot be individualized. The fat-formation process presents a final step in the formation — impregnated by the "Ego-organization" — of substances. Only that fat which carries this individual impression can be called "healthy". There is a constant interplay between the fat and warmth-formation processes. Warmth is transformed into fat, and fat, into warmth. But these processes occur in a "healthy" manner only when they occur under the direction of the "Ego-organization." Rudolf Steiner described this situation quite clearly. It is unfortunate that, although he did so over half a century ago, his insights have not been taken up by official nutritional research. "The healthy manner is when the human formative forces consume the existing fat reserves in developing warmth. An unhealthy manner is when fat is not used up by the Ego-organization in producing warmth but is brought into the organism unused."[1] The latter is thus a fat without master — or a warmth without master — within a person.

Just the opposite occurs, for instance, in the production of milk, to the extent that fat also appears here. The fat in mother's milk also proceeds from the mother's Ego-organization and carries its formative forces. "The forming power of milk rests upon this fact." The mother thus transfers the forming forces

117

of her own Ego-organization to the child. This is a further aspect of the process of milk production which we could only add here, after having become clear about the significance of human fat production. At a time when the Ego-organization of the child is not yet capable of independent activity, a warmth-formative force flows to him through the mother. Light is here again shed on the importance of breast-feeding.

With this introduction behind us, it will be easier to discuss the current recommendations regarding fat consumption. At the same time, we can consider the manifold problems of excessive fat consumption.

One apparent characteristic of the present-day research in this field is that one no longer can, or wish to, set specific quotas regarding fat consumption, a conclusion which is entirely justified. In the same way that experience has shown almost insurmountable difficulties in determining the need for protein, so, according to one modern presentation regarding the need for fat and carbohydrates, "an exact requirement cannot be determined."[3] Others who have addressed this theme — like H.A. Schweigart — have tried to give a detailed tabulation. Schweigart divides the daily fat requirement into the "physiological minimum requirement of 20 g", the "adequate minimum of 50 g and the optimum intake of 90 g." However, he mentions that this refers to "derived" values — i.e. they in no way correspond to reality.[8] Mohler writes that "70 g per day is usually considered tolerable."[9] Aign speaks of a recommended amount of 70-75 g total.[10] We shall explain why the determination of these values is so difficult. But first we would like to add some available figures regarding the actual consumption of fat. Mohler, for example, offers the following values, based on the year 1964. (The figures refer to grams per person and day):

Switzerland	136 g	Italy	87 g
Germany	133 g	Canada	140 g
Great Britain	142 g	USA	147 g
Denmark	159 g	Japan	44 g
Austria	119 g		

It follows from these figures that — with the exception of Japan and many other Asian countries — the fat consumption of

118

Western, affluent society is always too high. It sometimes reaches exactly double the "recommended amount." Also important in this regard is Ludwig's statement that fat consumption in Germany has risen from 10 kg per person per year in 1800, to 16 kg in 1900 and 26 kg in 1950. Since then it has risen even higher. Likewise, J.L. Mount writes in his book, *The Food and Health of Western Man* (1975): "Between 1910 and 1936, fat consumption has doubled, and in the last 50 years, it has increased 100%."[11] This applies to the western world.

If we assume that the values given for fat requirements are correct, it would follow that a great overconsumption of fat has appeared in our century, as various symptoms testify. Why, then, is it so difficult to make exact recommendations, or even determinations, regarding appropriate fat consumption?

The So-Called Essential Fatty Acids

We previously mentioned that, in researching fatty acids, scientists discovered their property of being either saturated or unsaturated. It was found that both properties have a particular relationship in the human organism. Moreover, modern nutritional research has coined the term "essential fatty acids". They are defined as those "which, in contrast to all others, cannot be produced by a person in his own metabolism." They "must therefore be taken in from outside" because they have "a quite specific, vitally essential function in the organism." This is how K. Lang put it in his book, *The Significance of Fat in Nutrition* (1970).[12] In fact, however, Lang bases his information on experiments with animals. He had to admit that "up to the present, symptoms of a large deficiency of essential fatty acids in human beings have not been observed." He thus comes to the conclusion that "the question of the level of fatty acids necessary for human beings . . . has not yet been satisfactorily answered today."

Even quite recently, a nutritional expert spoke of this problem in a similar way. In an essay on essential fatty acids, G. Wolfram wrote: "The individual essential fatty acids have differing abilities to prevent deficiencies in animal experiments . . . There has been no direct research regarding the biological value of different essential fatty acids for humans."[13] In fact, the most important experimental results here have been obtained by experimenting with rats. That "a human being is not a rat," how-

119

ever, is not only true, but we must also voice basic misgivings regarding the methodology of such animal experiments. The "laboratory rat" is a species specially bred by man. These rats are kept and fed under totally artificial conditions, and the result is thus not even typical for the species. The entire concept of "essential fatty acids" with regard to human beings thus stands, at best, on shaky ground. It is therefore not surprising that the amount required by human beings can be given only more or less hypothetically. Moreover, the same author says that, in general, "the effective mechanism of essential fatty acids has not been sufficiently researched."[13]

Linolic acid has been designated as the most important "essential" fatty acid for human beings. As such, it has been relatively well-researched up to today. It is an unsaturated fatty acid, which is found especially in thistle, sunflower, and corn oil, as well as in soya oil. As we mentioned, it plays an active role in the metabolism. Its "dynamic function"[13] has been described as having a "regulatory" action in many metabolic processes of cells. On the other hand, it combines with substances containing phosphorus and is thus related to certain structural elements in the organism.

Although in recent years there have been cases of individual infants whose symptoms disappeared after being given linolic acid, one cannot reach the general conclusion that it is "essential," based on these rare and extreme cases. What is true in an exceptional case need not be generally valid.

Nonetheless, the physiological significance of linolic acid in nutrition is evident. We should try, however, to consider the problem from other points of view.

Further Spiritual-Scientific Aspects

We have already mentioned that spiritual science has provided two facts regarding the relationship of human beings to fat. The first deals with the relative relatedness of fat to man, in that it proves to be the least foreign substance in nutrition. This relatedness, however, does not relieve the human organism of the necessity of relating to fat in the same way, basically, that it relates to protein. The much-researched processes of breaking down in the organs of digestion — which also take place with fat substances — point clearly in this direction. But we must consider

120

a second fact: the difference between plant and animal fats. It is amazing that natural science appears to be almost unaware of the different processes of these two substances in human digestion. In any case, one practically never meets with this question in the literature on the subject, though it is clearly posed with regard to protein. This is because chemically and analytically orientated research does not enable one to differentiate between fat of plant and animal origins. Moreover, the experiments here are almost exclusively done with animals and the results are then carried over to human beings. The only differences resulting from this investigative method are related to the different fatty acid samples which, as we said, are not basically different in plant and animal fats. Nevertheless it was discovered through such research that, for example, "infants absorb the fat from mother's milk better than that from cow's milk, although the fatty acid composition of both is essentially similar."[14] This difference has been attributed to the different arrangements of saturated and unsaturated fat portions of the fatty acid types of the two milks. With this differentiation, there is a corresponding structure of plant oils and fish oils, as opposed to other animal fats. We see that natural-scientific research does not get very far in this field.

On the other hand, we have already shown how human beings relate differently to plant and animal fats. As we mentioned in *The Dynamics of Nutrition,* both must be "destroyed" in order to be immediately built up anew. "With the fats he eats, he [man] develops a force, in that he destroys the substance. Fats are entirely his own product."[4] As with the processing of protein, a person does not process plant and animal fats in the same way. The latter are closer to him. Thus, he need not go as far in the process of destruction as with plant fats. Therefore "a person may be weaker than if he ate only plant fat". In this regard, animal fat is more digestible, as it is more similar to one's inner being. It is this point that appears to be of special significance regarding the question of plant and animal nutrition.

It is known — but perhaps too seldom considered in nutritional physiology — that fat makes food tasty. Without fat, animal as well as plant foods are less stimulating to the appetite and taste. In vegetables prepared with butter or some other fat, salad made with oil or mayonnaise, "cream sauces" of all sorts, meat dishes, or "browned butter" on fish — fat plays an impor-

121

tant role in strengthening and improving the tastiness of food. And even fatty meat as such is usually preferred to leaner meat. At the same time, fat allows the taste of the different foods to appear more strongly. In this regard, fat — including "bread and butter" — when used moderately, improves the taste and aids one's digestion. This certainly has its basis in the character of fat. It has a special relationship to man — to his warmth-organism and also to his life-organization — precisely because of its insolubility in water, i.e. its salt-alien character. In general, one derives more pleasure from eating foods with fat. This enjoyment also presents the danger of an over-consumption of fat, however.

Rudolf Steiner described this moment of enjoyment quite clearly: "When a person takes in the fat from an ox, or pig, or whatever . . . it goes into his body: it satisfies his desire . . . therefore he loves meat. Thus, one eats meat especially when the body loves meat."

The easy digestibility of animal food in itself combines with the easy digestibility of animal fat, and both intensify the enjoyment of the food.

However, we do not want to overlook the fact that fat is indispensable to man, even though its properties have contributed to an excess of fat consumption.

Before we go on to the question of obesity, let us characterize the individual plant and animal fats more closely.

The Real Essence of Fat

We can see from our previous considerations that we have to differentiate between fats of plant and animal origin. In keeping with our chapter on milk, we see that milk fat — although usually considered an animal fat — must be accorded a special position. Modern chemical analysis yields the further differentiation into saturated and unsaturated fatty acids. Finally, we have considered the question of the so-called "essential" fatty acids. In addition, there is the problem of excessive fat consumption.

A question now poses itself: are these criteria adequate for a qualitative evaluation of fat, or must we look for further new criteria? And how should we deal with the above-mentioned criteria?

We have already spoken of the basic differences between plant and animal fat. Let us again emphasize the fact that the

122

formation of plant fat — in the green leaves — presents a direct communication with the cosmic warmth forces. In contrast, the animal can form its fat substance only indirectly, out of these forces. In addition, the animal internalizes this warmth from the living organization at the level of its life-organization. On the path of this process of internalization, the saturated fatty acids appear to acquire their formative tendencies. We shall have to follow this problem further. In any case, we have here a basic difference between plant and animal fats. But this is not enough; the fact that the green leaf is the organ for original fat production raises another question: what about the process of fat formation in mushrooms, as well as in legumes which have already displayed a metabolism approaching that of animals? Moreover we must ask: is the process of fat formation similar over the entire earth, or are there qualitative differences in the tropical, temperate and cold zones?[2] Only an overall view of all these aspects can provide a yardstick for judging the quality of fat.

The fatty acids which appear as "unsaturated" are characterized by a more or less large amount of free — that is, not saturated with hydrogen — carbon. The chemical formula for saturated stearic acid, for example, is $C_{18}H_{36}O_2$. The hydrogen is completely bound to the carbon. Oleic acid, on the other hand, a so-called simple unsaturated fatty acid — the most common of its type — has the formula $C_{16}H_{34}O_2$. It thus has a free carbon double linkage. A polyunsaturated fat like linolic acid, mentioned above, has the formula $C_{18}H_{34}O_2$. It has two fewer parts hydrogen. The difference between saturated and unsaturated fatty acids is, on the one hand, not so great, and on the other hand can be clearly found in its relation to hydrogen. The unsaturated fatty acids are more active and busier. They are not yet fully consolidated and display a special bond to hydrogen.

What does this mean? This gas flees from the earth and is the lightest and most closely related to warmth. Rudolf Steiner characterized it as a substance "which, as far as possible, is related to the physical and, as far as possible, is related to the spiritual."[15] Hydrogen, which today is thought to constitute the sun, "actually negates everything." When hydrogen is internalized, it proves to be related to the human heart system. There it is related to the actual spiritualizing processes in man, to the phosphorus processes. "For in a certain respect, with the development of hydrogen,

123

that which is more animal-like in the lower part of man is transformed into something actually human in the upper part."[16]

The unsaturated fatty acids develop a bond with hydrogen. They are more related to movement and are dynamic. They stimulate the metabolism and develop a certain affinity for "their" organ, i e. the heart. In fact, green leaves — the organs of original fat formation — are especially rich in linolic acid, a polyunsaturated fatty acid. As Rudolf Steiner said of green leaves, "the greener they are, the more fat substance they give." And by means of these plant fats, "we make ourselves strong in the heart and lungs, in the middle man, the chest man."[4] In this way, we can discover a rational connection between these unsaturated fatty acids and human activities. The warmth contained in these fats serves to humanize the entire organism. It also appears as "warmth of heart" and forms the bridge between physical and soul-spiritual processes.

It is interesting in this light that an extreme consumption of highly unsaturated fatty acids can bring on inflammatory processes. On the other hand, the saturated fatty acids further the tendency toward hardening and sclerosis. We shall discuss this later on.

In fact, we find that plants are the organisms with the most unsaturated fatty acid types. These fatty acids remain liquid at room temperature. In the solid fats, like blubber and grease, we have mostly saturated fatty acids from animal organisms. But this does not yet adequately characterize the problem. Fat research has discovered something interesting here: the simplest forms of life in the sea exhibit the greatest variety in fatty acid types. Moreover, this varies between salt and fresh-water inhabitants. In the fresh-water plants and animals, the simple unsaturated fatty acids predominate. Among the salt-water beings, the C 20 and C 22 fatty acids are predominant. All organisms which live in water not only display such a variety but also a high level of unsaturation in their fatty acid types. However, the higher the level of organization in the animal kingdom, the more simple the composition of the fats. Thus, mammals have primarily only three essential fatty acids represented in their fat stores: palmitic, stearic and oleic acid. The first two are saturated and only the third is a simple, unsaturated fatty acid.

124

Such discoveries raise important and far-reaching questions which can only be alluded to here. They encompass the entire problem of evolution.

Fat Formation and Evolution

The lower forms of life — such as the lower aquatic plants and animals — have a basically different relationship towards warmth than do higher animals or even higher plants. Today, we differentiate between cold-blooded, varying and warm-blooded animals. The relationship of light to the different stages of life is also different. The present-day, warm-blooded animals are clearly close to man. Warm blood, however, is a fruit of earth evolution. "For warm blood was not in any kingdom of nature before the earth period."[17] The cold — and varying — blooded beings belong to an earlier stage of evolution — to the Old Moon, or even to an earlier stage which Rudolf Steiner called the Old Sun. (cf. Rudolf Steiner, *An Outline of Occult Science*). Descendants from such ancient stages of evolution still exist today in sea animals and plants. The sea thus reflects an earlier stage of evolution, whereas fresh water is more adapted to later earthly conditions. However, all these living beings are even more strongly related to the cosmic forces. Today, they still live as images of Old Moon or Old Sun forces. In their fat metabolism they are — and this is the interesting thing — more complicated than the higher forms of life. They contain primarily unsaturated fatty acids, i.e. they were not able to develop the saturated fatty acids — which tend toward the nerve-sense pole — in the way that the mammals did. The latter ensoul their bodies and come to an experience of their own warmth. But the lower aquatic animals still come into contact with soul forces externally and are thus similar to the flower-formation stage of higher plants. Thus, not only in the lower sea animals, but also in the fish, we find unsaturated fatty acids. But they are of an altogether different nature than the same fatty acids in higher plants: the fish remain confined in cold, watery surroundings. They there form, at the level of animals — but without a connection to earth evolution (except for lung fish which occasionally posses appendages, and can move on dry land) — unsaturated fatty acids. This is the expression of a pre-earthly, cosmic relationship to hydrogen (and to phosphorus as well, which is closely related to hydrogen). In contrast, the higher land

125

plants rise up to a level which is related entirely to earth evolution. They root in the earth and form chlorophyll in the green leaves. This chlorophyll is essential for the preparation of fat. Their unsaturated fatty acid products — e.g. linolic acid in green leaves — may be seen as an expression of the plant's cosmic-earthly relationship which reveals its solar origin in greening. The plant has a special relationship to man in its reversed, upright, threefold formation, as has been described in *The Dynamics of Nutrition*.

The fatty acid type also becomes simpler in seed plants, but it tends toward the unsaturated side, in contrast to its behavior in higher animals. In the fruit skins and seeds, palmitin oil and linolic acid hold sway. We should mention here that climate plays a decisive role *vis a vis* the fatty acid type. In plants which grow in colder climates, unsaturated fatty acids with low melting points predominate. Tropical plants further the formation of saturated fatty acids, although even here we find unsaturated fatty acid types in the seeds. This phenomenon proves to be important from a spiritual-scientific point of view.

In his second medical course (1921),[5] Rudolf Steiner spoke of how, in the tropics, "the earth sucks in the most from the extra-earthly", and lets the vegetation spring forth from it. Warmth and light, as cosmic forces, thereby obtain an earthly character. In contrast, these forces are most reflected back to the poles: "The earth shines the most at the poles." Light and warmth maintain their extra-earthly character. The same holds true for mountain plants which grow at high altitudes.

The warmer it is, the more oil tropical plants produce, but their oil is more earthly. The daily rhythm holds sway; there are no seasons. Tropical oils exhibit more saturated oil-formation, which tends toward solidification. "When the same plant can grow and flourish well in both hot and cold climates, it forms fat deposits with unsaturated fatty acids in cold climates. In warm climates, it forms deposits with saturated fatty acids."[3] In northern regions, plants produce less oil. The warmth is radiated more strongly back into the cosmos, rather than being substantially condensed. For all that, the unsaturated fatty acid types predominate. The palm and coconut trees — with their strong, primarily saturated oil products — stand in contrast to thistle oil, rape oil and other oils from northern lands. In the middle, between both —

in the Mediterranean — we find the olive tree. Its fruit has an oil containing c. 70% simple unsaturated oleic acid.

Within animal evolution, on the other hand, we find, among the mammals in polar regions, a copious fat formation which decreases among the animals in the tropics. But, as we saw, mammals tend toward saturated fatty acid types. In contrast, even the large aquatic creatures, like the whale and cod, produce many unsaturated fatty acids.

Ludwig put forth an evolutionary consideration in this regard: "In earlier evolutionary history, e.g. among the fish, the fat taken in with food is utilized and stored in the organism without any essential transformation. At this stage, animals are incapable of transforming carbohydrates and protein into fat. Among the amphibians, nutritional fat is indeed built into fat stores, but these animals can already synthesize fat. The ruminants form the end point of this development."[3]

Here, too, one sees that as the true terrestrial animals actually took hold of warmth — as they internalized their cosmic origin — a change took place in their fat metabolism. Only mammals and human beings are capable of producing fat within themselves from broken-down carbohydrates and even from proteins. They can, thereby, put all food substances at the service of warmth production and regulation.

This knowledge has long been used with regard to domestic animals, with the fattening of pigs or geese with carbohydrates, but the tendency has a largely negative effect in modern man. Additional fat is created from the excessive, refined carbohydrates eaten, and it contributes to overweight.

We have thus created the necessary basis for characterizing the specific types of fat and will now discuss the tropical oils, the legume oils — soy and peanut oils — and butter fat, to the extent that we have not already done so in the chapter on milk.

Tropical Oils: Coconut and Palm

Oil and fat have played an essential role in human nutrition in all cultures for thousands of years. In the tropical and subtropical regions of the earth, where the great early cultures developed, oil was of universal significance. It was used in the temple rituals and in medicine and hygiene. It always formed an important part of daily nourishment. In other words: people had insight

127

into the essence and character of oils. How, when, and for whom oil was used was never left to chance, for people saw, even if instinctively, into the patterns of this substance and its relation to man. In addition, the particular oil used was characteristic of the different human cultures. The northern, southern and Mediterranean cultures in part received their character from their oils.

Let us turn first to the tropical oils. We already mentioned the coconut and the palm, both of which play an important role as sources of fat.

The coconut tree grows as high as 30 meters, can reach the venerable age of 100 years, and thrives primarily in tropical coastal regions. From its probable home in Mexico, it has spread out over all tropical lands today, partly in large plantations. Up to one hundred fruits may ripen on a tree in a year. Their milk has been treasured since ancient times as a refreshing, tasty drink. These fruits take fifteen months to develop in the hot tropical sun and moist tropical air. They grow as big as a head and are surrounded by a water-tight skin. Only the seed inside, surrounded by the nutritive "milk", contains — in the seed tissue — the oil and the typical germ. This seed tissue supplies — after a process of boiling and drying — the so-called copra. This product is 60-75% fat and solidifies at 23° (c. 73°F). In temperate latitudes it is therefore solid, though it is liquid in its tropical origin. By pressing it cold, one obtains the white coconut fat with its nutty flavor. But the raw oil obtained in this way must first be deacidified and deodorized before being eaten. It contains up to more than 90% saturated fatty acids. The remainder is palmitic and oleic acid.

The palm tree — which grows more in the interior of tropical countries — plays a big role as a source of oil or fat. It grows to about twenty meters. The varying rain and scorching heat of the tropical jungles provide the atmosphere in which this tree produces its oil. The tree bears hundreds of orange to black fruits, the flesh of which is entirely filled with oil. This fruit flesh provides 30-70% palm oil, while the germs produce 45-55% of the so-called palm germ fat. The raw oil must be refined, whereas the palm germs are processed in various ways. Palm oil contains about 40% palmitic acid and about 50% oleic acid. It is used primarily to make soap, whereas palm germ fat is used in part for nutrition and has a predominantly saturated fatty acid pattern, similar to coconut fat. It is an important ingredient in margarine.

We have already mentioned something common to these two plants in pointing to the predominantly saturated fatty acid type of both. This is associated with the form pole of man, which tends toward hardening. The form of these plants confirms such a speculation. They were called *Principes,* i.e. princes, by Linné. The aristocratic, stiff and rigid carbon holds sway in such plants. It can produce the hardest substance — the diamond — and gives the palm leaves their formal dignity but also their inflexible shape. These plants rank fourth among the oil-producing plants in the world, so one can see the scope of the consumption of saturated fatty acids from this source alone.

The Soybean

Other oils which originated in warmer climates — soybean and peanut oils — offer an altogether different picture. Both plants belong to the larger family of legumes.

Let us first look at the soybean. It comes from the far east (China) and belongs to the oldest plants cultivated, having been used for thousands of years in human nutrition. The oldest existing records go back to 2800 B.C. It has since spread, from its original, far-eastern territory, over large parts of the world. Soybeans are often planted as monocultures in the U.S.A today but are rarely found in Europe. They play a leading role in nutrition, both as a source of oil (with a c. 20% oil content) and also as a source of protein (c. 40% protein content). They rank first with regard to the production of plant oils. Soy oil looks especially valuable because of its high (c. 60%) linolic acid content — a polyunsaturated fatty acid which is counted among the "essential" fatty acids. These considerations would lead one to see soy oil as one of the most valuable oils, which is just what the generally accepted treatments of this subject do. But in order to evaluate this plant in a realistic manner, we must consider criteria which are largely ignored today.

We have already said that, botanically, the soybean is a legume, a pod plant. The legumes are one of the largest plant families (with over 12,000 species) and are spread out over the entire world, except for the cold zones. Their special characteristic — of interest for our considerations — is their unique protein

129

formation, their relationship to nitrogen. They have special nitrogen-fixing bacteria in their fine root nodes. They are capable of taking in nitrogen from the air in the ground and using it for protein formation.

This symbiosis of the legumes and nodal bacteria occurs in a quite remarkable way. A small organism, today called *bacillus radicicola* (root-inhabiting bacillus), enters into the young roots of these plants. A kind of "infectious disease" takes place, which the legumes are immune to. In fact, the host plants are obviously prepared in their inner environment and they offer the bacteria an atmosphere in which they can thrive; then the plant begins to use the bacteria trapped in its root nodes and obtains nitrogen compounds from them. In fact, special channels are set up which provide the nodes with sugar and transport the nitrogen compounds synthesized by the bacteria to the interior of the plant. Virtanen was the first to show that these legume roots leave behind large amounts of amino acids in the ground. These plants thus provide not only themselves, but also the ground they are in, with nitrogen. This is especially important for agriculture. Rudolf Steiner emphasized this phenomenon in his lectures on agriculture and also shed light on the situation through spiritual-scientific research.[15]

We characterized hydrogen as that element which is lightest, least bound to the earth, and related to warmth. Similarly, nitrogen — the typical protein element — carries forces related not to the spiritual but rather to the soul world. Nitrogen (*Stickstoff* in German, a word which carries the connotation of suffocating or asphyxiating substance) is opposite to oxygen, the carrier of life, as the German name indicates. Animals and human beings internalize it and use it as a carrier of their soul forces. Plants cannot do this, but they are touched by it, "putting forth colorful crowns" in their blossoms and fruits. "The plant would not flower if the astral did not touch if from without."

As we have seen, legumes have a different relationship to nitrogen. They have already accomplished a process of internalization which is characteristic of soul qualities. It is thus understandable that legumes include sensitive plants like the *Mimosa pudica,* which responds to tactile stimulation with a closing-up movement. This beginning of "ensoulment" is just as clearly indicated by the red color in the active bacterial nodes. It is sim-

130

ilar in color to red blood and is called leghemoglobin. These plants are thus able to form and color a substance which otherwise appears only in higher animals and man as a carrier of soul qualities.

In the agricultural lectures mentioned above, Rudolf Steiner explains that we should pay attention to the tendency of the papilionaceous flowers to "want to bear fruit before they flower." That is to say, a "kind of stunting of the actual fruit of these plants takes place" which is expressed in a shortened ability to seed. This is all an expression of the fact that "with these plants, much more is held to the earth which lives in nitrogen." They are not only more earthly than the other green plants, but also more animal-like. They produce a protein which tastes much like meat, as is especially evident in the case of the soybean. These plants form poisons, a fact which must be considered when we use them as food.

The meat-like aroma of soy protein has been exploited by the modern food industry. The plant food is made to resemble meat through the use of TVP (Textured Vegetable Protein) which is made from soy flour. A modern treatise, cited in our chapter on protein, reads: "The vegetarian has here a pure plant product which affords him the pleasure others have in eating meat . . . It is as nutritious as meat and is totally comparable in taste."[19]

Here one can see quite clearly the characteristics actually incorporated in the soy plant, and it is interesting that modern research has utilized these characteristics to such perfection. When an alleged vegetarian allows himself to be deceived with such a "meat-like structure" — if the meat-like taste of the soy protein is not enough — this can only be seen as the expression of decadent nutritional instincts, combined with the refinement of modern technical practices. The perspectives thus opened for nutritional research are clearly spoken of by Cremer. He writes: "These foods can be easily adapted to any eating habits and to any religious or dietary prescriptions. They can be modified to correspond to the tastes of the population in any region." Western materialism here celebrates a calamitous triumph with an ancient, eastern, agricultural plant. With greater and lesser degrees of consciousness and unconsciousness, the spiritual knowledge of these connections in the mystery cultures which survived into Greek times is being ignored. Pythagoras — the

131

great philosopher of the Greek mysteries — was also the founder of a type of nutrition which his students were bound to follow. It included fruits, nuts, grains, milk, honey and vegetables. Beans were strictly forbidden.

Modern spiritual research is capable of filling such facts with the light of consciousness appropriate to the times. Here, in the significant words of Rudolf Steiner, we find our own observations regarding legumes confirmed by Steiner's spiritual observation. "Some plants are already strongly permeated with astrality, like the legumes, for instance. There, even the fruit remains in the lower regions . . . making sleep dull and thereby making the head dull when it awakens. The Pythagoreans wanted to remain pure thinkers. They did not want to bring in the digestion to assist the activity of the head. Therefore, they forebade eating beans."[20]

What is here expressed regarding legume fruits in general is naturally true of soybeans in particular. It holds true not only for the protein component but also for the process of oil formation. We thus see that the criterion of "unsaturated fatty acid" deals only with one aspect of quality. To make judgments in accordance with reality, we must learn to develop a much more comprehensive view; otherwise, we remain entangled in compulsive, materialistic thought — perhaps even in "bean thinking" itself, if we may use such a term. Such thinking draws a veil before the clear light of knowledge so desperately needed today.

We should at least be informed of the increasing amount of soy products in our daily food. Aside from the so-called "soy meat" and soy products developed from it, we find a great variety of "full soy products" offered today. These include whole soy flakes, cereal, groats, macaroni, paste and flour (often used as a soup base, but also found in baked goods). Soy lecithin is also used by the food industry. From the far east (especially from Japan) come soy sauce ("miso") and "natto" and "tofu", as so-called soy cheese. The soybean itself as a vegetable is, of course, also widely recommended in the east. Especially questionable, in this regard, is the discussion of macrobiotic nutrition for small children and infants in G. Ohsawa's *Zen Macrobiotics*.[21] In this book we read that cow milk or the milk of any other animal is not biologically intended for the human infant. Based on this serious error (dealt with in our chapter on milk) "Kokkoh" is recommended; this is a ready-made product of rice, oat flour, soybeans and sesame

132

which it is said "can nourish the child in cases where mother's milk is not available." Feeding people soybeans from the first day of their lives, and accompanying them with soy products through all stages of life — East and West here join hands in an ambiguous way. And, as Ohsawa writes at the end of his book, "Only then can there be a real union of West and East."[21]

The Peanut

The typical qualitative characteristics of soybeans are also applicable to peanuts — the second most important oil plant today. The peanut is also a legume, but it originated not in Asia, but in tropical Central America. It is thus an oil plant from the west which has spread out over the entire world. Today, the largest amounts of peanut oil are produced in Asia (60%) and Africa (30%). In Europe, only Spain has peanut production worth mentioning, while in the U.S.A., peanut farmers are becoming more significant. The peanut is similar to the soybean in its high protein content (26%) and high fat content (50%). The warmer and more constant the climate, the greater the amount of oil. The pattern of fatty acids is also similar to that of soybeans. Peanut oil is about 50% simple unsaturated oleic acids and up to about 30% linolic acid. This fact, along with its above average fat content as such, have given the peanut a leading role in the oil-processing industry. Peanut oil, the main product, is used both in margarine and as a table oil. In Switzerland, Spain and Italy, peanut fat is used to make "white chocolate". Peanut butter, from finely ground peanuts, is especially popular in the U.S.A. The seeds are eaten like nuts, both raw and roasted, and serve as an almond substitute in the baking industry. In the primary peanut-producing regions, peanuts are used as animal feed and fertilizer.

The essential quality of the peanut, however, is to be found not only in the high fat content, but also in the characteristic processes of growth and ripening which it displays. The dynamics of its oil-formation process speak in clear terms of its origin. One might wish to dismiss such a signature as a curiosity, but this would be to turn away from what is essential. If, in contrast, we try to proceed in the spirit of Goethe's *Metamorphosis of Plants* by remembering his words "Observe it becoming . . ." ("Werdend betrachte sie nun . . ."), we can begin to see its riddles unveiled.

133

After a relatively short germination period, the peanut sprout develops, with its typical leaf structure. Soon, the so-called sleep movement can be observed with the coming of darkness. It then does not strive upward toward the light, in typical fashion, but rather spreads out in bushy form. The developing tap-root has numerous secondary roots with bacterial nodes. The flower formation takes place in the leaf axils and exhibits the well known butterfly form with a gold-yellow color. Then the fruit nodes are formed with their ovules. And then comes an unexpected, dramatic development. During the night, the flower bud develops an impressive longitudinal growth. In the early morning, the flower develops; but in that same morning, the flower begins to wilt, after having undergone a self-pollination during the brief blossoming. Then a stem-like form comes out of the flower and grows, pushing the remains of the flower with it. This is the so-called fruit-bearer. However, this growth does not proceed upwards. On the contrary, the fruit-bearer tends to increase downwards, towards the earth, until it finally reaches the ground. Then the tip bores into the earth and grows a few more centimeters under the earth. Only then does the ovule expand, and it begins to grow horizontally under the earth's surface. The fruit-bearer now behaves like a root. It takes in nutrients from the earth — both water and substances. Calcium appears to play a large role here. As the bearer of the forces of animal desires, it has a significant influence on the ripening of the fruit underground. However, on the average, only one-fourth of the ovules sunk into the ground reach maturity.

We thus see how this plant brings three properties to expression. First, it has a weak relation to light, which we see in its lack of directed, horizontal growth — a property which it shares with many other legumes (beans, peas, etc.). Second, it is obviously overpowered by the gravitational forces of the earth, in that it actively penetrates into the earth with its fruit-bearer. Third, once the fruits come into the earth, they ultimately behave like roots — they deny their cosmic, solar, nature and turn to earthly forces. In the darkness of the earth, the moon forces are active, as we see in the formation of mushrooms. This relationship to the fungus world is clearly shown in the susceptibility of peanuts to fungi in the soil. If the shell is damaged, fungi easily penetrate into the peanuts and there produce the highly toxic "aflatoxin".

134

As is known, these poisoned peanuts have caused great damage when used as animal feed. In addition, the undamaged peanut produces a substance which promotes the coagulation of the blood. This can call forth thrombophilia, which shows a heaviness of the blood and the predominance of earthly forces.

The background outlined here should make comprehensible Rudolf Steiner's statement that "peanuts are to be completely avoided."[22]

Sunflower, Rape, Watercress, Linseed, Corn, Wheat Germ and Safflower as Oil Sources

Having looked at the tropical and sub-tropical oil plants, we shall now turn towards those of the northern temperate regions. Sunflowers, rape seed, linseed and safflowers should be mentioned here. Corn and wheat also belong, more or less, in this region, while sesame tends more strongly towards southern climates.

Sunflower seeds contain up to 65% linolic acid — quite a high proportion of unsaturated fatty acids. They are increasingly popular where the active nature of these oil forms (and its relation to the human heart and circulation) has been recognized. They stimulate tissue respiration. In fact, sunflower oil is formed in harmony with the rhythm of the sun. Anyone can see for himself how the flower tops of these plants are turned to the sun during the course of the day. They follow the movements of this cosmic star. From the gold-yellow color of the flowers, though, one might call it a Jupiter flower.

The fat content of the seeds is high (up to 50%). When pressed cold, they yield a mild-tasting table oil. However, sunflower oil is also used today for producing so-called "health food" margarine. At 10%, its content of saturated oils is quite small. Sunflower-seed oil serves well not only in cases of metabolic diseases, but also with skin diseases (e.g. eczema), because of its inner stimulation of respiration.

The cruciferous plants have a special place among the oil plants. Rape and rape-seed oil form one-sixth of all edible oils. Their relation to the sulfur process enables these plants to condense sufficient warmth-forces for abundant oil production, with predominately unsaturated fatty acids. These oils are thus especially popular.

Above all, it should be mentioned that this family includes watercress as well as horse radish and mustard. In watercress, too, the warmth-forming sulfur principle is at work. A juvenile oil is formed in the round, powerful leaves of this plant. It corresponds exactly to the process of oil formation described by Rudolf Steiner. He mentioned watercress specifically in this connection. A person "takes in more fat when he eats watercress, for example — this small plant with the tiny leaves — than when he eats bread."[4]

It appears to us that light is shed here upon the process of oil formation, especially among the cruciferous plants. They produce an especially valuable oil in their abundant seeds — full of unsaturated oils — by means of the sulfur process.

Oil formation in linseed brings us to the northern unsaturated fatty acids. Linseeds stimulate the digestion, e.g. when used to season bread. It has been shown that linseeds work against cramps and inflammations and that they stimulate the intestinal flora. Linseed oil has recently become known as a dietary help in cases of skin diseases, such as eczema, furunculosis and cradle cap.

J. Budwig has made especially praiseworthy contributions to the research into linseed oil. In her writings, she emphasizes the dietetic and healing value of linseed oil. "Budwig-Muesli" is a well known special combination of curds and linseed oil, from an old Silesian recipe. She has used it successfully in a diet against cancer. The old term *Linum utilisatissimum* — i.e. the highly useful linseed — has proven itself anew in our time.

Rudolf Steiner also pointed to linseed with regard to its nutritive effects.[15] Linseed today is usually planted and threshed like grain. It is characterized by its high content of unsaturated linolic acid. It provides an example of this type of oil formation, typical among the plants in northern regions. This is in contrast to the animals in northern climates, who produce more saturated fats. Of course, such plant oils easily become rancid, as they are very sensitive to the oxidation processes. This limits their use as food oils.

However, corn oil has become increasingly significant in the last decades. Although the oil content of corn is low (3-7%), it is valued today because it is rich in phosphides. Wheat germ oil is similar.

The advantages we mentioned for linseed oil also apply to these two grain-germ oils. They have recently come to the fore because of research into the so-called "fat-soluble vitamins." We shall deal with this matter in our chapter on vitamins.

The safflower ranks first among plants with regard to linolic acid content. It contains 75% linolic acid and only 10% saturated fatty acids. This puts it at the extreme opposite to the palm oils, which have primarily fatty acid types. Although safflower oil is especially recommended in health food circles today, we should consider its one-sidedness with regard to its stimulation of inflammatory processes. Its one-sided structure makes it more valuable as a remedy than as a food.

We have not mentioned all the important oils here — e.g. such oils as sesame, poppy and cottonseed. But we have given enough characteristic examples for an informed consideration. Before turning to the most important oil of the human middle region — olive oil — we should like to look at one more indication regarding nut oils.

Nuts as a Source of Oil

Nuts are an extraordinarily valuable source of nutrition and deserve special consideration. Here, however, we shall speak only of their significance for fat in the diet. The three most important nuts in this regard are the hazelnut, the walnut and the almond. All three have a pattern of fatty acids in which the unsaturated part is modest, so we can speak of the high dynamic metabolic reaction potential of these nuts.

The proportion of fat in hazelnuts is quite high; at 62% it is the highest of the three nuts mentioned. Walnuts with 58% and almonds with 53% fat are, however, not far behind. This high fat content is often not considered enough when people consume the various nut products. In Europe, hazelnuts are available as a puree, fruit paste and nut butter. Rudolf Steiner especially recommended hazelnut butter in the above-mentioned lecture of 1904.[22]

These nuts offer a great advantage for our nutrition in that, with them, we do not consume isolated fat (as we do with the above-mentioned oils) but rather enjoy it in a natural composition with protein, carbohydrates, minerals, etc. It is just this completeness which makes hazelnuts valuable.

137

As we have seen, walnuts are only slightly less rich in fat than hazelnuts, but they have a different character which we shall consider later.

Almonds present an altogether different picture. They belong to the rosaceous plants. Their fat is accompanied by an especially high protein content (12%) which makes these nuts nutritious but also hard to digest. Marzipan — a popular almond treat — makes this obvious. Also of great importance is almond milk, which Rudolf Steiner strongly recommended; he suggested adding a bitter almond to the sweet almonds in preparing this milk. The cyanide process is here at work, giving the almond a specific tone. But here, too, moderation is called for in the eating of almonds.

Finally there is the Cyprian almond which is not actually a nut, but which plays a certain role in the oil production of unsaturated fatty acids. In many regards, it is similar to the most important fruit oil, which stands in the middle between the tropical/sub-tropical and the northern oil plants: olive oil. Since olive oil is of special significance, we will devote special consideration to it.

The Olive Tree

The olive tree, first mentioned in the near east, was cultivated thousands of years ago. From there, it spread throughout the entire Mediterranean region. It appears to have grown originally in Abyssinia and Arabia, both as a tree and as a wild shrub. At the beginning of Greek culture in the seventh century, it covered the hills and coasts of the mainland and islands with its evergreen woods.

The olive tree was highly regarded in the Jewish culture of the Old Testament, as well as in Greek culture. Olive oil was in general use for sacrifices in the temple, for food, for annointing the body, and for oil lamps. Quite early on, this tree was called "holy". It was dedicated to the Goddess Athena, and her olive trees on the Acropolis were untouchable, as symbols of spiritual clarity and peace. In Olympia, the victorious competitors were decorated with olive branches. A Greek myth relates that Jupiter gave preference to the gift of Minerva, who brought him an olive branch; its fruit was not only good to eat, but it also yielded a miracle juice which seasoned the food of men, healed their

138

wounds, gave strength to their bodies and gave light to the night. According to biblical tradition, the "oil of mercy" comes from an olive tree growing from one of the seeds which Seth placed in the mouth of his father, Adam. For these cultures, olive oil was simply oil, as the Latin word *oliva-oleum* — synonomous with oil — shows.

The olive tree does, indeed, belong to the Mediterranean region and is characteristic of this climate. It is protected from extreme cold in the north by the Alps, and borders the hot deserts of the African coastal lands. The extremes are moderated because the multifaceted ocean surface reflects back light and warmth, thus preparing the atmosphere of this region from which 90% of all olives come. It is as if an image of both human poles — the cool brain and the fiery metabolism — comes to a mercurial balance in the Mediterranean region. The heart forces — the human "middle" — seem to be incarnated in this olive tree landscape. The forces of earth and sun are reconciled, and earthly and cosmic warmth interpenetrate one another. In his *Heilpflanzenkunde* Wilhelm Pelikan described the noble character of olive oil as follows: "In it, hard knowledge is purified upwards, into the grace and peace of the sun life. It gave strength to food and provided a balancing mildness to the polarities of sharp, sour, and salty."[24]

The olive ripens slowly and constantly in the sun-filled summer and fall. The harvest begins only in the mild winter time. For oil production, the fruit must have reached a certain degree of ripeness. Olives harvested too early contain less oil.

Even the so-called green olives can hardly be eaten freshly harvested. Only after careful storage and aging do they achieve their desired quality. The ripe black olives, however, are the most valuable. "Virgin oil" or "first pressing, cold-pressed," yield the highest quality.

Let us look at the composition of olive oil. We see at once that it is rich in the oleic acids called "simple unsaturated." Its extraordinarily high content of these oleic acids — 70%-80% — differentiates it from all other plant oils. It contains hardly even 10% linolic acid. On the other hand, it contains an even smaller percentage of saturated oleic acids. Here again we see a clear central position between the two extremes of saturated and highly unsaturated elements. In fact, we may call olive oil the oil of the middle. Its mild aroma and taste also bear witness to this. It has a clear relationship to man, in that its melting point is close to human fat formation. Furthermore the composition of subcutaneous human fatty tissue roughly corresponds to that of olive oil with regard to its fatty acid pattern.

It is known that fats are more easily digested the closer their melting point is to the human body temperature. From this point of view, olive oil is almost entirely digested by the human body, closely followed by butter, which also melts at c. 37°C (c. 99°F). Olive oil easily forms emulsions, another fact which explains its digestibility. In addition, it stimulates the appetite, especially when used with salads or vegetables. The green leaf — the primary organ of fat production — is especially suited to nourishing man's middle region, as we have seen; olive oil is especially suited in this regard. In addition, Italian researchers have determined that olive oil provides the best known cholagoic and choleretic factor, whereby the effect of pure oil is superior to that of the usually refined products on the market. For this reason, olive oil forms an important part of a liver-gall diet.[25]

Other therapeutic effects of olive oil have been known for some time now. Its "basic therapeutic effect" has been described as "mild, supple, enveloping, gentle, opening and effective against cramps." Internally, it is effective against infections, the bites and stings of poisonous animals, and catarrhic conditions in the organs of respiration and digestion. It is also helpful against constipation and hemorrhoids, that is, against blockages and stagnation. Externally its effect is also loosening, soothing and tension-relieving, in cases of burns, etc.[26] Olive oil massages are also effective in cases of gout and rheumatism. Further, olive oil can protect one against freezing when it is applied as a coating. We shall see that this external effect, in its enveloping, protecting and warming capacity, was perceived by an old wisdom already traditional in ancient Greece.

In ancient Greek times, the special quality of olive oil and its effect on the human organism were known. "There are two liquids," says Pliny, "which are agreeable to the human body. Inside, wine, and outside, oil. Both come from trees, but the oil is necessary." And Democrates of Abdera responded to the question of how one could remain healthy, and live to an old age, with this dietary rule: "internally honey, externally oil."

140

A Roman gave a similar answer to the emperor Augustus, when he asked for the means of living to be over a hundred years old. This Roman answered, "internally with wine and honey, externally with oil." *Intus mulso, foris oleo,* goes the saying.[27]

Rudolf Steiner said that this saying originated from the Mysteries. In his first medical course (1920),[16] he says: "It is interesting that this method of establishing an archetypal phenomenon played a large role just at the time when the cultivation of the medical art proceeded more from the Mysteries..." For example, he said, "If you take in honey or wine internally, you strengthen from within the forces which work out of the cosmos into you." One could also say that "you thus strengthen the actual Ego-forces — for that would be the same. If you rub your body with an oily substance, however, you weaken the harmful effects of the earth-forces in you, forces which stand opposed to Ego-activity in the organism. And if one finds the right balance between sweet strengthening from within and oily weakening from without, then one will live to be old, according to the ancient physicians. Let the harmful effects of the earth in your organism be taken from you by the effect of oil, in that you rub yourself with oil. And, when you are able, when you are not too weak in your organization, let the Ego-forces be strengthened with wine or honey, for you then strengthen the forces which lead you into old age."

This refers, on the one hand, to the "sweet strengthening" by internal means and, on the other, to the "oily weakening" from without, i.e. the ability of oil to protect people from adverse earth forces. All this is related to the nature of fat, which forms warmth, stimulates the individual warmth-process and, even from without, spreads a protective and warming sheath over the human skin. We also see the important cosmetic significance of oil, wherein olive is especially appropriate. Even the early Greeks used it in their oil salves.

Thus, olive oil proves to be the oil of the middle, of balance, of mildness, of the soothing of heat and cold. It is, in fact, a truly mercurial oil.

About Butter and Margarine

At this point we should say a word about butter, which we have already mentioned in our discussion of milk.

Butter is an old food. It was produced in ancient Greece, though not highly valued there. The word "butyron" — from which the English word "butter" comes — was probably a word borrowed from Scythian. The Thracians were called the "butyrophagio", the "butter eaters." Among the Scythians, horse butter was also popular. The making of butter from milk is more likely an invention of northern peoples, who were directed more towards a concentrated warmth-formation.

We can see that butter is a food which arose through human art and manipulation; it is not a directly natural product, as are, say, the various oils. But we must say, however, that the production of butter originated in an ancient, instinctive but certain, knowledge of the secrets of substance and their relationship to man.

Butter was made according to traditional recipes throughout many centuries. Among the essential and noble tasks of the farmer was the production of butter — as well as of cheese and other milk products — by himself. Only recently has this activity again been taken up on individual farms, as a response to the problem of the quality of our food. Coming in between, historically, is the factory production of butter which began in the last century.

The formation of butter is based on a unique phenomenon of milk fat, its globular structure. We have discussed this in the chapter on milk. The structure of butter comes from the natural emulsion of the milk globules. Milk protein as well as the so-called phospholipoids, cholesterol and other substances are involved as much here as the fat is. Here, the corpuscular structure of the milk fat plays an important role, though the so-called granular structure of butter is not identical to the original. Nonetheless, this structure plays a large role in the reabsorption of butter by the body. We shall return to this idea later.

To evaluate butter, it is first important to look at its fatty acid composition. We come across the fact that, to date, 76 fatty acids have been identified in butter. No other edible fat comes even close to this.[8] About 50% are saturated fatty acids. The rest are simple, double or even 3, 4, or 5-fold unsaturated fatty acids. Among the saturated are butyric acid (3-4%), myristic acid in a higher concentration and palmitic acid. Among the unsaturated fatty acids, the simple ones, at 25%, make up the largest portion.

142

In this respect, milk fat bears a certain resemblance to olive oil. The double unsaturated linolic acid varies between 2-4.5%, and the more highly unsaturated fatty acids appear in qualtities of about more highly unsaturated fatty acids appear in qualities of about 1%.

Here we have a peculiar, perhaps even a unique, phenomenon. Beginning with natural fat, a many-sided fatty acid composition is created. Though in man himself the unsaturated component is greater, we must nevertheless say that butter fat has a univeral character. One should also consider the degree to which the dynamic, highly unsaturated fatty acids compensate for the quantitatively more plentiful lower and middle unsaturated fatty acids. In any case, we could not say that its fatty acid composition justifies any serious concern regarding butter. The total composition of butter is, as we mentioned, a "fat emulsion" in milk and water and yields the following picture:

Fat (minimum)	82.0%
Water (maximum)	16.0%
Fat-free dry milk substance	1.5-1.8%
Protein (from above)	0.3-0.9%
Lactose	0.5-0.9%
Salts	0.1-0.16%

(source: Ludwig, 3)

We can see that butter is very concentrated fat food, a fact that is perhaps not often enough considered.

The wholesomeness, digestibility and intake of butter into the organism can be considered, to begin with, by using the criteria put forth in the description of fat. There are, however, a number of additional, special considerations. First, we must consider that butter (as was noted in the chapter on milk) has a plant-like character. This is significant especially with regard to the argument of margarine manufacturers that their product comes from "pure plant oil." Also important is the melting point of butter. It is somewhat below human body temperature. And fats with a melting point close to 37°C (98.6°F) are absorbed better than those with higher melting points. There appears to be an inverse relationship between the digestibility and the melting point of a fat. In this respect butter — along with olive oil — belongs to the group of best and most easily digested fats. In contrast, animal fats often have high melting points: e.g. pig fat (c.42°C), chicken fat (c.40°C), beef grease (c.48°C), and mutton grease (c.50°C).

The fat structure of butter also plays a role in its absorption. Schweigart writes: "Nature has arranged it so that the fat globules of milk ... pass over directly to the lymph."[8] In the intestines, the individual fats needed in the organism are already built up anew. Due to the plant-like character of milk, this process is more difficult than it is for actual animal fats. However it is therefore all the more valuable. We may here mention Rudolf Steiner's advice: "When it comes to fats, we should give preference to butter made from milk ..."[22]

We can, today, support this recommendation. However, we must do so with a limitation, in that the quality of milk — as the starting point of butter production — has suffered from the influence of modern agricultural practices. Moreover, the technical processes in the dairy are no longer unobjectionable. Butter available from a bio-dynamic source, however, can be valuable and commendable even today.

Our recommendation of butter also applies to something often put forth as one of its disadvantages — its cholesterol content. According to Schweigart, this content comes to 180-280 mg/100g. For some time, cholesterol has been the focus of much research, and of even more interpretation and opinion; often it is simply a catch-word for anything to be avoided.

We tried, in *The Dynamics of Nutrition,* to characterize this problem and to put it in its proper perspective. We saw that cholesterol can be seen properly only if a view is given to the entire metabolism. Thus Ludwig, for example, relates the results of some of his research and observations: "Among the lower social classes, with their low-calorie diet, primarily from cheap carbohydrates, the serum cholesterol values were low. The higher the social level, and the more butter and more calorie-rich the diet, the higher rises the cholesterol concentrations in the blood."[3] Among these "cheap carbohydrates", however, are refined products such as flour products and sugar. We shall return to consider the extent to which a qualitatively inadequate and exaggerated consumption of carbohydrates stimulates the over-production of fat. The cholesterol problem cannot be solved in a one-sided way, especially in light of the fact that we ourselves produce cholesterol in the body and that, as we have shown, this cholesterol production is necessary within limits. The widespread rise in the cholesterol level must, in any case, be seen as a question of one's entire nutri-

144

tion. The average consumption of cholesterol today is given at 500-800 mg. daily. This average holds only for a mixed diet, however, since plants produce no cholesterol; nor does it stress the importance of the fact that a person produces much cholesterol himself. It has been shown experimentally that with a fully cholesterol-free diet, the cholesterol level was lowered only 24 mg %. (K. Lang).

Lang touches on something even more important: "The consumption of large amounts of polyunsaturates caused a large breaking-down of cholesterol into bile acids, as well as an increased excretion of cholesterol and its metabolic products."[12]

Kuehnau has recently presented this fact in an impressive way. He points to the "cholesterol-lowering effect of these fatty acids," and to the same effect of raw plant fibers.[28] Similarly, H. Cremer has determined that "serum cholesterol values are significantly lower among vegetarians than among meat and fish eaters."[19]

The cholesterol problem is thus clearly a problem of the entire diet. Can anyone still say that 100 g of butter per day — a generous amount — with less than 300 mg of cholesterol, could play a negative role as part of a reasonably formed diet? Whoever eats too much, or has a wrong or one-sided diet, will be confronted with the cholesterol problem — and we don't want to underestimate this fact. But least of all should we eliminate butter, or replace it with margarine, in a "lactovegetarian" diet.

There are other reasons, as well, for not attributing the significance to this "artificial fat", margarine, that is frequently done today. For example, we have already mentioned which plant oils are used to produce margarine. Coconut fat is one important raw product. Peanut oil is also used. We have already described these oils. We must also consider the many technical processes used to produce margarine, e.g. the hydrogenation (hardening) of fats. Ludwig argues: "Hydrogenation is a process which constantly takes place in the metabolism of men and animals." Therefore it is physiological. And what takes place in "the autoclave with the help of pure hydrogen and a nickel catalyst . . . is the same chemical process that takes place in animal and man."

We here confront the disastrous, abstract thinking that still largely holds sway over modern science. People honestly believe that a process in an inorganic environment, and with altogether different technical requirements, is the "same" as an analogous process taking place in a totally different way, in a living environment. Until we see that inorganic formative forces are not capable of being bearers of life within the organism, and can have only the character of the appearance of life, we shall not learn to form a realistic evaluation of this problem.

The same holds true for the addition of synthetically produced vitamins in the oils. So why is it emphasized that certain "health food" margarines are made "exclusively from unhardened plant oils and fats," if it is contended that hydrogenation is physiological?

The arguments of the margarine industry are hardly convincing. The reasons Rudolf Steiner put forth for preferring butter are certainly still valid today, probably even more than they were in his time. However, even here, one must still be wise in considering certain limitations.

Animal Fats

It now remains for us to have a quick look at animal fat. Apart from the so-called invisible fats in meat, sausage, ham, etc., beef and pork lard play the greatest role in the human diet.

Beef lard is a fat with a relatively high melting point and overwhelmingly saturated fatty acids. Today, only a small portion of it is used directly in food. Earlier, it served as the basic fat in margarine. Today it is used mostly in producing soap and candles and to some extent in making sausage.

Pork fat, on the other hand, is one of the most important dietary fats. It is also overwhelmingly made up of saturated fatty acids, but its melting point is lower than that of beef fat. It is of varying quality, depending on where it originated in the pig's body. With a fat content of 99%, it is extremely concentrated. Interestingly, it easily takes on the smell of the dried fish powder used to feed the pig, as well as the typical sexual odor of the male animal.

In bacon, pork fat undergoes a curing process, whereby the often-used nitrate salts become a cause for concern. With ham, smoking is added to the curing process, and this, too, can damage one's health.

Goose fat, in contrast, has a high proportion of oleic acid (75%). One can see that the bird-organization is clearly different

146

from that of the mammals. The bird's organization is much less oriented toward the earth's heaviness. Their warmth-organization is also different: they are more cosmically oriented.

Finally, we have already noted that sea-creature oils have a primarily unsaturated fatty acid content. In this respect, whale and fish oils are quite similar, although they are at different evolutionary stages. Herring, sardine and salmon oils (which can form up to 20% of the fish) can be used only after hydrogenation, because of their strong odor. Similarly, whale blubber is used only in certain margarines after refinement and hydrogenation.

We would be deceiving ourselves if we ascribed a high value to sea-animal oils because of their high unsaturated fat content. Rudolf Steiner described fish in a way that can help us to consider these creatures in a spiritual-scientific manner. "That which is connected with human reproduction — which first appeared, germinally, at the very end of the Moon period and which first really came about during the earth period — the fish are related to that, the fish and even lower animals."[29] This is important in evaluating nutrition which includes fish and even such foods as caviar. Another of Steiner's indications, from an earlier lecture on nutrition (1904), is worth mentioning: "With fish, one eats the entire world — kama as well."[22] "Kama," for the old Indians, meant the desire for existence.

Our consideration of the fats and oils important in human nutrition has thus come to an end. We may now turn to the question of "fat addiction" — the problem of obesity.

But before turning to this problem, we should point briefly to the important question of the effect of heated fats. Much research has shown that certain chemical changes — which can be harmful to the health — go hand in hand with the strong heating of fats. The frying fats present a special problem, especially when high temperatures (over 200°C) are used. Regarding this, A.L. Prabuck says: "For this reason, the common practice of reusing the frying oil, and simply replacing the lost amounts with fresh oil, is thoroughly objectionable; the production of substances hazardous to the health is furthered in this way."[50] It has also been shown that charcoal grilling forms hydrocarbons which are today called carcinogenic. The same holds true for the production of smoked meats.

The Problem of Obesity

The question of overweight or obesity presents a central problem in the west today. According to a number of different studies, in Switzerland about one-third of the men over thirty-five are overweight. In West Germany, according to the so-called *Hessen-Studie,* about 50% of the present-day population is overweight. Anyone who has visited the United States cannot help but notice the number of people, often young, with enormous bodies. In his book *Food and the Health of Western Man,* James Lambert Mount writes about this situation: "50% of the men in their thirties are overweight. Among men in their fifties, 60% are overweight." Mount confirms other authors in pointing out that overweight reduces life expectancy and furthers a predisposition toward degenerative diseases. The significance of this fact can be seen in a study by J.C. Somogyi:[31] "Among the overweight, heart attacks are three times as frequent and the mortality rate is twice as high. And 85% of all diabetics are overweight. A number of other diseases — for example all forms of arteriosclerosis, gout, cholelithiasis, arthritis, etc. — are caused or furthered by overweight."

From these indications alone we can see what a significant role obesity plays in modern civilization. We also see the multiple threats to human health connected with it. Yet as much as this situation seems to be clarified, it is difficult to see what the causes are. Equally complicated are the possibilities for preventing and treating overweight. As Somogyi points out in the above-mentioned essay: "Much about its origin still lies in the dark." Let us first attempt to create a picture of the present state of research in this field, insofar as it is of significance for our study.

In most discussions, an obvious fact about the inner human metabolism plays an important role. We have hardly touched on this important aspect: the possibility of transforming carbohydrates and protein into fat substances. Within our organism — i.e. from our own protein — we can construct our own sugar (glucose). Modern calculations (Mehnert-Forster) estimate that 1 g of glucose is produced from 2 g of protein. On the other hand, fatty acids cannot be converted to glucose. And yet the conversion of carbohydrates into fats apparently plays a big role. According to Ludwig, "the carbohydrates taken in with food are primarily used

148

protein ——→ gFAT
↘ sugar

for triglyceride synthesis. Only a fraction is used for glycogen storage." Stetten and Boxer say that 30% of all dietary carbohydrates are converted into fats. Indeed, the fat and carbohydrate metabolisms are closely intertwined. Mehnert and Foster speak here of a "kind of interplay which is of great significance for the entire metabolism." On the other hand, the organism can produce protein neither from carbohydrates nor from fats.[3]

We can thus see the importance of the unique position of protein: in the human being, protein proceeds only from protein. On the other hand, we have a new factor to consider with regard to fat: both protein and carbohydrates can be transformed into fat. Of course the question remains open as to whether the production of fat from protein is — in the strictest sense of the word — a physiological process. With all of these transformations, however, the above-mentioned sequence of facts plays a role described by Rudolf Steiner and Ita Wegman in *Fundamentals of Therapy:* "In a healthy organism, the animal [astral] forces produce or take in only as much fat as the Ego-organization can convert into warmth processes . ." For "it is healthy when the human formative forces consume the body fat in the process of warmth production." This is a clear description of the physiological path which fat should take in the human organism. In the chapter on protein, we showed that failure to use protein, as such, comes from a kind of "luxury consumption." This leads to an alienation of protein from its actual task as a building substance. Because protein is hard to store, it is pushed back when too much is present and is converted to carbohydrates or fats. This is possible only with an irrational expenditure of energy. For this reason, Aebi coined the term "luxury calories."

Something else also occurs. "When protein is used as a calorie source in this way, the result is that the accompanying fats and carbohydrates are all the more readily stored."[31] In other words: the forced alienation of protein — and its conversion into carbohydrates or fat — also causes a pathological deposit in the organism. The latter becomes overwarmed and helps itself by depositing substances which go beyond the physiological need. The metabolism runs into a dead end, i.e. it becomes ill. "It is unhealthy when fat is not used up by the Ego-organization in warmth processes but is, instead, brought into the organism unused."[1] On the other hand, if one's consumption of carbohydrates is suffi-

∴ enhance warmth org in bm

149

cient and — especially important — of high quality, the organism is enabled to conserve protein.

The third possibility — an excessive consumption of protein and an avoidance of carbohydrates — is often discussed today. It has recently gained a lot of attention in the U.S.A. through *Dr. Atkins' Diet Revolution*,[33] a book which has sold over a million copies and has been translated into German. It was written by a physician and is a classical example of the total lack of understanding of the reality of nutrition. "Throw everything you've known about overweight overboard," he says, and goes on to recommend a fully one-sided protein diet — up to 170 g per day, which is possible only with animal protein. At the same time, the consumption of carbohydrates is severely limited to a maximum of 35 g daily, since modern man suffers from "chronic carbohydrate poisoning" or "carbohydratis." This "anti-carbohydrate diet" is offered, therefore, with the guarantee that it will rid you of your excess pounds. Without the benefit of any power of qualitative judgment, a diet has been created — and is indeed practiced by millions — which is suited to the complete animalization of mankind. Pure materialism, and the corruption of the powers of thought, thrive in a way of thinking which may be intellectually convincing but totally unspiritual, based on prejudices and antipathy ("man owes the animal world for his nutrition"[34]). For this reason, Steiner warned that "the consumption of protein substances should be kept within definite limits."

Instead, Atkins recommends this menu to his clients: "1st day: 4 lamb chops, salad. 2nd day: 7 frankfurters, sauerkraut. 3rd day: ½ pound lobster with green beans. 4th day: two dozen spare ribs, 1 steak, cheese, salad. 5th day: three eggs, cottage cheese, 1 pound of chicken, 1 dozen spare ribs. 6th: day 1½ pounds of steak with baked onions . . . And, in general, eat as much and as often as you want, eat sumptuously, and take off up to nine pounds in the first week, five pounds in the second week, etc."

Even Atkins knows that such a diet is very injurious to the health. He therefore speaks of "possible complications," recommends high-potency multiple vitamins, and warns of possible "gastroenterological and cholecystcholangiopathic complaints." But the harm done is much more profound and extensive. We have already described it — both in this book and in *The Dynamics of Nutrition* — from various points of view. This diet "strictly for-

150

bids" bread and all baked goods, cereals, fruit juices, honey, milk, yogurt, etc., a regimen which shows all too clearly what would become of man if Dr.Atkins' prescriptions were followed.

Nonetheless, this book does contain some truth. The over-consumption of refined carbohydrates, together with the overuse of fats, has indeed made obesity a considerable problem. But Atkins would replace one evil with another, perhaps even worse in its effects. The solution to this problem can only come about by a complete rethinking — by taking up a "dynamics of nutrition" which exists and can be utilized today.

The immoderate consumption of carbohydrates has a devastating effect. Eating enormous amounts of fat — especially from animals — undermines human health. On the other hand, crude fibers — which are to be found abundantly in grains, fruits and vegetables — are necessary helpers for our health. These facts, and many more, are clearly known today. We know that modern man's lack of movement plays a big role in corpulence, that over-consumption disrupts the natural senses of hunger and thirst — which are already soul-factors — and that the relationship of the soul-factor to obesity should gain increasing attention.

For example, Pudel describes a "behavioral psychological disturbance"[30] of the adipose tissue, in that it shows an increased external sensitivity: "For the adipose tissue, we see that external stimuli affect the subjective feelings more strongly than do inner stimuli." This means that the packaging, selection, taste and smell of food strongly stimulate the appetite and may lead to unnecessary eating. We see here the beginnings of a "fat psychology" which has deeper roots than one might at first think. Rudolf Steiner also referred to such matters when he described, for example, how "when a person eats the fat from an ox or a pig, it goes into his body and satisfies his sense of well-being . . . He thereby loves meat . . ."[4] In the case, described by Pudel, of an increased dependence on external stimuli, we can see that there is a clear weakening of the Ego-organization in the organism. Animal behavior can gain the upper hand, and a compulsive dependence on the environment is typical of such behavior.

slim, astral forces

The Fats

1. Rudolf Steiner/Ita Wegman, *Grundlegendes für eine Erweiterung der Heilkunst nach geisteswissenschaftlichen Erkenntnissen*, Dornach 1977 (GA 27). English translation, *Fundamentals of Therapy*, London 1967.
2. Rudolf Steiner, Three lectures given in Dornach 17 - 19 December 1920, published in *Die Brücke zwischen der Weltgeistigkeit und dem Physischen des Menschen. Die Suche nach der neuen Isis, der göttlichen Sophia*, Dornach 1980 (GA 202). English translation of above three lectures appeared as *The Bridge Between Universal Spirituality and Physical Man*, Spring Valley 1979.
3. L. Ludwig, *Fett und Ernährung*, Hamburg 1968.
4. Rudolf Steiner, Lecture given in Dornach 31 July 1924 under the title "Über das Verhältnis der Nahrungsmittel zum Menschen — Rohkost und Vegetarismus," published in *Die Schöpfung der Welt und des Menschen. Erdenleben und Sternenwirken*, Dornach 1977 (GA 351).
5. Rudolf Steiner, *Geisteswissenschaftliche Gesichtspunkte zur Therapie*, Dornach 1963 (GA 313).
6. Rudolf Steiner, Lecture given in Dornach 22 September 1923 under the title "Ernährungsfragen," published in *Rhythmen im Kosmos und im Menschenwesen. Wie kommt man zum Schauen der geistigen Welt?*, Dornach 1980 (GA 350).
7. L.A. Cioffi, "Diätetische, physiologische und soziale Aspekte des Übergewichts," Symposium in Zürich, 8/9 September 1976.
8. H.A. Schweigart, *Butter und Margarine*, Hanover 1966.
9. W. Mohler, *Sinn und Unsinn unserer Ernährung*, 1972.
10. Aign, "Übergewicht und Ernährung" in *Schriftenreihe der Schweiz. Vereinigung für Ernährung*, Heft 7, Bern 1970.
11. J.L. Mount, *The Food and Health of Western Man*, London 1975.
12. K. Lang, *Die Bedeutung der Fette in der Ernährung*, 1970.
13. G. Wolfram, "Essentielle Fettsäuren," in *Ernährungs-Umschau*, Heft 9, Frankfurt/M. 1976.
14. K. Lang, *Biochemie der Ernährung*, Darmstadt 1974.
15. Rudolf Steiner, *Geisteswissenschaftliche Grundlagen zum Gedeihen der Landwirtschaft*, Dornach 1979 (GA 327). English translation, *Agriculture*, London 1977.
16. Rudolf Steiner, *Geisteswissenschaft und Medizin*, Dornach 1976 (GA 312). English translation, *Spiritual Science and Medicine*, London 1975.
17. Rudolf Steiner, *Aus der Akasha-Chronik*, Dornach 1973 (GA 11). English translation, *Cosmic Memory*, Englewood 1971.

18. Rudolf Steiner, *Die Geheimwissenschaft im Umriss*, Dornach 1977 (GA 13). English translation, *Occult Science— An Outline*, Spring Valley 1972.
19. H.D. Cremer, "Die Bedeutung des pflanzlichen Eiweisses für die menschliche Ernährung," in *Ernährungs-Umschau* 3/76, Frankfurt/M.
20. Rudolf Steiner, *Der Mensch als Zusammenklang des schaffenden, bildenden und gestaltenden Weltenwortes*, Dornach 1978 (GA 230). English translation, *Man as a Symphony of the Creative Word*, London 1970.
21. G. Ohsawa, *Zen Makrobiotik*, Hamburg 1971.
22. Rudolf Steiner, Lecture on Nutrition, 1905.
23. J. Budwig, *Krebs — ein Fettproblem?*, 1956.
24. W. Pelikan, *Heilpflanzenkunde*, Vol. II, Dornach 1962.
25. P. Viola, *Die Fette in der menschlichen Ernährung. Das Olivenöl*, 1971.
26. A. Michaelis, *Die Oele*, 1894.
27. V. Hehn, *Kulturpflanzen und Haustiere*, 1963.
28. J. Kühnau, in *Ernährungs-Umschau*, 5/76, Frankfurt/M.
29. Rudolf Steiner, *Der Mensch als Zusammenklang des schaffenden, bildenden und gestaltenden Weltenwortes*, Dornach 1978 (GA 230). Reference is here made to the sixth lecture given 28 October 1923 in Dornach. English translation, *Man as Symphony of the Creative Word*, London 1970.
30. A.L. Prabucki, "Wissenswertes über die Herkunft und Verarbeitung von Fetten und Oelen," in *Schriftenreihe der Schweiz. Vereinigung für Ernährung*, Heft 5, Bern 1970.
31. J.C. Somogyi, "Vorbeugung und Behandlung des Uebergewichts," during a symposium on "Diätetische, physiologische und soziale Aspekte des Uebergewichts," 8/9 September 1976 in Zürich.
32. H. Aebi, "Eiweiss, Ernährungsfaktor Nummer Eins," in *Schriftenreihe der Schweiz. Vereinigung für Ernährung*, Heft 17, Bern 1971.
33. R.C. Atkins, *Dr. Atkins' Diet Revolution*, McKay 1972.
34. Rudolf Steiner, Lecture given in Berlin, 17 December 1908 under the title "Ernährungsfragen im Lichte der Geisteswissenschaft," published in *Wo und Wie findet man den Geist?*, Dornach 1961 (GA 57).
35. V. Pudel, *Verhaltenspsychologische Aspekte der Adipositas*.

The publication dates mentioned refer to the latest editions available in German and English.

Chapter IV

Carbohydrates (Sugar) as Mediators
of Form and Consciousness

The Form and Nature of Carbohydrates

"The human organism engages with all of its members in
activities, the impulses for which can only be within the organism
itself." With these words, Rudolf Steiner and Ita Wegman begin
the chapter on sugar in their book *Fundamentals of Therapy*.[1]
This statement points to two important aspects of sugar. On the
one hand, it is capable of bringing on activity in the organism.
But, on the other hand, this activity must arise from the organism itself. Modern nutritional research points to the first aspect
in speaking of carbohydrates (a group to which sugar belongs,
chemically) as "energy sources," as opposed to the "building
material" of protein. However, it is difficult for modern science
to find a realistic relationship to the second aspect. Nonetheless,
an important fact is well-known: the metabolism of carbohydrates in the human organism proceeds in a direction exactly
opposite to that of plants. Thus there is clearly a polarity between
these two. We mentioned these facts in *The Dynamics of Nutrition*
and shall enter into a deeper discussion of them here.

We begin our presentation by looking especially at the nature
and significance of sugar. We thereby hope to emphasize that,
in human nutrition, this form of carbohydrate occupies an un-
contested central point, around which all other types of carbohydrate group themselves. It therefore appears justified to begin
our consideration with the following questions: What is sugar?
How is it formed? What is its relationship to man? Although

154

sugar has been known and consumed for millenia, research into this question began only relatively recently: not until the time of Goethe were the natural-scientific methods advanced enough to make a fundamental statement with certainty about sugar formation in plants: the formation of sugar or sap proceeds from water and carbon dioxide, with the help of sunlight. One of the most fundamental life-processes was thus recognized. At the same time, the creative activity of plants — in making organic substances from inorganic matter — was also seen. Human beings — as well as the animals — are incapable of doing this. Their activity proceeds in a higher direction, turning toward what is soul-spiritual.

A modern plant physiologist described this process as follows: "The transformation of inorganic, mineral carbon dioxide into organic compounds is one of the most important biochemical processes in nature. It is the basic reaction which makes life on this planet possible."[2] Today, the basic chemical equation for this reaction is written as follows: $6\ CO_2 + 6\ H_2O = C_6H_{12}O_6 + 6\ O_2$.

Of course this is only a formula for what really happens. "Photosynthesis" actually takes place under only three conditions: the presence of carbon dioxide, the activity of sunlight and the working of chlorophyll, the green colorant in the leaves. The important role in photosynthesis of the "green" in plants was first discovered by Willstaetter in 1910. Shortly thereafter, the significance of chlorophyll for human blood-formation was recognized, mainly through the work of Buergi, in Bern, who was stimulated in this work by Rudolf Steiner. However, it was not until 1939 that Hans Fischer penetrated to an exact understanding of the similarity between chlorophyll and hemoglobin, the red colorant in blood. He showed that just as chlorophyll has magnesium in the central position, so hemoglobin has iron at its center. It has since come to light that chlorophyll also requires the iron process, but from the periphery. Moreover, copper is at work, both in green leaves and in red blood, in the formation of their colorants.

In *Fundamentals of Therapy*[1] Rudolf Steiner and Ita Wegman described this process from a spiritual-scientific point of view. In the third chapter, on the phenomena of life, we read: "In the plant, the substances of the earth are raised up, out of the realm of terrestrial effects."

They thus come to the realm of the "raying-in forces." "In the transition to life, matter must withdraw from the 'outraying' (earthly) forces and join with the 'in-raying' forces . . . And from the working together of the 'earthly' and 'cosmic' forces, the being of the plant arises. The out-raying physical forces are taken hold of by the in-raying, etheric/cosmic forces. Thus, the form and organization of the plant are the unique result of both spheres of force." Nonetheless, "the plant allows the physical to rule in it when the etheric no longer actively works on it from cosmic space. This is the case at night, when the sun ether stops its activity." We shall see the effect of this rhythm of night and day on the formative processes of sugar and starch.

Despite intensive research, natural science still has not succeeded in following exactly the formation of starch in green plant leaves. One may assume, however, that in the green chloroplast of the leaf cell, sugar is formed at first and is then immediately changed into starch. The subsequent working of the plant has been described with the following calculation: 20,000 beech leaves, for example, have a surface area of about 40 m². However, if their chloroplasts could be laid next to one another, they would have a surface area of 15,000 m². In other words, a huge surface is created in order to allow for the optimal effect of light, the assimilation of carbon dioxide and the excretion of oxygen through the thin fissures in the leaves. According to the American researcher Rabinovich, the plants on the earth convert about 200 billion tons of carbon into carbohydrates (including sugars) every year. This is the enormous, incomparable achievement of the plant world — it produces life forces on the earth with the help of the cosmic sun forces.

We must keep in mind here that all dead organic materials — such as wood, peat, coal and petroleum — also originate from the plant's assimilatory capacity. These products, in turn, form the basis for the development of human culture and civilization. In fact, almost all sources of energy and food have a common starting point: sugar. Not only does all food on earth stem from plants, but we also owe to them the oxygen — formed in the process of photosynthesis — which we breathe and by which we live. Considering this tremendous formative-force process taking place in the plant world, we can understand why merely natural-scientific research must admit to the following conclusion: "What

156

really goes on within a plant is, for us, to a great extent still a mysterious, unknown process."[3]

The polarity between plant and man — which is so impressive in this process — is tremendously significant for the understanding of both plant and man. "If there were no plants, all organisms breathing oxygen would have to die out in a short time." Rudolf Steiner took this truth as a point of departure in his description of these processes.[4] Even though they lacked a knowledge of modern chemistry, medieval seekers of wisdom knew the profound significance of these processes and related them to the concept of the "Philosopher's Stone."

What is thereby formed in the plant is dextrose or fructose. However it may also be cane sugar, starch, cellulose, pectin, plant rubber or mucilage, all of which are basically carbohydrates. CHO_s

The starch formed in the plant by means of photosynthesis is, however, at first converted back into sugar. This "migrant" sugar then streams through the plants' capillaries in the night. It goes to the reserve organs — to the cotyledons and nutritive tissue in the seeds, to the nodes and roots — and it is there newly built up as starch. Leaf starch is an original formation: i.e. it is still totally cosmically oriented. "Reserve starch" is a secondary formation which comes anew under the influence of the in-raying forces. In between, forces which are primarily earthly bring forth the "migrant" sugar during the night. Modern botanists have researched this daily rhythm quite exactly.[5] One expression of these opposite forces can be seen in the difference between the spherical structure of starch and the crystal-mineral structure of sugar. The old Sanscrit word *sarcara* or *sacara* — from which the Greek word *saccharon* (sugar) arose — actually means "crystalline." This points to an important relationship which we shall deal with later.

Here, however, we wish to add that there are a large number of "sugar plants" which are characterized by the fact that they store sugar ("sucrose" or cane sugar) in various organs. Sugar cane and sugar beets should be especially mentioned here, since they are the raw materials for our modern factory sugar production. However, carrots, onions and many other plants also fall into this category. Why do these plants store such large amounts of sugar? Modern botany teaches us that "in all cases, this reserve is stored up for the formation of large flower clusters." There-

157

fore, the harvest must "take place before the formation of blossoms."[2] This means that the crystalline sugar wants to turn again to the cosmic forces of the periphery in the process of blossom formation.

Functions of Carbohydrates in Man

Through the industrial processing of such reserve sugar, man anticipates the natural process and hence can consume either this manufactured sugar, or else the starch, in his nutrition. However, he must break these products down, by means of his digestion, into simple sugar — into glucose. For "in this state, starch is a foreign body."[1] This glucose, formed in the small intestine, is taken into the human blood as "transport" sugar — analagous to the "migrant" sugar in plants. "Glucose is a substance which stimulates activities which are of the same nature as the activities of the human organism itself."[1] However, it is built up into human starch — glycogen — in the liver, and is stored there, a process corresponding to the storage of sugar in the plant's "reserve organs".

The liver is thus a kind of storage organ for glycogen. Human sugar formation is thereby included in the 24-hour rhythm of the liver, i.e. in the actual human rhythmical organization. We spoke of this in detail in *The Dynamics of Nutrition* and will continue our discussion here. This circadian rhythm is synchronized with the earth's respiration. Through the latter, this human rhythm is connected to the cosmic rhythm of the Platonic "world year". During the inbreathing phase of the earth — until 3 A.M. — the liver stores up glycogen. Then in the morning hours — until 3 P.M. in the afternoon — it releases it into the blood as sugar. Thus, as we have seen, this liver function stamps the process of sugar formation with the seal of its own individual Ego-rhythm. When glycogen is formed from the glucose in food, the glucose is really taken up by the organism for the first time. It now belongs to the person but is still connected to its original, cosmic, sun-rhythm. Sugar as such flows in human blood with great consistency; its concentration can vary only within very narrow limits (between 60 and 120 mg%). Through the above-mentioned process, it becomes a substance "which can work in the realm of the Ego-organization."[1]

158

These words contain modern spiritual science's most significant insight into the nature of sugar. In *The Dynamics of Nutrition* we spoke of the important role of the liver in the human warmth-organization. We also pointed out that it is precisely in warmth that the highest member of man's being can exist. The warmth ether — which is so powerfully active in the liver — reaches the height of its activity in the liver with the transformation of plant sugar into human glycogen. Then "it gives over this inner sugar to the entire body, which thereby has its inner warmth."[6] Thus, one can in fact "follow the Ego-organization within the realm of the material by looking for the presence of sugar."[1] At the same time, this sugar "corresponds to the taste of sweetness, which exists within the Ego-organization."[1] In other words: the human Ego experiences itself not only in the warmth nature of sugar, not only in its mineral structure, but also in its (either apparent or hidden) sweet taste.

We thus touch upon another secret of sugar and its significance for man. Its sweet taste is a force of attraction for the Ego. Even when this experience of sweetness is no longer in man's consciousness — for example, when glucose is produced from starch, etc. in the small intestine — the Ego-organization unfolds its activity. The experience of sweetness "penetrates into the unconscious regions of the human body." And the Ego-organization, in another language, in Sanskrit, has the root word *sud* — which also means sweet — and which has become "sweet" or "süss" in more modern vocabularies.

We must emphasize here, however, that the sweet taste alone, without a connection to the structure of sugar, does not create a field of activity for the human Ego. In other words, the so-called artificial sweeteners are definitely not substitutes for sugar. They simply deceive one with their sweet taste.

Another comment is also appropriate here. The strict limits of human blood-sugar concentration show quite clearly that the activity of the Ego-organization through sugar is subject to clear and fast limits. Too much or too little sugar in the blood bring forth illness; man may consume only a certain measure of sugar, and he may not go beyond this measure without danger. The present-day abuse of sugar (which we shall speak of in more detail) can be understood only as stemming from a lack of knowledge, and a misdirection, of the nature and function of sugar.

The liver stores up to 150 g of glycogen and transforms it back into the blood. By the same token there are three primary fields of activity into which this stream of sugar flows: the brain, the heart, and the muscles in the limbs.

It has long been known that the human nervous system, and especially the brain, is "exclusively dependent upon sugar as a source of energy".[7] The brain needs about 120 g of sugar in 24 hours in order to be active as the instrument for the formation of our consciousness during every moment of our waking life. Sugar here serves the development of Ego-consciousness in thinking. Conversely, glucose flows from the blood into the muscles, thus transmitting the activity of our will into the movement of our limbs. Finally, the heart muscle needs a daily supply of sugar of about 30-40 g in order to accomplish its work. Sugar thus prepares the way for our feeling. We thereby see how the human organization needs and makes use of sugar in all three realms of its activity within the soul forces.

In this way, sugar is "consumed". Carbon dioxide and water are produced, the former being exhaled and the latter excreted. This is just the point which gives rise to so many illusions and errors. One might believe that the cycle of substances is closed here, and that man is bound to this inescapable ring. However, modern research is unequivocal in speaking about energy. "Although energy cannot be lost, this form of energy is no longer usable. With regard to energy, there is no circulation."[3] This means that the products excreted by man — CO_2 and H_2O — are worthless with regard to energy. They require a new, original fructification with "energy" from the cosmic sun-forces, mediated through the process of photosynthesis.

In reality, this zero point with regard to force and matter is to be found in man. (cf. Chapter 3 in *The Dynamics of Nutrition*). The reader is reminded of Gigon's words: "The life process can never be considered from the point of view of energy . . ." We see that, through man, a new, higher activity of forces is ignited in the soul-spiritual organization. Through this activity, the human organism is not only formed as an individuality physically, but it can also become individually active in its higher forces — in thinking, feeling and willing.

It has become clear that "the organism is a relationship of activities." It now becomes even clearer that it is precisely through sugar that the human organization "develops activities in all its members, which can only have their impulses in [the person] himself." We thus return to our point of departure for this chapter and may now turn to other aspects of the question of sugar.

Sugar Consumption in West and East

In his small treatise *Betrachtungen ueber den saekulaeren Wandel der Ernaehrung* (Considerations on the Change in Nutrition),[8] E. Ziegler has shown that the daily consumption of sugar from 1850 to the early 1970's has risen from 7 g to 140 g per person. The sugar consumption of the Swiss population increased about twenty-fold. This enormous increase, however, is not exceptional — on the contrary, it points to a certain consistency in the world. Looking at the figures available for the consumption of sugar in the world, we come across the following facts.

The Republic of Ireland — Europe's most western country — stands at the top of the list with an annual consumption of 63.6 kg of sugar per person. A number of European countries follow close behind: Great Britain and Denmark, both with 56.0 kg, Holland with 58.6 kg and Switzerland with 54.0 kg. In contrast, West Germany with 34.8 kg, France with 31.4 kg, Italy with 24.0 kg and Spain with 18.3 kg are at present quite far behind. We find a remarkable similarity in the U.S.A., 48.0 kg; Canada, 43.6 kg; South Africa, 45.8 kg; Australia, 53.2 kg; New Zealand, 50.4 kg.

Let us now compare these statistics with the figures from eastern Europe. We see that East Germany, Poland and the USSR — all between 30 and 33 kg — are similar to some west European countries. In the far east, however, things are much different. We find that Japan, with 16.5 kg, and Iran with 21.3 kg, have a relatively high consumption. On the other hand, Communist China uses only 3.6 kg and the average annual sugar consumption for all of Asia comes to only 4.8 kg per person.

Of course, all these figures fluctuate. Most are taken from Geerde's table[3], based on data in 1961. Others are as recent as 1975. The main thing is not the absolute figures but the tendencies which the figures reveal. These are manifold. The tremendous increase in sugar consumption since the middle of the last century

161

is shown unequivocally. This has taken hold most in the western — or, rather, in the western-oriented — countries. In contrast, the far eastern countries have so clearly remained behind the "western" group that this tendency cannot be overlooked. A question is thus raised: has the western mentality — the materialistically oriented western civilization — developed a need for sugar, especially for refined factory sugar? The research of Cleave and Campbell is significant here.[9] They compared the sugar consumption of Indians in India to that of Indians in the South African province of Natal, an area strongly influenced by western civilization. The results are quite clear: the latter consumed c. 50.0 kg per capita annually, while the people in their native India consumed only 5.5 kg. The sugar consumption of the Indians in Natal is thus about nine times higher than that of their brothers in India. The researchers found a similar situation among black people. Rural blacks in southern Africa consume 2.7 kg per capita annually; those in the cities of the same countries, about 40 kg. The blacks in the USA consume c. 45 kg of sugar per capita annually.

Sugar and the Development of Consciousness

We shall speak later of the conclusions drawn by the above-mentioned researchers. We first wish to use these figures to clarify the tendencies in world-wide sugar consumption already outlined. Rudolf Steiner made a significant contribution regarding this matter in pointing out that when one investigates the western-oriented nations (e.g. the English), one finds a high level of sugar consumption. Among the eastern nations, however (Steiner then used the Russians as an example), one finds a relatively low level of sugar consumption. This is related to the fact that the western peoples have developed more self-consciousness, more Ego-consciousness, than have the eastern peoples. In English, for example, the word "I" — referring to one's self — is always capitalized, whereas the Russian peasant, at the time of Steiner's remarks, always avoided speaking about himself whenever possible. He wanted to extinguish his egoity; it was not very developed.[10]

What we see here as a pattern seems to be fading because of the spread of western materialistic tendencies over the entire earth. This phenomenon, nonetheless, leads us back to the above-

162

mentioned characteristic of sugar: namely, the human personality can reveal itself through sugar. "Where sugar arises, there appears the Ego-organization in order to orient the sub-human [vegetative and animal] corporeality toward the human."[1] In this regard, man reverses the plant-formation process and overcomes the animal process by consuming sugar; sugar, therefore, mediates "a kind of innocent Ego-consciousness" — i.e., it endows man with a natural "personality character".

Although such insights admittedly depart from the realm of the natural-scientific, analytic method, a method based on observation will not fail to notice how clearly sugar consumption affects people in the above-mentioned way. This aspect of sugar activity comes to expression through the activity of the brain. Still, we should emphasize what Rudolf Steiner said in this regard: "Of course, this must all be kept within healthy limits."[11] Meanwhile, these "healthy limits" have long been abandoned. We saw this clearly reflected in the figures for sugar consumption cited above. In 1913, sugar consumption in Switzerland was about 70 g daily per person — about half of what it is today. And even that level of consumption was too high. One might ask about the possible causes for this almost unbelievable increase in sugar consumption. We may conjecture that the evolution of modern man, with his overly intense and one-sided development of personality, leads him to unconsciously search for support in the physical realm. He thus succumbs to a kind of addiction which forces him to eat more and more sugar to get the same effect. A pathological condition has long since come about which has been impressively diagnosed today. And there is yet another error with serious consequences stemming from the fact that sugar consumption makes possible and stimulates the development of the human forces of consciousness. But if a person does not do this — if one does not sufficiently use the instrument thus prepared — development in a false direction takes place.

On the other hand, the form in which sugar usually appears — in refinement — is also extremely significant. It gives us cause to consider the problem of sugar from the point of view of cultural history.

Sugar and the Will

Before entering into this discussion, let us examine the other side of sugar: the will-side. We have already pointed out that sugar has a direct effect upon the limbs. It is necessary in large quantities for the movement of the musculature, i.e. for the activation of the will. Rudolf Steiner described this aspect of sugar as clearly as he did its consciousness-forming aspect. In a lecture to workers on July 31, 1924,[12] he clearly said that "If he [man] could not produce sugar, through and through, gentlemen, do you have any strength. The moment you are not full of sweetness, through and through, you have no more strength — you would collapse."

This description is of interest from many points of view. On the one hand, strength in the physical sense is clearly spoken of — that is, the development of strength by means of the physical body, of the limbs. Rudolf Steiner proceeds to describe a new polarity which exists between those peoples who eat a lot of sugar and those who eat little. Those who use little sugar, "those are the weak peoples, with regard to their physical strength." The others are "strong peoples." Is this not another indication of the primieval polarity between eastern and western peoples? In the east, sugar is used more moderately but in such a way as to best further the spiritual forces. In the west, people develop their forces much more in the earthly sphere, in the physical world. We see this idea expressed again in the words: "Food which has carbohydrates gives the body forces which it needs for work, for movement."[12]

We must keep in mind that Rudolf Steiner expressly spoke of "carbohydrates" here and said "if man could not produce sugar ..." What is essential is the human process of sugar-formation, not the ready-made sugar. Hence Steiner wrote, in the *Fundamentals of Therapy,* that the Ego-organization appears whereever sugar arises."[1] And at another point in the above-mentioned lecture he said, "When I chop wood — when I apply force externally — I become weak. But if, inwardly, a force is built in me that can transform carbohydrates into sugar . . . then I become strong."[12]

Here is expressed what Rudolf Steiner called "The Secret of Man". "The point is not that one is filled up by food, but rather that food develops forces within the body." Food can only do this if it contains such forces itself — and it is just these forces which have been stripped from refined sugar. It provides "empty calories" in the sense of modern nutritional research.

So we can ask ourselves: what is the best sugar for man? The answer is: that sugar which he produces himself, which he allows to arise within himself.

164

Man must produce glucose from cane sugar, to the extent that he can still exert his own forces in this production. Above all, he must convert starch into sugar. In addition, Steiner said that "wheat, rye etc. — they have carbohydrates in them in such a form that man can produce sugar in a favorable way. Actually, he can make himself as strong as possible by means of the carbohydrates in cereals."[12]

From these words, we have an indication of how Rudolf Steiner grasped the problem of sugar refinement, even if he did not express it directly. At the same time, we can see the significance in this regard of grain in our nutrition.

However, we must not become one-sided and banish sugar as a direct bearer of sweetness. We mentioned in *The Dynamics of Nutrition* that sweetness is immediately perceived on the tip of the tongue, and that a sweet taste requires quite a bit more dissolved sugar than the salty, sour and bitter tastes need from the appropriate substance. We see that we need this direct experience of sweetness, just as we need the sugar produced in the stomach and intestines.

We shall see that in earlier times — actually not so long ago — sugar was almost always used as a stimulant (in a way similar to table salt) or even as a medicament, as well as a flavoring, because sugar, in small quantities, intensifies the taste of many foods. "Sugar releases hidden aromas."[3] Similarly, it stimulates the functions of the liver. Rudolf Steiner recommended it as a special dietary stimulant for melancholic children. And when children take sugar on the sly, one should look to see if their liver functions are in order, i.e. if the will is developing properly.

Such indications clearly show the significance of the experience of sweetness as such. But they must be evaluated differently today. Even small children today have quite often lost their natural nutritional instincts because of the bad examples set by parents and educators. Instead, they are enslaved by an uninhibited addiction to sweets.

Cultural - Historical Aspects

Modern research into the history of plants has shown that the sugarcane — probably the oldest sugar plant — is indigenous to the far east, where many small and large islands are spread out from India to Australia. This was once the site of the ancient continent of Lemuria, the theater of earlier human history. Rudolf Steiner has communicated much about Lemuria from his spiritual research. Neither the earth nor man were as hardened then as they became in historical times. The plant world had only reached stages of development which were "similar to our palms and similar vegetation." The plants, too, were much less solidly anchored. Through various types of cultivation and breeding, they could be made of service. "The transformative power of man over nature was, compared with modern conditions, immeasurably large."[13] Baxa and Bruhns write, in their comprehensive study on "sugar in the life of peoples" *(Zucker im Leben der Voelker)*[14]: "According to the most recent botanical and geographical studies, the origin of cultivated sugarcane in pre-historic times was in Malaysia. Nonetheless, in historical times, India is the origin of cane sugar cultivation and sugar extraction from cane." The earliest use of *Saccharum officinarum* is put at the time between 15,000 and 8000 B.C. In reality, it may have been much earlier.

It is interesting that Rudolf Steiner describes this stage of human evolution — the Lemurian epoch — as the time of the first appearance of Ego-consciousness in the experience of the most advanced people. The "spark" of the Ego began to ignite itself on the earthly corporeality of the human being. The cultivation of cane sugar falls just at the time of this epoch-making stage of development. May we not assume that sugar itself — with its "sweet" experience so essential to mankind — was put into the service of this powerful progress, that it ignited the "Ego sparks" of man in order to awaken a still innocent egoity, a capacity which we have already seen as a property of sugar?

Along with sugarcane, the date palm may also have proceeded from the palm flora of that time. It was also cultivated in many ancient cultures as a source of sugar. Even in historical times, it is known that the Sumerians, Babylonians and Egyptians planted date palms as early as 3000 B.C.

Similarly, honey was also known in pre-historic times. Cave paintings dated at 10,000 B.C. point to this fact. The cultivation of honey was widespread in ancient Egypt. On the American continent, maple and corn sugar were being extracted by the

Indians even in ancient times. We can thus see that the possibility of producing sugar goes back to a very early stage of human evolution, that sugar is a primal food of humanity, and that the desire for sweetness is a primal need of human evolution. Later on, in historical times, the relation of man to sugar corresponds to this fact. We shall consider this in the following section.

The Relation of Man to Sugar in Historical Times

Very little is known of the cultural history of sugarcane in ancient India. A traditional text from the *Atharva-Veda* serves as a reminder of the high Indian culture with the words: "I have crowned you with interlaced sugarcane . . ."

A traditional Indian legend tells how Vishvamitra created the sugarcane as a food for the gods. Only in later historical times do we find that man learned to concentrate sugar sap and to make a thick syrup. Then, finally, a crystallized mass of sugar called *gur* was produced. The oft-mentioned name *sakkara* also appears in a number of writings. Pliny, the Roman historian who died at the eruption of Vesuvius in 79 B.C., wrote: "Sakcharon comes from Arabia, but that from India is superior. It is a 'honey' made from cane, white like rubber, and breaks between the teeth. It is never larger than a hazelnut, and is only used as medicine." In fact, Dioskurides, writing at the same time, in his theory of medicine, also mentions "Sakcharon" as "a kind of extracted honey from India" which is used for medicinal purposes.

In both cases here, cane sugar is referred to as honey. This points to the fact that, in ancient Greece and Rome, honey was at first the only sweetener known. It is thus no wonder that fleet commander Nearchos, upon discovering the sugarcane in India in 325 B.C., described to Alexander the Great a plant which "produces honey without bees."

This discovery marks a turning point in the history of cane sugar. Alexander at once ordered this plant brought into his kingdom and cultivated in Egypt and Sicily. Sugarcane thus came into occidental culture. From there, it began a victorious march all over the world — in the service of the development of human personality.

Up to the time of Buddha, sugar was still woven into the legends of people. It then entered into the historical evolution

167

of humanity. A typical legend tells of how Buddha met a thief who had just been led to the place of execution. The thief there gave the holy one his last meal — four pieces of sugar and a drink of water. As a reward for his deed, he was born again as a tree-divinity in a sugarcane grove.

The time of Alexander the Great marked a stage in human evolution which served the formation of the individuality and the development of personal abilities. The Persian culture also developed in this direction, and it later provided the base for the Arabic culture. Sugarcane also spread to Arabia. Indeed, according to Indian and Persian tradition, it was left to the Arabs to develop a process for producing refined sugar. *Kurat al milh* — a "ball of sweet salt" — was the name the Arabs gave to this sticky product extracted from thickened cane syrup, a designation echoed in our word "caramel".

In the domain of the Arab caliphs, sugar was highly valued and much used. A description of the opulent wedding of the Caliph of Baghdad, Harun al Raschid, in 807 A.D., tells us that 40,000 kg of sugar were used for this festival alone. We may thus assume that, at the flowering of Arab culture, high sugar consumption and the tremendous desire for sugar, so common in our time, already had their precedents.

However, sugar remained relatively unknown outside of the Arab world for several centuries. The crusaders were the first to bring news of sugarcane back to Europe. A contemporary account of the first crusade (1096 -- 1099) under Gottfried von Boullion reports: "In the fields of the plains of Tripol, there was an abundance of a honey-reed called Zucra. The people sucked out the reeds with great delight, enjoyed the pleasant sap, and because of its sweetness, they never became satisfied with this drink..." The German order of knights took over both the extensive sugarcane plantations and the techniques of sugar extraction from the defeated Arabs. As early as 1166, the Sicilian King William II donated a mill for squeezing sugarcane to the monastery of St. Benedict of Monreale. Sugar came to Europe by way of oriental trade. As a legacy of the Arab empire, which pursued sugar cultivation as far as Rhodesia, there was trade in sugar pieces from Babylon, white sugar from Alexandria, powdered sugar from Rhodesia and sugar loaf from Cypress. However, sugar was at this time only used as a spice and medicament — or at most a

168

treat for the well-to-do — because it was tremendously expensive.

In 1492, news of sugarcane finally reached the new world. Columbus took it from Madeira (where it had been brought by the Arabs) to Cuba, which became the "new sugar island,"[9] from whence it quickly spread over large portions of Central America.

It was significant for European development that a personality like Emperor Friedrich II had already issued a decree in 1232 to promote sugarcane cultivation on the island of Sicily. He also saw to it that experts were sent from Jerusalem to Palermo to teach the art of sugar production to the Sicilians. Friedrich himself was a great lover of sugar. His Master of Philosophy had to prepare syrup, and even violet sugar, for him.

Mention of sugar in medieval Germany appears for the first time around 1205, in Wolfram von Eschenbach's *Parzifal.* In a writing from 1485, called *Guest of Health,* there is a contrived picture of sugarcane, based on descriptions by Galenos of Pergamon (200 AD) and the Arabian physician and philosopher Avicenna (980-1037). Here, however, sugar is described primarily as a medicament, although it is mentioned that pastries with sugar can strengthen people.

Thus we can see that sugar entered only gradually into central Europe, in spite of the fact that the world empire of the Portuguese contributed much to the knowledge and availability of sugar. Henry the Seaman had sugarcane brought from Sicily to Madeira. From there, it went not only to America, but also to western Africa. by the 15th century, sugar from Madeira was already competing in Europe with that from the Levant. In 1500 there were over 120 sugarcane mills driven by negro slaves.

We thus come to another chapter in the history of sugar: the cultivation of sugarcane and the extraction of sugar were, to a large extent, the cause of an extensive slave trade. Many contracts are known that brought black men and women to America to be used for sugar production. The indigenous Indian population was almost exterminated, and the new Spanish rulers brought more and more slaves into their new territories. Baxa and Bruhns write: "The extention of sugarcane cultivation into the wide and fertile, but sparsely populated, regions of America made the slave trade — which lasted until the 19th century — expand tremendously. The increasing desire for sugar in Europe contributed significantly to the increased demand for slaves in

America."[14] In 1600 there were already 120 sugar factories (with innumerable negro slaves) in Brazil. Thus, the increasing need for sugar in Europe contributed to a very dark chapter in history.

Nonetheless, sugar consumption remained limited to the upper strata of society. At this time, people gave in to gluttony for sugar, although only on special occasions. One example is a report of a duke's wedding in Perugia on June 28, 1500. "After the great festivals came the early meal. It was so opulent as to hardly be believed. Every kind of fruit was there made out of sugar. In addition, there were frogs, crabs, snakes, birds . . . all out of sugar, as well as every other type of confection." In 1513 the King of Portugal sent the newly elected Pope Leo X "a pope with 12 cardinals, all made of sugar and as large as real men. There were also 300 candles made of sugar, each 3 yards long, and 100 crates of sugar . . ." In 1505 there appeared, in a tract on "the Teutonic larder," a condemnation of the "sweet-tooths who wish to have or know nothing, unless it is salted with sugar." However, it also gives various indications for the use of sugar. Finally, in 1544, Ryff stated that "sugar now has come to such acclaim and universal usage that it is no longer restricted to the pharmacy, but has found its way into the kitchen. It is used in nearly every food and drink because it flatters and enhances the taste. A special saying has thereby arisen: Sugar spoils no dish."[14]

We see that with the dawn of modernity — the beginning of the development of the human consciousness-soul in our cultural epoch — sugar consumption went far beyond the limits in which it had been kept for millenia. Sugar has become an increasingly normal part of our diet, and everyone wants to take part in its consumption, since everyone wants to develop the awakening personality forces it carries.

From the 16th to the 18th centuries, sugar consumption among the general population was not considerable; it was coming into increasing use, however, and occupying the arts of healing and medicine, which appeared then as precursors of a natural-scientific orientation. In 1637, a *Saccharologia* appeared, written by a German physician, Angelus Sala. In a medical dissertation from 1701, we read that pure sugar is a digestible and easily assimilated food. Finally, the famous physician and contemporary of Goethe, Hufeland — in his book *Die Kunst, das menschliche Leben zu verlängern (The Art of Extending Human*

Life) — recommended sugar as cooling, loosening and purifying. However, he warned of the consequences for the teeth which result from eating sugar: "Do not chew sugar and avoid baked things with sugar, as they contain many soft sticky particles." This is truly modern advice from the year 1795.

Something new entered into the evolution of sugar consumption with the discovery of the sugar content in beets. People were already aware of their sweet taste. Indeed, the Ancient Greeks prized them as vegetables. However, as the result of systematic research, the German pharmacist Andreas Sigismund Markgraf was the first to extract a "salt" from beets which in no way differed from "true perfect sugar." In 1749, Markgraf published his *Chemische Untersuchungen* on the subject. This book was met with interest but did not lead to large-scale production of beet sugar. His pupil, Franz Karl Achard, was the first to bring such production about. In 1799, large-scale experiments were begun involving the cultivation of beets and the extraction of beet sugar. Achard was a brilliant man, involved in other forward-looking experiments. He soon became famous in Europe, but he by no means lacked opposition. The cane sugar monopoly feared undesirable competition. In 1799, Achard anonymously published a small pamphlet with the bold title: *The Newest German Replacement for Indian Sugar, or Sugar from Beets, the Most Important and Beneficial Discovery of the 18th Century.* In this pamphlet he mentioned that by means of beet sugar, mankind would be freed from the "eternal tyranny" of slavery "caused by something from an unfortunate cane, desired by millions of Europeans." With this publication, the polemic really became hot. A political event of a different nature brought about a resolution. In 1806, Napoleon blockaded Europe, thus stopping the sugar trade from European ports. The resulting sugar shortage brought victory to the discovery of Markgraf and Achard. After the fall of Napoleon's empire, the market was flooded with cane sugar. But the sugar beet industry had already gotten a firm footing. The sugar content of beets was increased, the process of extraction was made cheaper, and beet sugar thus became competitive. Not until 1890, however, did beet sugar finally become dominant over cane sugar. At the turn of the century, over 50% of the sugar produced in the world came from beets. In 1903, an international agreement regulating the relationship of beet and cane sugar was reached.

171

At the same time, something else had occurred: a leap in the world-wide production of sugar.

From Sugar as Medicine to the "Pathogenetic Factor"

In 1850, world-wide production of sugar was about 1.8 million (metric) tons. By the turn of the century, it approached eight million tons. In 1930, the 25 million ton mark was reached, and by 1960, production was over 50 million tons. In a little over a century, sugar production had increased 35-fold. In 1975 it was up to 81.6 million tons. (*Ernaehrungs Umschau*-4/75).[15]

A comparison with two agricultural products, wheat and potatoes, is offered in the following chart (according to Geerdes):[3]

	Wheat		Potatoes		Sugar Beats	
	t	in %	t	in %	t	in %
1903/04	88, 059, 875.	100	117, 123, 170.	100	11, 345. 208.	100
1959/60	248, 900, 000.	283	276, 000, 000.	235	50, 180, 000.	448

From these figures we see that sugar beet cultivation has had the greatest increase in production, even though it is the lowest of the three in terms of quantity produced.

The tremendous increase in world sugar-production has been interrupted only by the two world wars. In both cases, it quickly recovered from the set-back and proceeded to climb to new heights.

The enormous increase in sugar consumption is certainly a social question as well. The price of sugar was lowered considerably, thanks to modern industrial production. This made it possible for ever wider segments of the population to use sugar as a general food. In 1447 in Germany, a kilogram of sugar cost 5 gold Marks. Goethe paid 2.70 gold Marks in 1793. Compared to the enormous increase in sugar production, the price today is still relatively high. And, as recent events have shown, it is subject to considerable fluctuation.

We are therefore inclined to believe that the developments here outlined are the expression of a certain development of consciousness. Sugar — especially crystallized, inorganic sugar — served to stimulate man to separate his Ego-consciousness, his personal character, from the old group consciousness. It served
172

his independence, bestowing "inner solidity" upon him. "In this regard, one may, in a sense, praise sugar," said Rudolf Steiner.[1] In the same connection, we find the above-mentioned indication: "In countries where statistically little sugar is consumed, people have less of a personality development than those in countries where statistically more sugar is consumed." In consuming less sugar, people remain "less personal." "Where there is sugar, there is the Ego-organization"; this concise statement clearly shows that the sugar process — as a process of mineralization, as a development of sweetness — must be active within the human being. However, we must not only be able to build up our own bodily sugar. We must also be able to break it down again. It is precisely with these two activities that the Ego-organization develops itself. Building up and breaking down are in a constant interplay with one another. They must balance out one another.

Man wants to experience this sugar process directly, through his taste of sweetness, because this process is thereby immediately accessible to his consciousness. To the extent that this holds true, man has lost the healthy moderation necessary for the above-mentioned balance. On the one hand, western man eats much too much sugar. On the other hand, he has produced and preferred a sugar which cannot fulfill this task because it has been refined.

We may ask anew: has man not turned the task which he can and should accomplish, with the help of sugar, into its opposite? On the one hand, we see an increasingly unrestrained increase in sugar consumption, without the corresponding development of conscious activity. On the other hand, we have the bringing of sugar itself to an extreme mineralization process, an isolation process. It thus does not meet with the corresponding physiological capacity in man, who cannot overcome it in such proportions. Sugar today has thereby become a "pathogenetic factor," as modern researchers call it. It makes people sick more than it furthers their health. The extent to which it influences the consciousness has hardly been researched.

It is thus especially important that we can find in the work of Rudolf Steiner an indication of the direction we can take to heal this pathological degeneration.

We have already mentioned the production of one's sugar which plays an essential role: the sugarization of starch in the process of digestion, which may come with eating grains. In fact, humanity has taken this path, as it has placed grain at the center of its nutrition for millenia. It has drawn strength from this sugarizing process. The direct consumption of sugar, in contrast, has played only a minor role, as we have seen.

In *Fundamentals of Therapy,* Rudolf Steiner clearly expresses this theme. He differentiates between "sugar consumed directly" and "starch, consumed and converted into sugar . . ." We shall return to this distinction in our discussion of diabetes.

First, however, we will offer a further description of this problem by Rudolf Steiner. In his second medical course (1921)[16], while discussing a particular remedy, he spoke of "starch flour". With it, we "in a sense appeal to those forces which work intensively when sugar is being worked upon . . ." That is to say that when sugarizing starch, the inner forces are more active than in the mere digestion of sugar. Thereby, more forces are brought to the inner man. Basically, the sugarization of starch — and even the production of glucose from cane sugar — is a kind of "refinement process". But in this case the organism must do the "refining" itself — and with physiological means.

Spiritual-scientific observation shows that in the digestion of starch, both the Ego-organization and the astral body are active. The former works in the mouth, the latter in the deeper regions of the digestion-organization. The cooperation of these two obviously must be more intensive when it is a case of sugarizing starch. This can be seen in the well-researched effect of consuming factory sugar. Refined sugar goes quickly into the blood, so that one speaks of a "shock to the system" which brings on a rash increase of insulin secretion. In contrast, starch products are converted only very slowly into soluble sugar. "They only cause a mild shock to the system and thus are less taxing." (Bircher-Benner, *Handbook for Diabetics*).[17] The different rates of decomposition reveal one of two things: either a shock to the organism or an activity controlled by the inner forces, by means of the increased resistance offered by the intensified activity of the two higher members of the human organization. The effects of sugar digestion clearly continue in the blood. We see, therefore, that it is precisely in the blood where the balance between the two higher and the two lower members of man's organization is

174

disrupted. As we shall see later, this is the essential cause of diabetes.

Carbohydrates in General

We here include a section — which fits in organically with our presentation — which the reader has perhaps thought was left out. We have not yet given an overview of carbohydrates in general, as they are formed in the plant world and confront man in his nutrition. This omission was intentional, however, as we wanted first to speak of the nature and significance of sugar. As we have seen, sugar achieves a central place regarding the relationship to man. From there, we can realistically grasp the entire spectrum of carbohydrates.

Today, the polysaccharides are divided into di-and mono-saccharides. Starch belongs to the former. It is so-called "storage carbohydrate", and we have already described something of its formation. It has a colloidal structure which changes drastically upon absorbing water. It can be made especially accessible to human digestion by cooking. Another storage carbohydrate is lichenin, which is active in the "slime" of oats.

On the other hand, the "structural carbohydrates" play a big role in the construction of the plant. Most important is cellulose, then comes pectin, and then hemicellulose, e.g. lignin, and plant rubber. We have already emphasized their importance as "roughage" in *The Dynamics of Nutrition*. We shall return to them in our discussion of grain.

Practically speaking, there are only three di-saccharides significant in human nutrition: sucrose, lactose, maltose. None of these can be used directly. They must, as we have said, be broken down into monosaccharides, i.e. into glucose, fructose or galactose.

Among these, glucose (also called "grape sugar") is the most important, to the extent that most carbohydrates are broken down into glucose with digestion. Fructose, found in fruit and honey, goes another way in the human metabolism. This is especially significant for an understanding of diabetes. Galactose plays a role in the digestion of milk sugar or lactose.

Interestingly the sucroses — cane sugar and beet sugar — are chemically identical. Today, no difference is made between them, although just such a difference is essential for a qualitative consideration.

175

Maltose or malt sugar is found in malt extract, but has only a limited significance.

We might also mention chitin, a structural carbohydrate found in lower animals. In human beings, we find the so-called mucopoly saccharides, protein sugars, which serve as important building blocks for cartilage, tendons and ligaments. In the subcutaneous connective tissue, we have so-called muco-polysaccharides which account for the elasticity of skin, blood vessels and tendons.

This short overview makes it clear that "our whole extistence is dependent upon the sugars, and that the process of photosynthesis is a prerequisite for life on our earth.[3]

Sugar as Understood Through Spiritual Science

This brings us back to a process connected with photosynthesis and assimilation. A spiritual-scientific deepening of our understanding can lead us to a broader knowledge of the significance of sugar formation.

We may ask: to which of the three members of the human being is the process of photosynthesis related? The answer is the rhythmic organization, midway between the metabolic and nervous systems. This "chest-torso" system (as Rudolf Steiner called it) is, indeed, related to the plant world. We have seen how the plant takes carbon dioxide from the air and — with the help of the cosmic forces of light and warmth — builds up sugar. In contrast, man has developed the process counter to this in his breathing. He takes in the oxygen which the plants give off during the day and combines it within himself with carbon to make carbon dioxide. The carbon, however, comes into him through his food. Not only carbohydrates, but also proteins and fats, bring it in. We use this carbon in order to build up our own substances. Oxygen mediates the life forces; it is the bearer of the etheric formative forces on the earth. Carbon is the basis for all shape, form and substance-formation in the realm of the living — thus we have organic chemistry based on carbon. It is the "bearer of all processes of formation in nature", the "great sculptor" as Rudolf Steiner called it in his agricultural course.[18] However, the carbon framework in man is not lasting. It has no tendency toward rigidifying. It is thus unlike the plant, which produces wood and coal. Indeed, it is characteristically human "that it can always immediately

176

destroy the form which just arose, in that man excretes carbon, combined with oxygen, as carbon dioxide" in the process of breathing.[18] Man builds up within himself a carbohydrate with carbon which constantly forms and then dissolves itself. This is the glycogen in the liver, which man breaks down into human sugar, glucose. He then allows it to circulate in his blood, carrying sugar all around. The human Ego makes use of a physical carrier in this carbon which moves in the blood. "The human Ego lives as the actual spirit in man in carbon,"[18] and finds its highest expression in the formation of sugar. "Where there is sugar, there is the Ego-organization."

What would happen, though, if carbon were not constantly combined with oxygen in the breathing process of the human middle region? What would happen if this dissolution process did not occur? Then, a process of becoming plant-like would in fact take hold of man. "All vegetation would suddenly grow in man." As Rudolf Steiner put it in his *Study of Man:*[19] "Man has this capacity: he could always produce a plant world . . . his torso-system has a strong and constant tendency to produce the plant world . . ." This would mean that man would become ill. To remain healthy, he must constantly hold back this process. Indeed, he must produce a counter-process — the formation and exhalation of carbon dioxide. "With respect to his chest-torso system, man is capable of creating a realm counter to that of the plants." And we accomplish in ourselves the process of becoming human in that we overcome this process of becoming plant-like, in that we bring forth a counter-process against outer nature.

In our metabolism — through our nutrition — this plant-formation process is at first constantly offered to us. However, by means of our breathing, we constantly dissolve it. This occurs in that we bring forth a consciousness-forming counter-force from our "upper man", from our nerve-sense region. We overcome the process of becoming plant-like in our lungs. Thus, at the same time, we heal ourselves of the tendencies to disease which enter into us. For — as Rudolf Steiner was able to discover — "in a certain sense, we have an image of all of our diseases in the plant world." At the same time, however, these plants carry within them the forces to heal such sicknesses. Novalis had already intuited this and spoke of it in his *Fragments*. Indeed, man brings forth an "anti-plant kingdom" within himself. It is "the counter-

177

part to everything which happens outside in the plant world." This process represents a pushing back of the outer plant tendencies. It is also an inner process of permeation by the soul. For the force which works in man's rhythmic organization against becoming plant-like — i.e. the extension of the life-formation force as such — is of a higher nature, of a soul nature. "Man ensouls these processes of nature in his process of breathing."

However, this is possible only because the inner process of breathing is not the imitation of a natural process. That is, it is not really a "process of combustion", as was first assumed. Modern nutritional theory has modified this view but has still not penetrated to the reality of the situation. Thus Mohler, for example, writes: "The earlier equating of biological oxidation to a burning process is valid only with regard to the gross equation and the end products, CO_2 and H_2O."[20] The human organism is here understood as an accumulator which charges and discharges itself. We have shown in the *Dynamics of Nutrition* how little reality is grasped with such a conception. Here we would like to add what can be gained, practically, by learning to view such processes in accordance with reality.

In his *Study of Man*,[19] mentioned above, Rudolf Steiner points out that such a "combustion process" does not take place in man — not even in small steps, as is often believed today. Rather, it is a "combustion process where the beginning and end are missing." The natural process of "combustion" can be seen, for example, in the first formation of fruit or in the formation of seeds in grains and legumes. Man, however, is not up to this beginning combustion process. If he eats unripe fruits or seeds — some are even poisonous — he cannot handle them with his digestion. They make him ill. It is the same when outer "combustion processes" go too far. When food rots or ferments, it is then similarly unsuitable. In other words: "In fact, man does not carry out the natural processes in the same way that they are carried out in his environment. Rather, he only carries out the middle part." He joins himself bodily only with the middle part of the natural processes, and it is precisely for this reason that he can overcome, ensoul and humanize them. This plays an important role in the quality of nutrition: food must have reached the proper degree of ripeness. This fact, in turn, is related to the activity of the sun, especially to the warmth power of the sun. The sun's

178

warmth brings about sugar formation in the fruits, seeds etc. — i.e. it brings about the proper sweetening. The natural process thus comes to meet the human formative process, so that the latter can take hold of substance with the higher organization, ensouling it and permeating it with man's Ego.

We have seen that the process of plant formation — which is also a threefold process — proceeds from the root pole to the leaf organism. The latter is the actual place of photosynthesis and assimilation. The growth process then develops further to the formation of flower and fruit. Thus, the plant grows from below upward.

The human formation is the polar opposite of this process. The root pole moves upward as the head organization, and the flower and fruit pole — the metabolism — moves downward. The rhythmical balance of these processes of building up and breaking down takes place at the same level as in the plants — i.e. in the respiratory region. Thus we see how man, in taking in the process of plant formation in his nutrition, works "against the upward-striving plant nature with the downward-striving human nature." Man must hold in check — or work against — these plant processes. "That which the plant develops upwards, man develops from above downwards." Man permeates himself with consciousness forces from above in his nerve-sense formation. He bears his higher organization, soul and spirit, into the lower organization and there lets it submerge in the enlivened corporeality (whereby it loses the forces of waking consciousness). On the other hand, the plant grows into a process from below. It does not reach this process, but touches upon it in the formation of flowers and fruits, which corresponds to a process of ensoulment. "The plant grows toward the Ego-activity, toward the astral activity."[21]

We have seen that human blood-sugar fills both the upper and the lower man and is expressed in its strictly constant concentration in the blood. By means of this sugar content, the human Ego establishes its balance among the other members of the human being. In other words, by means of blood sugar, the Ego-organization regulates its activity toward both the consciousness-forming and the vegetative poles. It harmonizes the upper and lower processes by holding the process of plant formation in check in the appropriate way, and by bringing forth a counter-process.

179

In this way, the Ego-organization can stimulate sugar to the threefold activity we have mentioned: nerve-sense activity as a function of thinking, metabolic-limb activity as the expression of the will, and heart activity as the organic basis of human feeling. If this harmonious balance is achieved, man uses up the sugar in his organism. If the balance is disturbed, the resulting condition finds expression in the excretion of sugar in the urine: *Diabetes mellitus* sets in.

We have thus come to a point which opens our understanding to the most significant disease related to sugar metabolism. Before going further in this direction, we should add a section on the refinement of sugar, as this is important for evaluating sugar. We shall see that the refined sugar furthers the incidence of *Diabetes mellitus* in a special way.

The Refinement of Sugar

The tremendous increase in sugar consumption recently is surely related to the fact that sugar is available in such an easily accessible, soluble, preservable and at the same time concentrated form. This is brought about by modern refining.

We have already mentioned that the process of refinement was discovered many centuries ago. A kind of crystal sugar was already produced in ancient India and Egypt. During the early middle ages, the Arabs developed a fine art of sugar refinement. This leads us to believe that the striving to consume sugar in the greatest possible concentration — i.e. with the greatest sweetness — has been around since ancient times. In keeping with our thesis, we may see something justified in this striving. But this justification is based on two premises: first, that sugar was eaten only in very small quantities, and second, that the degree of purity was not as great as it has been since the 19th century.

One of the first exact descriptions of sugar refining comes from an anonymous author. His *Natural History of Sugar* was published in 1719 in Amsterdam and is based on years of observation on the Island of Martinique. The actual sugar "factory" was comprised of five cauldrons, and lime was already being used. As early as the 18th century, the number of European refineries was contantly growing. Previously, these refineries were in the countries which produced the sugar. The French scientist Du

180

Monceau first revealed the carefully guarded secret of sugar refinement in 1764, in his book *Art de Raffiner le Sucre*. One year later it was translated into German. This work — complete with illustrations — offers an exact description of sugar refining at that time. However, the methods of sugar refinement did not improve until the discovery of beet sugar and the cultivation of sugar beets in Europe.

The English chemist Howard obtained two patents in 1812 and 1813. His process was the first thickening of sugar syrup in the absence of air by means of low pressure. By 1818, the first vacuum cooker was set up on the continent. In 1862, one report read: "The sugar industry has reached a remarkable degree of perfection." In fact, the sugar industry has been the school-master of many other industries — especially the chemical industry.

Let us turn to a brief description of the modern process of sugar refinement, as described by Geerdes.[3]

He begins by saying that "The production of sugar is a comprehensive process." This points to the fact that modern sugar production uses all technical possibilities. However, cultivation has not decreased. Quite to the contrary, it has become more and more of a monoculture, with all of the attendant advantages and disadvantages. Mineral fertilizers and pesticides play a large role here.

The actual refining takes place in eight major processes: washing, shredding, leaching, pressing, separating, saturating, evaporating and centrifuging. Each step is determined by the most modern technical means. By leaching (extraction), the so-called raw syrup is produced. This takes place today through the use of a process of diffusion discovered in 1840. In large leaching towers, the raw syrup — a 12-14% sugar solution — is left behind. Since this solution has many natural elements, both organic and inorganic, which are considered undesirable, they are removed through further procedures. This latter purification uses quick-lime and carbonic acid. Then the syrup is thickened by evaporation, filtered and brought to a cooking station, where the thick syrup is boiled in a vacuum until it becomes supersaturated. The first sugar crystals thus begin to form. Finally, the sugar mass is put in powerful centrifuges which run at 1000-1500 r.p.m. and separate the red-brown syrup from the colorless crystals. After several centrifugings, refined sugar emerges. This clear and pure

181

sugar solution is then thickened again and processed into the various sugar products.

These processes — right up to the packaging — are extensively automated. Regarding the final product, it is no doubt true that, "untouched by human hands, free of dust, clean and hygienic, sugar goes directly from the factory into the hands of the consumer."[3]

Even from such a short overview, one can see what a profound alteration takes place with the refinement of sugar. Such a processing is practically unheard of for any other food. Even compared to refined flour, refined sugar — with respect both to the techniques used and the degree of refinement — is subjected to a much more extensive processing. Even a 70% white flour has a degree of refinement of only 30%, whereas sugar is about 80-85% refined. Factory sugar is thus the most highly refined food.

Moreover, the techniques used give rise to the questions: what actually happens during refinement, and what is the quality of the resulting sugar? These questions are not easily answered. However, some important aspects arise from the physiological-pathological viewpoint when we ask the question: what is the effect of factory sugar on man? Today we have a large and important *dossier* on this subject which ought not be overlooked. It is so comprehensive that we can only summarize it and point out the most important facts and aspects.

The Effects of Refined Sugar on Man

Many researchers have studied the effects of refined sugar on man, and it is amazing how relatively early certain important observations were made. We already mentioned Hufeland, who expressed concern over the consumption of sugar, even though the refinement techniques were not very thorough. Bunge expressed this in more concrete terms and his description is surprisingly modern. In his work on *Increasing Sugar Consumption and its Dangers*[22] (1904), he begins with the basic insight that "all of our natural nutrients are not chemical individualities but mixtures." If a substance in them is chemically isolated, "the organism does not receive enough of the other necessary nutrients." This is especially true of inorganic salts. The lack of calcium in particular, "which is often already too scarce in our diet,

182

is quite serious." Further, "it must be considered that fruit" —
which Bunge called the natural sugar carrier — "contains organic
iron compounds without which deficiencies and iron-poor blood
easily come about."

Bunge gives the calcium and iron content of various foods in
a table. Some examples are:

In 100 g dry substances are:	mg Calcium	mg Iron
Sugar	0	0
Honey	6.7	1.2
Graham Bread	77	5.6
Dates	108	2.1
Plums	166	2.8
Human Milk	243	2.3—3.1
Figs	400	4.0
Strawberries	483	8.6—9.3

With these indications, Bunge hoped to show that eating
sugar-rich fruit not only satisfies the desire for sugar but is also
good for the health. "On the other hand, when one takes to unnatural foods — to an individual chemical produced artificially,
to pure sugar — we must expect, *a priori,* that this deviation from
the norm will have harmful effects on the health."[22] As the danger
of an insufficient intake of calcium salts and iron is especially
great in the growing organism, in children, "one should give
them, above all, ripe grapes and, additionally, figs, dates, pears,
apricots and plums which are available all year round, either
fresh or dried. As far as possible, children should be kept from
all products made with pure sugar and little else, e.g. candies,
confections of all kinds . . . The use of pure sugar should be limited
to the greatest possible extent . . ."

Important results of the lack of calcium in sugar are described
by the Japanese researcher Katase in his book on the influence
of nutrition on the human constitution,[23] where he describes
impressive research on the effects of isolated sugar on the growing body. He fed a rabbit an amount of isolated sugar equivalent
to 40-60 g/day for a child of 20-30 kg. He observed severe pathological changes in the whole skeletal system, in the form of softening, bending, cracking, and breaking. The microscope revealed
a leaching out of calcium from the bones. In further experiments,
he determined that this damage took place on the 7th day, when
the rabbit was given ½ g sugar/day, and on the 3rd day when it
was fed 1.5 g/day. "If the tolerance of man is exactly the same
as that of these rabbits, children of 5.6 years and 20 kg body

183

weight can only take 6 g of sugar without harm." Such experiments confirm Bunge's indications even if they address only one aspect of the problem.

Isolated sugar has occupied the work of vitamin reasearch even more during the last decades. Two works stand out here: *Vitamins and Their Clinical Applications*[24] by Stepp, Kuhnau and Schroeder (1952) and *Sugar as Vitamin B Robber*[25] by Stepp (1956). The multifaceted work of these authors leads to the conclusion that an increased consumption of isolated sugar brings about a more or less severe thiamine deficiency. This danger is increased by the overwhelming consumption of refined cereal products. Because it is a case of national nutritional habits, the danger of the results of a relative thiamine deficiency is about the same for all social classes.

At a symposium on "Tendencies in Nutrition and Diatetics" (Zurich, 29 March, 1973), H.R. Muehlemann[26] put the consumption of isolated sugar in Switzerland at 132 g per capita daily, i.e. 48.18 kg per year.

Finally, we point to the presentation of T.L. Cleave and G.D. Campbell in *Saccharidosis*[9] (1970). Cleave and Campbell have made a whole catalog of pathological symptoms which they relate to the present overconsumption of refined sugar and other carbohydrates. Among them is the rapid increase in diabetes. Even the German Society for Nutrition has (according to E. Ziegler), in its report of 1969, recommended that sugar consumption should not be more than 60 g daily[8] — a figure probably still too high. The research of Bunge, however, is still valuable in this regard. It would indicate that a much greater reduction of isolated sugar in favor of fresh or dried fruit and whole grains is in order. A. Roos, in particular, has supported such a nutritional restructuring. He writes: "Without a massive reduction in sugar consumption, an increase in fruit consumption cannot be achieved."[27] Without referring directly to Bunge, Roos deals similarly with the problem of tooth decay.

Bunge also posed the question of the caries-promoting effect of isolated sugar. However, too little concrete research had been completed at that time for him to reach any objective conclusions. The decrease of calcium salts through the eating of sugar — which also lowers the consumption of calcium-rich vegetables — was one possibility he cited for the degeneration of teeth which had

184

already begun. However, the latter has reached catastrophic proportions only in the last fifty years. Thus, its causes are better known today, although research in this area is still in process.

Roos has done a service with his important treatise, *The Degeneration of Culture and the Decay of Teeth*. He does not deal with this problem only from the limited standpoint of caries. Rather, he writes: "I am of the opinion that present-day man eats much too much sugar, and that this one-sided nutrition will have consequences which will only appear later. The entire person is altered by this 'modern nutrition'. His development is not harmonious but disturbed. Tooth decay in young children is a visible manifestation of this."

The material collected by Roos in his extensive studies is so unequivocal that it seems impossible to doubt his conclusions. He makes a basic proposal: "If the Swiss people are interested in overcoming the present crisis to their teeth . . . then all forms of propaganda must be used to encourage a much greater consumption of fresh fruit." He shows convincingly that this can come about, however, only with a "massive reduction in sugar consumption". This can be achieved, on one hand, through a "fight against sugar mania" — i.e. against the senseless consumption of sugary candy, baked goods, ice cream, chocolate, etc. — and on the other hand, by a turning back toward wholegrain products.

At this point, we quote from A. Fleisch's[15] *Nutritional Problems in Times of Want*.[28] He writes: "Statistics and interviews examined by A. Roos regarding the development of tooth diseases during the war yielded a favorable result. The number of fillings per 100 school pupils dropped by half, the number of root fillings dropped to one-sixth of what they were. All school dental clinics reported a sharp decline in caries. This improvement of the teeth is attributed to the beneficial influence of the war-time nutrition, and especially to the restriction of sugar and baked goods and the substitution of wholegrain bread for white. Ninety percent of the dentists consider dark bread beneficial for building up teeth."

Thus, it has already been proven that such a diet has the effect of preventing dental caries. It is interesting that Bunge had already pointed out the relative inexpensiveness of sugar as compared to bread. He attributed the increase in sugar consumption to this fact. The same argument has been brought forth today, e.g. by H.R. Muehlemann in his lecture on "Sugar and

185

Sweets" at the above-mentioned nutritional symposium in Zurich. He suggested that a one-percent luxury tax on "sweets" would mobilize about five million Swiss Francs per year in Switzerland. Bunge, in his discussion of sugar, wrote: "Sugar should be taxed as heavily as possible. All import tariffs on southern fruits should be lifted. All means should be used to promote gardening and fruit cultivation." Such a statement shows how realistic and yet how universal were Bunge's thoughts.

Finally, we should mention that E. Ziegler[8] has studied the relation between modern nutritional forms and caries. He not only focused on this problem but also — along with Roos — discovered the connection between increased sugar consumption and developmental conditions, or disruptions, of the entire human being. Bunge himself did not look at sugar as a substance with a limited or localized effect. Indeed, he didn't even attribute further significance to the carcinogenic effects of isolated sugar. He thought in terms of a disruption of the entire metabolism and of all human development. This is reflected in a letter to his brother, Alexander, wherein he wrote: "Along with these lines, I send you my phillipic against sugar . . . When one is constantly surrounded by disgustingly degenerate people, one searches for all causes, and finally comes upon sugar."[29]

H.R. Muehlemann was absolutely right when, in the above-mentioned lecture, he said, "it will be the task of preventive medicine . . . to stigmatize the abuse of sugar as much as the misuse of nicotine and alcohol."

M.D. Bruker should be credited with having presented many of the above-mentioned ideas with comprehensive documentation. In *Sugar as a Pathogenetic Factor*[23] he says clearly that all of these negative effects are related to "chemically isolated sucrose" which "of course has other physiological effects than does a natural food." This is just what we have repeatedly said here. We must differentiate between sugar as such — which the human being has a legitimate need for — and the present-day form of factory sugar. Trying to make an adequate distinction between these two has caused much confusion and misunderstanding.

However, on the whole, we can recognize the pathological effects of modern-day factory sugar, both from its being refined as well as from its being over-consumed. These effects are entirely

186

comprehensive, as the previously mentioned researchers, Cleave and Campbell, tried to show in *Saccharidosis*.[9] We shall first consider the results of their research, as related to *Diabetes mellitus*.

On the Problem of Diabetes

We have already come to Rudolf Steiner's spiritual-scientific findings, which shed a new light not only on this threatening disease but also on the problem of sugar in general.

Man expresses a polarity between the nerve-sense system and the metabolic organization. Between them, the rhythmical activities must constantly hold the balance. The plant — also threefold — is the opposite of this. The root-pole is oriented toward the earth and corresponds to the human head-organization. Conversely, the human metabolic organism corresponds to the flower, fruit and seed formations. In this respect, the plant grows toward a process which it does not reach but which it approaches in the fruit: the process of ensouling, as incorporated in animals and man. "The plant grows toward the Ego-activity, toward the astral activity." The sugar content of human blood harmonizes both poles in that it creates an "anti-plant process," i.e. a process counter to the plant process streaming into man with its sugar. Therefore, man is capable of properly utilizing sugar to the extent that he doesn't excrete it through the kidneys, as is the case with *Diabetes mellitus*.

In the case of diabetes, it comes about that "the Ego-organization, upon submerging into the astral and etheric region, is so weakened that it is no longer effective in its working upon sugar substances."[1] This condition is prepared in the organism and can then appear suddenly and spontaneously. Among such causal moments, Rudolf Steiner mentions especially "excitement or upset which is not singular, but repeated; intellectual overwork; hereditary burdens." These three causes are also known to modern medicine, although they are evaluated differently and others are added to them.

The fact that these psychological moments are an expression of the "weakening" of the mastery of the Ego-organization in its submerging into the body is most enlightening. It is often observed today that psychological shock in particular can bring on diabetes. However, one must keep in mind here that the disease

187

had already prepared itself in the person, and that certainly not every shock works in this way. "Intellectual overwork" is also important; it is a characteristic of modern man which buries the harmonious activity of his three soul forces — thinking, feeling and willing — with a resulting weakening of the Ego-organization. Equally evident — but also as little persuasive — is the "hereditary burden." Rudolf Steiner said, quite clearly, that because of such burdens "a normal integration of the Ego-organization into the total organism is prevented." The predisposition of the Jewish people to diabetes is a case in point.

Today, however, there are two other factors which can bring on *Diabetes mellitus*. They are the over-consumption of sugar itself and the equally immoderate consumption of alcohol. Rudolf Steiner mentioned both in 1925, relating them to a temporary derailing of healthy sugar metabolism. They have, in the meantime, long since become pathogenetic factors. Cleave and Campbell[9], using extensive statistical material, conclude the following: "This over-consumption, especially of sugar, burdens the pancreas and is the actual cause of the incidence of diabetes." This "over-consumption" refers to the refined carbohydrates. The unrefined carbohydrates have exactly the opposite effect: they work against the arising of diabetes. On the other hand, these two researchers reveal a onesidedness, since the pancreas must be considered only as an organ through which diabetes appears. Inadequate insulin production by the pancreas is itself a result of the above-mentioned causes. Therefore, one cannot cure diabetes with insulin. In his description of diabetes, Rudolf Steiner did not even mention the pancreas. This point will have to be clarified later. It is nonetheless true that the function of the pancreas can be buried by the immoderate consumption of refined carbohydrates. However, Cleave and Campbell also write: "It must be assumed that what burdens the pancreas also harms other parts of the organism." It should especially be kept in mind that refined sugar is an unnatural concentration of that substance, as we have already seen. In being absorbed so quickly by the organism, it does, indeed, bring about repeated shocks.[5] In other words: "They are brought on either by over-consumption, by the speed of the intake and absorption, or by both." The same situation applies to the consumption of alcohol.

Among the interesting studies of Indians and Blacks con-

188

ducted by Cleave and Campbell, we shall mention only the following.[9] The sugar consumption of Indians in their homeland rarely reaches 30 g per capita daily and is usually under 15 g. The present average for the whole country is 15 g per person daily, or about 5½ kg yearly. These figures from the mid-1960's correspond roughly to the sugar consumption in Europe one hundred years ago. In contrast, the sugar consumption of Indians who have lived for generations in the South African province of Natal is about nine times as high. On the average they consume about 50 kg per person yearly. Correspondingly, they experience a "leap in the incidence of diabetes. This disease may be more frequent here than anywhere else in the world . . ." In contrast, only about 1% of the population of India are so afflicted.

A comparison of the Bantus in South Africa with black Americans reveals a similar situation. Among the genuine rural Bantus, "diabetes is extraordinarily rare," in spite of the fact that they "eat large quantities of natural sugar cane." However, they eat only small amounts of refined sugar.

The situation has been altogether different among the Zulus in the cities of South Africa. They receive 16% of their calories from sugar, as opposed to 1% for the rural Zulus, and the respective consumptions of sugar are 40 and 2.7 kg per capita yearly. The incidence of diabetes among the city Zulus is correspondingly more frequent. Blacks in America consume over 45 kg per capita yearly, and their frequency of diabetes is the same as in the rest of the population.

This research seems to indicate that the sudden increase in the consumption of carbohydrates does, in fact, undermine the ability of the human Ego-organization to actively master and harmonize the total personality, a conclusion which holds true for all peoples and races. The researchers have tried to take a comprehensive look at the problem and have concluded that the immoderate consumption of refined carbohydrates has a widespread and profound effect on the human organism. They therefore coined the term "saccharidosis" to describe the only illness which has as its cause the consumption of refined carbohydrates. It is manifest not only in *Diabetes mellitus*, but also in obesity, tooth decay and the increase of gastric and intestinal ulcers.

The results in the human organism of over-consuming refined carbohydrates are, without a doubt, extensive. We know that not

189

only the carbohydrate metabolism, but also the fat and protein metabolisms, are disturbed. Rudolf Steiner had an even more comprehensive viewpoint. He said that the insufficient use of the digestive forces in the organism is "really the same factor which brings on gout, rheumatism, diabetes, etc."[18] This is certainly the case when one eats refined carbohydrates, although Steiner was here speaking of the consumption of animal products. "If one eats animals, these forces are deposited in the organism. They remain unused, and thus begin to use themselves in that they deposit metabolic products ... or drive out necessary things ... such as happens with diabetes ..."

So we see that a very comprehensive outlook is necessary in order to understand diabetes. Out of his insight into these processes in the entire human being, Rudolf Steiner was able to develop a new therapeutic idea for *Diabetes mellitus.* This is described in his first medical course (1930)[10] and in a lecture of October 9, 1920,[21] both of which have been mentioned already. In both cases, attention is drawn to the polarity between the processes in man and in the plant. The plant grows from below upward, toward a higher process. It forms substances which are an expression of the world attained by animals and man, the etheric oils — substances which are easily burned (i.e. which are close to the element of warmth), volatile and characterized by special aromatic forces. We encountered them in *The Dynamics of Nutrition,* in the discussion of aroma in Chapter 4. And "when we see etheric oils arising in certain plants, then the result of such a consideration is . . . that it is the activity opposite to the Ego activity as it is forced into the human organism which leads to diabetes . . ." In this way, one can work against diabetes. In the medical course, Steiner mentioned rosemary oil, specifically, as an oil which can be used, highly dispersed, in a bath. This therapy with etheric oils has been realized today in the so-called "oil-dispersion bath." (Developed by W. Junge, D-7321 Birenbach, West Germany).

Of course, this therapy does not touch upon the necessary dietary treatment of diabetes. We shall return to that question later.

A Spiritual-Scientific View of Sugar Quality

We owe the reader another explanation in relation to the proper quality of refined sugar. Numerous inquiries have been made into the effect of sugar on man, and we have mentioned some of the important ones. They all indicate that, when sugar is over-consumed, it undermines and hollows out the actual core of man's being. In this regard, it is similar to alcohol, which can also bring on diabetes.

Sugar is the substance which the human Ego-organization needs in order to unfold its activity in the organism. In the case of diabetes, this substance inundates the blood and tissue, without being sufficiently taken up by the highest functions of the human organism, and so brings on the degeneration of this organism. The diabetic coma is brought on by hyperglycemia, i.e. by an increase in blood sugar to 500 mg. % or more. Sugar then appears uncontrolled — the Ego can no longer take hold of it in the organism. Blood pressure drops; apathy and sleepiness appear, followed, finally, by complete unconsciousness. This is a disturbing counter-image to the awake, self-conscious man, who uses sugar to be active in his organism.

Is there something that has happened to the sugar itself which enables it to further the incidence of the disease? We suspect that there is when, for example, we look at the processes used in modern sugar refinement, described earlier. Two processes stand out: vacuum extraction and the centrifuging of the sugar syrup. Both processes are used so often today that their application appears to be taken for granted. Nonetheless, the alteration of substances subjected to these processes extends not only to the physiological-chemical level, but also to the qualitative level.

Without a doubt, the ability to create an ever more perfect vacuum — an air-free space — represents a large step forward in technology. In ancient times, when many people still had a spiritual view of things, it was taken for granted that a vacuum could arise in the physical world only, but that in reality the whole world is filled with beings. The presence of these beings in the world was experienced as just as real as — even as more real than — the presence of gases and the like in the atmosphere. A mere which brought the whole question into the field of technology. echo of this concept lived in the views of Descartes, Pascal, Torricelli and others who considered this question in the 17th century. Then came Otto von Guericke with his "spheres of Magdeburg"

A scholarly Catholic cleric, Pierre Gassend, gave the natural philosophy of the 17th century an impulse toward the later, mechanical, atomistic, world-view. He spoke of three types of vacuum: The *vacuum separatum* is the infinite space in which God created the finite world. The *vacuum disseminatum* is a collective of empty spaces between the "corpuscles" in which they move. A third vacuum, called *coacervatum,* can only be created artificially. Guericke succeeded in doing this.

The old view avoided the nature of nothingness or emptiness. But the *horror vacui* was dealt a severe blow by Torricelli's experiments. No less a figure than Blaise Pascal sought to explain the vacuum phenomena which occurred during the measurement of atmospheric pressure by means of quicksilver. However, the traditional idea persisted, that an empty space is filled with "heavenly matter". Numerous theories were put forth to harmonize the new physical knowledge with the traditions of the spiritual conception. Finally, however, the *horror vacui* was largely overcome, and Guericke contributed much to this outcome. Then the theory was put forth that nature abhors a vacuum, but that this abhorrence can be overcome. As this process became apparently possible, through technical means, the old idea — that the vacuum is filled with "esprit" or "spirits" — was forgotten. It was suggested that interstellar space is an absolute vacuum, which can be technically reproduced on earth.

The first technical application, in the true sense, came with the construction of the steam engine. One can easily see the profound change caused in the entire life of the earth by James Watt's invention in the eighteenth century.

Rudolf Steiner also spoke of this immensely important development in a lecture of November, 1916, in Dornach.[30] "What really happens when one uses space devoid of air — that is, when one drives the air out of space?" asked Rudolf Steiner. In a certain sense, Goethe had already answered this question in his *Faust,* written just about the time when Watt constructed his steam engine. At the end of the second part of *Faust,* referring to Faust's recent death, Mephistopheles speaks the highly significant words:

Gone, to sheer Nothing, past with null made one!
What matters our creative endless toil,
When, at a snatch, oblivion ends the coil?
'It is by-gone' — How shall this riddle run?
As good as if things never had begun,
Yet circle back, existence to possess:
I'd rather have Eternal Emptiness.

Goethe has given these words to Mephistopheles — the incarnated power of evil which works against the divine. With his spiritual vision, Rudolf Steiner recognized that "when one constructs a steam engine, one gives demons a chance to incarnate. One doesn't have to believe in them if one doesn't want to: that is negative superstition. Positive superstition is to see spirits where there are none. In steam engines, however, Ahrimanic demons are real, and they are brought right into a physical body."

We cite these words in full consciousness of how strong, even today, is the "superstition" that recognizes the spirit only when it manifests itself in the material world as "spiritualism" or some such thing; otherwise, such a concept is rejected. It is seldom recognized that the misfortune of our time lies precisely in this fact. However, the intention of a work like our *Dynamics of Nutrition* can never be realized without entering into such questions about the true nature of things.

For now, this indication is sufficient to allow us to draw a picture of the sugar-refining process. Sugar, as we have seen, is the bearer of the forces of human personality, a function which is grossly caricatured, in essence, in the production of factory sugar.

Here we can only indicate the effect of the centrifugal process on the inner quality of sugar. By means of the centrifuge — which has become a necessity in modern food processing — centrifugal forces are brought to bear on the substance. As high speeds of circular motion are reached, the earth forces in matter are overcome. At the same time, condensed substance is led back into a pre-earthly condition. This process also concretely affects the quality of substance, but it works in a direction opposite to that of vacuum production. It is interesting that Rudolf Steiner used this process to bring out the medicinal properties of certain plant substances. Its justification in the producing of foodstuffs, however, is a whole different story.

These examples should give some idea of how, today and in the future, trained insight must be applied to the processes used in modern food production which are currently judged only according to purely technical criteria. However, these criteria are insufficient for genuine qualitative research.

About Honey: Cultural and Historical Aspects

We cannot end this chapter without speaking about honey, a substance which, for many years, was perhaps man's only source of sweets.

As we see, for example, in the famous Avana Cave paintings in Spain — dated at 10,000 B.C. — honey was already known in prehistoric times. Ancient Egyptian and Greek mythology also shows this, and speaks of the divine origin of the honey bee. An Egyptian myth tells of how the tears of the sun god, Re, fell to the earth and became bees. In this way, honey and wax arose from divine tears.

The people of Israel also knew about honey. It is mentioned more than fifty times in the Old Testament, where it is spoken of as a sweet food.

Even more information about honey has been handed down from the ancient Greek culture. Plato complimented the delicious honey from Hymettus, a mountain ridge near Athens, which is still tasty today. And Plutarch writes: "We call the bees wise, and value them as creators of yellow honey — an honor bestowed solely because of the physical sweetness which pleases our palates."

In Greece, sweet foods, like honey cake, were often used in the temple services, in the cultic ritual, as a sacrificial substance. This was especially true in the shrines of Demeter. It is reported that in the shrine of Askelepios, in Epidaurus, the holy snakes were fed with honey.

Let us add a few more characteristics about honey and its original use in ritual. It is interesting to note that the cultivation of honey seems to have preceded that of wine. Plutarch, in an after-dinner speech, writes: "Before man got to know the grape, honey was used, both in drinks and sacrificial drinks." In the *Iliad,* Homer speaks of sacrifice where "yellow honey and ground holy barley" were used. Pindar, the Greek lyricist, compares his song to a sparkling drink made from milk and honey. In his

194

Pythian hymn, he mentions the Delphic bee in referring to the priestess Pythia; this reminds us of the ancient connection between the bee, held holy because of her purity, and the cult of Demeter; it also explains the use of honey to placate Pluto in the cult of Ceres, for "many such proofs have shown, and many examples have taught, that part of the divine and the ethereal breath lives in the bees." Pindar also relates that Plato, left by his wet nurse, was visited by a swarm of bees, who fed him hymettian honey. And Ovid describes the golden age with the words:

> All around were streams of milk,
> All around flowed streams of nectar,
> And all around yellow honey dripped from green oaks.

The motif of the paradisal land of human origin, where milk and honey flow, is also found in the *Bible,* where it is referred to twenty-one times. Equally important, this concept is found in the Orphic mysteries, where we hear of a sacrifice of four cows and four steers, from whose flesh a generation of bees arises. The same motif is also found in the Mithras mysteries.

We see here many indications of the original relationship of man to the sweet element. In milk this sweetness is entirely of cosmic origin; in honey, it brings the cosmic Ego-forces to man.

This perception is mirrored in the cult of the Indian god Homa, which first made use of a honey drink, later replaced by an alcoholic drink. In this way, the Homa drink became a Soma drink, which then led into the Dionysian mysteries. In another instance we see the element of honey — in the form of the beeswax candle — enter into the Christian ritual. According to one legend, God the Father bestowed his blessing on the bees as they left Paradise and, therefore, no Mass may be sung without beeswax. The apostles gave Christ honeycomb to eat. And at Easter, milk and honey were poured into the holy chalice, to signify rebirth out of death.

The Homa drink in India was the "meth" of the Germanic peoples. The *Edda* says that the dew which falls from the cosmic ash tree, Yggdrasil, is called "honey fall." And in Valhalla, the gods and heros drink the sweet meth from the great Heidrun, "from whose udder so much meth flows, that all in heaven have plenty." Here again we see the connection of milk and honey as the primal nutrition.

195

The root word "meth" is itself multi-faceted. In Sanskrit, it was *madhu* and it appears in Greek as *methy,* meaning sweet. On the other hand, the root word *sud* originally meant fragrant. It reappears in the language of the Goths as *suts* and in German as *suess,* i.e., "sweet". We may assume that both forms for expressing sweetness suggest what we mentioned earlier: "Nothing else is as appropriate for, and corresponds as well to, human nature as sweetness."

Thus, in ancient India, honey had to be present when one greeted the birth of a human soul. "Virgin honey I bring you to celebrate. With gifts from the generous Savitar, blessed in old age, protected by the Gods, may you live a hundred autumns in this world."

That honey has been recognized as preserving the force of life is shown in the words of Democrites, a contemporary of Hippocrates. When asked how one could live to be a hundred years old, remain healthy, and extend one's life, he answered: "Inside, with honey, outside with oil."

In his first medical course, held in 1920, Rudolf Steiner spoke of this medical "primal phenomenon" as he called it, saying: "If one finds the proper balance between sweet strengthening from within and oily weakening from without, one can live to a ripe age. If you take honey internally, you strengthen the forces coming to you from the cosmos from within outwards. One could say, you strengthen the actual Ego-forces."[10]

Thus, the circle is closed which leads the inspirations of the ancient myths to modern spiritual science. We can again recognize the inner nature of foods from spiritual sources. To the above words, Steiner added: "It is interesting that this method of presenting a sort of primal phenomenon played a large role at the time when the cultivation of medicine etc. came from the mysteries." For "one wanted to use facts, and not theories, to show people the path. We must again return to this approach." Rudolf Steiner thus pointed to the fact that the knowledge and importance of honey originated in the mysteries. He also said, at the same time, that, for modern human consciousness, access to a rational penetration of the inner properties of food comes from the same source.

The ancient mystery wisdom became decadent, and the wisdom of honey — and of sweets in general — was therefore forgotten. We see this clearly in the transition from Greek to Roman

196

culture. Among the Greeks, cultivation of honey was mentioned in the seventh century B.C., and honey cakes and breads were counted among the most delicious foods. On the other hand, the Romans began to use honey more as a luxury. Especially during the reign of the Caesars, honey-cake bakers were much beloved, and the so-called "sweet market" *(forum cupedines)* where honey, flowers and fruits were sold, soon played a leading role in city life. The craving for tasty foods led to the progressive improvement of sweet drinks, and people learned to make honey wine with violets, roses and spices.

In this way, the old medicinal uses of honey were lost. With Hippocrates, we find 265 different honey remedies, all prepared with the most select ingredients. These were made for centuries according to his indications, but they went more and more from the realm of medicine to daily use and finally became luxuries. Finally Rudolf Steiner was able to find a connection to the old mystery wisdom and could then, out of new insight, point to the role of honey in present-day nutrition. He said, "When a person adds honey to his food, he wants to work on his soul element in such a way that the soul, in turn, works on the body in the right way," thus indicating an appropriate direction for the use of honey in our time.

Spiritual-Scientific Evaluation of Honey

All of these indications lead us to an evaluation of honey. Furthermore, we shall see that the results of modern spiritual research point out a path to us.

Modern discussions of honey begin by calling it "a product of both plant and animal origin." The process of honey formation is, in fact, unique in this regard, and spiritual science may help us to better understand it.

Seen from the perspective of nutritional chemistry, honey at first appears to be a natural mixture of various sugars: about 45% glucose, 50% fructose and 5% sucrose. Like the real sugars, honey is a composition in which almost all nutrients are represented: mineral substances (0.3-1%), proteins (0.3-2.5%), organic acids, enzymes, fragrance and vitamins. Characteristically, only one substance is missing: fat[32]. We thus see a certain one-sidedness in honey.

197

Rudolf Steiner pointed to other processes as well. It is essential for honey production that the bee be permeated with poison. This typical poison is a necessary prerequisite for the bee's activity in producing honey.

This leads us to the dynamic approach to understanding that Rudolf Steiner was able to cultivate, especially with respect to honey. In his *Nine Lectures on Bees*[31] (Dornach, 1923) we find an extraordinary and comprehensive discussion, revealing the significance of honey more fully than he has done for any other food. We can mention only a few points here, but we strongly recommend these lectures to the reader. A nutritional-physiological study from the pen of Werner Christian Simonis also gives us a living picture of this substance.[33]

The clear predominance in honey of different sugars already points to where we must look for its activity in the human organism. Honey speaks to the formative forces in man and shows its formative force in its tendency to crystallize. These forces orient themselves toward the Ego-organization, the dominant formative principle in man. This makes honey especially suitable for aged people, where the formative forces — as opposed to the deforming tendencies — stand in the foreground.

In this regard, Rudolf Steiner has designated honey as a food for a special diet or as a medicament. "Therefore, honey is especially to be recommended to people who have grown old, for it gives our body real firmness." Honey has the force to give man form and firmness. Especially in old age, one needs the structural forces that honey can give. However "we surely don't need to eat it in large quantities, since it is only a question of getting the forces from it." This indicates that Steiner thought of honey primarily for special diets, or as a medicament, although he did say: "It is an exceptionally healthy food." However, he immediately added, "one should not eat too much of it," otherwise "too much formation comes about which can bring on pathological conditions."

It is significant that Rudolf Steiner used honey in one of his "typical remedies" — in "Scleron" (available from Weleda, Inc., Spring Valley, New York). In *Fundamentals of Therapy*,[1] we find an important discussion of this subject. Among other things, he writes: "All healing of sclerosis can only consist of opening a path to the outside for the salt-forming processes which other-

198

wise remain in the body." This takes place, at first, by means of lead. Then, however, "it is further necessary that these processes, as they run their course, are kept, so to speak, fleeting — are not allowed to persist. This comes about with the addition of honey." Here, Rudolf Steiner comes to an exact, specific evaluation of honey and of sugar as such. "Honey puts the Ego-organization in a position to exercise the necessary mastery over the astral body. It thus takes away the relative independence of the astral body which comes about with sclerosis." In other words, "honey transfers the breaking-down effect of the astral body to the Ego-organization. And sugar puts the Ego-organization in a position to fulfill its specific task," namely, sugar is able "to work directly on the Ego-organization."

This presentation is a classic example of how exactly and precisely the modern spiritual research of Rudolf Steiner is able to penetrate and explore the world of substance with the light of knowledge. We may use it to develop our own power of judgment. Moreover, we can experience how necessary it is for us, today, to have a power of knowledge that does not remain in generalities, but which — like natural science — is able to see into particulars.

According to Steiner, honey given to a child as early as nine or ten months, "up to the third or fourth year," can help to prevent rickets — but only if given in the proper dosage.

Finally, Rudolf Steiner mentions another application: we may use honey as a remedy "not for very small children, but rather for children who are at their change of teeth, or not far beyond the change." Here, the general formative power of honey, proceeding from the nerve-sense pole, stands at the fore.

At this point, Rudolf Steiner said something which has given rise to certain misunderstandings. He said that honey is most effective for small children "when it is in moderately hot milk." One should "put only a little honey in the milk," although for older people "primarily the honey — and not the milk — is what helps." One could conclude that milk is appropriate for children and honey for older people, and that milk plays no further role for old people. However, as we showed in our chapter on milk, this is not the case. On the contrary, milk can be drunk in old age with full justification. The indication here of "lots of honey and a little milk" has a more dietary-therapeutic character, whereas beginning with the lecture of January 8, 1909,[34] Rudolf Steiner said that "one can obtain positive results among old people if one gives them honey without any milk."

It is not for nothing that honey and milk are spoken of together, or that it has been said: "One must not say that Nature is a bungler, because she makes only milk but not honey in a woman's breast. Rather, one must say: this shows us that, for the small child, milk is the main thing, and that more honey should be given to the child as he grows."

Honey has a forming force which is related to the crystallization force of silicon, to the "hexagonal force." This property also brings it into relationship with the human formative-force. This force is found in the nerve sense organization, and it permeates the entire person from there.

For this reason, silicic acid can "prepare the way for honey" in people who have trouble with it. One can give "to adults some very highly diluted silicic acid in honey. Then the honey will be effective in the person."

One sees how honey can be effective in man. In reality, it is one of the most wholesome foods and has always been among those substances deemed necessary for man. This is confirmed both by so-called folk medicine, based on ancient insights, and by recent experience. Its blood-forming effect, its disinfectant power and its significance in liver diets have all been justifiably pointed out. With its high fructose concentration, it is far more easily tolerated by diabetics than other sugary foods. One must remember, however, that honey is a very concentrated sugar and can be recommended only in small doses. This was certainly the case even in ancient times, when honey was the only sweetener.

Honey represents one of man's greatest achievements in "breeding". As Rudolf Steiner mentions, the honey bee was bred from the wasp during the ancient Atlantean period. The process of honey formation itself points to an element which makes honey appear as a plant product and not as an animal product at all. This process begins in the plant. The life of the worker bees, who sacrifice their reproductive drive — an essential element in animals — puts the process of honey formation in the realm of plant formation.

We can end this discussion of honey with a quote from Rudolf Steiner which emphasizes the value of this substance to the extent that it is pure and unadulterated. "This extraordinarily healthy honey could play a much greater role in human nutrition than it does today, if people could really and fully comprehend how tremendously important the consumption of honey is."[31] These words, spoken in 1923, are certainly still valid today.

A Summarizing Description of Sugar

As a conclusion to this chapter, we will attempt to offer a comprehensive characterization of sugar and its significance for man. The most important thing we encounter is its relation to the highest member of man's being, the member most actually human: the Ego-organization. No other food substance brings us as close to the forces which actually make man human.

In the processes of plant breeding — as in the case of sugar-cane and sugar beets — as well as in the process of animal formation, which brought forth the honey bee, there lived a lofty ancient wisdom which could see the purpose and goal of humanity with intuitive certainty. These processes stand worthily beside ancient man's two other great acts of cultivation, which also opened sources of sugar — the cultivation of grains and of fruits, such as apples, pears, plums, apricots, peaches, etc. Their sweet fruit, in turn, forms a basis for the production of honey. We shall return to these indispensible sources of nourishment in another volume.

Civilized man has harvested the fruits of this wisdom for centuries. Even in those places where other sources of sugar were used for the experience of sweetness — dates, corn sugar, maple syrup, etc. — these served the same purpose, the development of the Ego-organization.

Sweet substances were first taken from the flower and fruit region of the plant. Then they came from the leaf region. Finally, man learned to release the sugar forces in the root formations. Thus the entire threefold man was brought, step by step, into the formative power of the Ego-force.

Through all this, one was always mindful of, and connected to, the great, cosmic, creative power of the sun. Its light and warmth accomplish the tremendous miracle of sugar production in the plant kingdom anew, every day. We may gain an inkling of the inexhaustible power at work here by looking at the sober figures used by modern nutritional science. According to these indications, the total production of carbohydrates by green plants

201

is about 2.7×10^{11} metric tons per year, although only about 1% of the sunlight is actually utilized.[20]

However, what is done with sugar which arises in this way is an altogether different story. Mankind has succumbed, here, to a powerful temptation which continues every day. A thick veil is being woven over the true value of sugar. Mankind vacillates between fear and seduction, either worshipping sugar or defaming it.

Cleave and Campbell[9] point to a result of modern research which throws some light on this situation. They say that diabetics have a weakened sensitivity to the taste of sweetness. They develop a reduced sensitivity to this substance which can bestow upon them the "personality". The "healthy ability to judge earthly conditions," which sugar can mediate, eludes their human potential. In this regard, Rudolf Steiner explained that sugar goes down the path from the organic to the inorganic. It thus approaches the working of the mineral world. This means that sugar "unburdens the sense organs"; it supports the specific nerve and sense activities.[35]

This mineral character of sugar makes it necessary that, in the inner digestion, it be temporarily transformed "to the volatile nature of the warmth-ether."[36] It must leave the realm of weight entirely. In this way, sugar tends to open itself again to the forces of the cosmos, from whose widths it originally received its formative forces while still in the plant. Modern man, however, has so alienated sugar from its origin that he goes down many a false path, e.g. in forcing sugar to convert to fat, etc.

We could say that it is tremendously fortunate that part of the carbohydrates, formed out of the cosmic forces, become starch. Especially with grain starch, this gives man the possibility of learning to make his own sugar. This is still the surest way of leading the sugar process to the process appopriate to man: the use of sugar as an instrument for the development of the Ego-organization.

References
Carbohydrates

1. Rudolf Steiner/Ita Wegman, *Grundlegendes für eine Erweiterung der Heilkunst nach geisteswissenschaftlichen Erkenntnissen*, Dornach 1977 (GA 27). English translation, *Fundamentals of Therapy*, London 1967.

2. A. Frey-Wyssling, *Stoffwechsel der Pflanze*, Zürich 1949.
3. Thomas Geerdes, *Zucker — ein Grundnahrungsmittel und seine Geschichte*, Stuttgart 1963.
4. Rudolf Steiner, *Menschheitsentwicklung und Christus-Erkenntnis. Theosophie und Rosenkreuzertum. Das Johannes-Evangelium*, Dornach 1967 (GA 100).
5. Konrad Mengel, *Ernährung und Stoffwechsel der Pflanze*, Jena 1965.
6. Rudolf Steiner, Lecture given in Dornach, 23 February 1924 under the title "Aufbau und Abbau im menschlichen Organismus. - Die Bedeutung der Absonderung," published in *Natur und Mensch in geisteswissenschaftlicher Betrachtung*, Dornach 1967 (GA 352).
7. H. Aebi, "Eiweiss, Ernährungsfaktor Nummer Eins," in *Schriftenreihe der Schweiz. Vereinigung für Ernährung*, Heft 17, Bern 1971.
8. E. Ziegler, "Betrachtungen über den säkulären Wandel der Ernährung," in *Schriftenreihe der Schweiz. Vereinigung für Ernährung*, Heft 12, Bern 1975.
9. T.L. Cleave/G.D. Campbell, *Die Saccharidose*, Zürich.
10. Rudolf Steiner, *Geisteswissenschaft und Medizin*, Dornach 1976 (GA 312). Reference is here made to the thirteenth lecture. English translation, *Spiritual Science and Medicine*, London 1975.
11. Rudolf Steiner, *Welche Bedeutung hat die okkulte Entwicklung des Menschen für seine Hüllen - Physicher Leib, Ätherleib, Astralleib — und sein Selbst?*, Dornach 1976 (GA 145). English translation, *The Effects of Spiritual Development*, London 1978.
12. Rudolf Steiner, Lecture given in Dornach, 31 July 1924 under the title "Ueber das Verhältnis der Nahrungsmittel zum Menschen — Rohkost und Vegetarismus," published in *Die Schöpfung der Welt und des Menschen. Erdenleben und Sternenwirken*, Dornach 1977 (GA 354).
13. Rudolf Steiner, *Aus der Akasha-Chronik*, Dornach 1973 (GA 11). English translation, *Cosmic Memory*, Englewood 1971.
14. J. Baxa/G. Bruhns, *Zucker im Leben der Völker*, Berlin 1967.
15. "Zucker und Zuckeraustauschstoffe," in *Ernährungs-Umschau*, 4/1975, Frankfurt/M.
16. Rudolf Steiner, *Geisteswissenschaftliche Gesichtspunkte zur Therapie*, Dornach 1963 (GA 313).
17. Bircher-Benner, *Handbuch für Diabetiker*, Zürich 1967.
18. Rudolf Steiner, *Geisteswissenschaftlich Grundlagen zum Gedeihen der Landwirtshcaft*, Dornach 1979 (GA 327). English translation, *Agriculture*, London 1977.

19. Rudolf Steiner, *Allgemeine Menschenkunde als Grundlage der Pädagogik*, Dornach 1980 (GA 293). English translation, *Study of Man*, London 1975.
20. H. Mohler, *Sinn und Unsinn unserer Ernährung*, 1972.
21. Rudolf Steiner, *Physiologisch-Therapeutisches auf Grundlage der Geisteswissenschaft*, Dornach 1975 (GA 314). Reference is here made to a lecture given 9 October 1920.
22. G. v.Bunge, *Der wachsende Zuckerkonsum und seine Gefahren*, 1904.
23. A. Katase, "Der Einfluss der Ernährung auf die Konstitution des Organismus," quoted from M.O. Bruker, *Der Zucker als pathogenetischer Faktor*, Bad Homburg 1962.
24. Stepp/Kühnau/Schröder, *Die Vitamine und ihre klinische Anwendung*, Stuttgart 1952.
25. Stepp, "Zucker als Vitamin B Räuber," in *Med. Klinik*, Vol. 51, 17/1956.
26. H.R. Mühlemann, "Zucker und Süss-Stoffe," given at a "Symposium für Entwicklungstendenzen in der Ernährung," Zürich 29 March 1973.
27. Ad. Roos, *Kulturzerfall und Zahnverderbnis*, Bern 1962.
28. A. Fleisch, *Ernährungsprobleme in Mangelzeiten*, Basel 1947.
29. G. Schmidt, *Das Geistige Vermächtnis von Gustav v.Bunge* Zürich, 1973.
30. Rudolf Steiner, *Das Karma des Berufes des Menschen in Anknüpfung an Goethes Leben*, Dornach 1980 (GA 172). English translation, *The Karma of Human Vocation*, New York 1944. Reference is here made to the ninth lecture, given 26 November 1916.
31. Rudolf Steiner, "Ueber das Wesen der Bienen," published in *Mensch und Welt. Das Wirken des Geistes in der Natur. Ueber das Wesen der Bienen*, Dornach 1978 (GA 351). English translation, *Nine Lectures on Bees*, Spring Valley 1975.
32. B. F. Beck/D. Smedley, *Honey Your Health*, New York 1971.
33. W. Chr. Simonis, *Milch und Honig*, Stuttgart 1965.
34. Rudolf Steiner, Lecture given in Munich, 8 January 1909 under the title, "Ernährungsfragen im Lichte der Geisteswissenschaft".
35. Rudolf Steiner, Lecture given in Stuttgart, 28 October 1922 to an audience of physicians, published in *Physiologisch-Therapeutisches auf Grundlage der Geisteswissenschaft*, Dornach 1975 (GA 314).
36. Rudolf Steiner, *Der Mensch als Zusammenklang des schaffenden, bildenden und gestaltenden Weltenwortes*, Dornach 1978 (GA 230). English translation, *Man as Symphony of the Creative Word*, London 1979.

The publication dates mentioned refer to the latest editions available in German and English.

Chapter V

The Mineral World in Nutrition: Spirit Activity in Earthly Matter

Introductory Considerations

The discovery of minerals in foodstuffs did not occur until the last century. If, for example, we open a book on human physiology written by R. Tigerstedt in 1897[1], we find "inorganic nutrients" dealt with in less than two pages. Tigerstedt does indeed assert that "the mineral components of nutrition are just as important for the preservation of the body as are the organic nutrients," but aside from table salt he doesn't mention any minerals in particular. In a discussion on the theory of metabolism, he puts forward the assumption that, in order to fulfill its task, "the tissue fluid needs a certain ash component." Aside from these interesting indications, he does not mention minerals at all.

In G. von Bunge's comprehensive *Human Physiology*[2], however, the "inorganic nutrients" are presented to a much greater extent. Bunge proceeded from his own analysis of milk. He names seven mineral substances — K, Na, Ca, Mg, Fe, P and Cl — which he found and measured in mother's milk. He compares this analysis to a series of analyses of other foodstuffs — honey, wheat, potatoes, beef, egg yolks, etc. — in an attempt to investigate whether or not these minerals, which are indispensible for the infant, are contained in the same amounts as in mother's milk. Thus, the spectrum of mineral substances is here broadened, and specific questions are possible.

205

Nonetheless, his treatment of this subject is modest. When we compare it to a presentation developed out of modern nutritional theory, we can easily see how much progress has been made in this field. In K. Lang's book on the biochemistry of nutrition, written in 1974[3], the chapter on water and minerals covers nearly seventy-five pages. In addition, in order to do justice to the current state of research, he includes another fifty pages on trace elements. We mention this only to point out the scope of mineral research today. This breadth of knowledge is an indication of the significance accorded to mineral substances in nutrition today.

Of course nineteenth century scientists came to this knowledge by means of the analysis and dissection of living tissue. As a result, this research created a great obstacle to the understanding of reality — an obstacle which has been only partly overcome today. The character and nature of mineral substances could not be discovered in this way. Thus, the true significance of these substances for our nutrition remains hidden.

Strange as it might at first seem, it remained for spiritual science to discover this significance. We shall see that Rudolf Steiner actually discovered the significance of minerals and that he became the founder of a realistic mineral research which includes research into nutrition.

In order to do justice to our theme, we must necessarily take full notice of results of spiritual-scientific research. We shall, of course, have to stay within certain limits, and my presentation here will not be a handbook. I shall proceed, however, from some of the information given in *The Dynamics of Nutrition* which should make an understanding of this theme somewhat easier. At the same time, one sees a change in modern bio-chemical research which moves closer to our viewpoint.

The Necessity of a Dynamic Approach to Modern Mineral Research

The classical nutritional theory of the nineteenth century used, as the basis of its research, the caloric values of the nutrients it discovered. When faced with minerals, it no longer had this support. How could it judge and evaluate these substances without the apparently indispensible foundation of its entire method?

206

To express this dilemma — as well as to obtain a view of new perspectives in the conception of nutrition in general — we may look at such statements as the following. In the book by H.D. Cremer on minerals as components of nutrition (Basel, 1953)[4], we read: "In recent years, nutritional research has, in general, increasingly abandoned the static conception in favor of a dynamic conception. It was held to be less important to determine what food consists of than how it works on the organism. The utilization of all substances and their effect on the organism are dependent upon the relationship of the substances to one another: on the one hand, of the minerals to each other, and on the other hand, of their relationship to the type and amount of primary nutrients."

In fact, this mode of conception had already been established by Rudolf Steiner in the 1920's. He said, for example, "that the main thing is not an ordering according to weight in the metabolism. Rather, it is a question of whether we can take in the vitality of the forces in our food in the right way."[5] This research method not only fulfills Cremer's criterion, but it also goes beyond it to establish a true "dynamics of nutrition." Thus we see that we cannot understand the role of minerals in nutrition unless we adopt a method which has been recognized as essential for nutritional research in general. It is significant that it is precisely the mineral metabolism — apparently an inorganic process — which can, in reality, be comprehended only with such a mode of consideration. We shall also consider the actual formative forces, within which the mineral appears as an expression of the world of substance.

We must make a special attempt to grasp the mineral, specifically, in its becoming, in its process of formation. What appears today as mineral substance is, in reality, an end product — an excretion out of the life processes of the organic world. The truth is just the opposite of what materialistically oriented natural research assumes. The mineral was the last thing to appear in evolution, as something dead which was separated from the living. Just as coal originated in living plants, so is the entire mineral realm the result of a hardening of the plant kingdom. In an earlier condition of earth evolution, the plant world could exist without the mineral kingdom. What today appears as mineral substance was at that time still part of the life processes of plants.

We see this condition represented in living substance today, when we look at protein — the building material of the living — which is filled with a mineral composition. There is no living protein without a mineral composition, and this fact is significant for our considerations. Indeed, modern research has established that, without the symbiosis of protein and minerals, protein loses its living formative force. G.A. Schmid[6] points to this fact, in his book, *Sound Nutrition and Health,* when he writes that "proteins without mineral content — i.e. chemically pure proteins — are known only in a dead condition."

The mineral composition typical for protein contains sulfur, in addition to the seven elements mentioned above, as a characteristic substance. We pointed this out in our chapter on protein.

Rudolf Steiner described the developmental process of this mineral-plant creation in a wonderful way, also giving the exact point in time when this development took place. This was during the early Lemurian epoch — a time which is also of special significance for the evolution of man.[7] At this early stage in the development of the earth, man did not have any mineral substance in him. That which later condensed into his skeleton and that which permeates the blood and tissues as a human element were, at that time, not pervaded by death processes, but rather were filled with pure life processes. Only when the mineral kingdom was formed — when the solid, mineral earth as such came about — did man, as a physical being, incorporate mineral substance into himself. In this way, he actually became an earthly being. "Our earth progressed to the formation of the mineral kingdom. And with this, man at the same time took in the mineral realm."[8] This statement by Rudolf Steiner can lead us to the understanding of a basic relationship between man and the mineral kingdom. Because man incorporated the dead mineral into himself, he became connected to this earthly element. "At the moment when the mineral kingdom formed itself, man entered into his first incarnation. The mineral element developed through long periods of time. And since that time, we go through our earth embodiment. Previously, we were substantively different beings." The progress of earth evolution to the point where the mineral kingdom was formed not only brought about an essential restructuring of human corporeality; an important change in nutritional conditions must also have occurred. Both the plant and animal king-

208

doms had acquired the capacity to fit their living protein into the mineral element. This means that they became capable of living under different conditions. Man had to attain the strength to deal with this mineral element in his nutrition — to work it into his own organization; hence, the necessity of death entered into the human being, as well as the power to overcome this element of death — i.e. the power of rebirth. In addition, man began to deal with the mineral as such, and to overcome dead earthly matter — albeit only to a small degree, even today — by taking in table salt.

To do this, however, man needed a new organ — a higher force — than he had been able to take into his organism until that time. We call this force our "I" or Ego. It is able to take hold of our bodily nature. "For this reason, the Ego could go through the first incarnation there, where the mineral element had formed itself."

We have looked at this fact from other points of view in *The Dynamics of Nutrition*. We turn to it here in order to understand the nature of the mineral world as such, as well as its relationship to man through his processes of nutrition.

The present-day human organization is dependent upon the direct intake of mineral substance. Table salt — more aptly called rock salt — serves this purpose. Among other reasons, this is because this chemical substance has a definite effect within man. It has a unique taste which plays a special role in our experience, and it has become a "seasoning" for food. At the same time, however, it is water-soluble, so that even on the tongue its mineral-formative processes can be reversed. Thus, rock salt can be overcome by man, and when this occurs, the mineralization process within man is worked against. Man, who has descended to the earth, thereby combats becoming earthly by means of his Ego-organization. If he did not do so, he would harden into a pillar of salt — he would become completely sclerotic. As is well known, however, this process of overcoming the earthly has definite limits. An oversalting of food — as is common today — brings on pathological conditions.

Apart from his use of rock salt, man today is dependent on the ability of plants to absorb minerals. Since the plant learned to root itself in the earth, its organization not only developed these organs for the earth, whereby the roots themselves are enriched, but also the flow of sap in the plant dissolves the minerals in a fluid element and carries them to the entire plant organization. In this way, they are connected to the proteins and also accompany the other nutrients. The root itself, as the salt pole, is associated with that organization in man which is itself most mineralized and which opposes the process of mineralization. This is the head, the nerve-sense organization. This explains why rock salt is indispensible for the forming of thoughts, as Rudolf Steiner often pointed out. The reader is reminded here of our study of the carrot in *The Dynamics of Nutrition*.

The Crystallization Capacity of Minerals

A general discussion of minerals brings us to yet another problem. Among the most salient characteristics of these substances is their ability to crystallize, i.e. to construct and enter into specific forms. The mineral world — at least in its foremost representatives — thereby possesses a quality which sets it apart from the other kingdoms of nature. Minerals have two forms in which they appear. On the one hand, they can be amorphous — that is, without form. On the other hand, under certain conditions each mineral takes on a typical form. Whether the transparent columns of quartz (a silicon compound) or the bundles of rays of antimonite, or the round forms of bloodstone — the peculiarities of the individual types of minerals are always revealed in their crystals.

We find this crystallization capacity in living beings in a variety of ways. Consider the iron crystal, which appears in the erythrocyte — the red blood corpuscle — and also in the so-called "brain sand", deposited in the pineal gland, which is chemically a crystalline form of calcium carbonate ($CaCo^3$). These are only a few examples of how man is permeated by the crystal-forming forces which he evidently needs.

Thus the question arises: what does this crystal-forming force express? What force gives rise to these crystalline formations? Rudolf Steiner gave a new approach to this subject in his book *Theosophy*[9]. When we look at a crystal formation, we may experience how the ability to crystallize reveals a higher formative force than is found in amorphous substances. If we then conjecture that the crystal brings the mineral a step closer to the plant kingdom, we find our assumption confirmed by spiritual-scientific research. In fact, with the formation of crystals, amorphous rock is taken hold of by a formative force which, at a higher level, penetrates the plant as an "etheric body". It there lives in the variety of forms of the plant world. To the extent that the human organization also displays such crystal formations, we may assume that these also bear witness to a living organism of formative forces. We might also put it this way: the human organism cannot tolerate a purely mineral structure of an amorphous sort which has entirely fallen out of the life organization within it. The organism must constantly dissolve these crystals and thus bring them into the stream of its life. Only out of this stream can it then form its own crystals. If the organism cannot do this sufficiently, these crystals form deposits which are symptoms of a weakening of the Ego-organization. We see this, for example, in the formation of various "stones" and also in uric acid crystals; these are pathological within the life conditions of the human organism.

One might also say: the formation of crystals bears witness to the organization of formative forces which even the mineral cannot do without, although they merely put their stamp on the mineral from outside. One such formative force is seen in the spiralling tendency of the plant, as discovered and described by Goethe. Significantly, such a spiralling tendency has recently been discovered in the formation of quartz crystals.

The Character of Minerals

In the formation of minerals and their ability to crystallize, we have a property of this lowest kingdom of nature which we have already touched upon. We said that the mineral was released from the higher realms of life — beginning with the plant kingdom — in the course of evolution. Thereby, it did without an independent life of its own, such as the plant has by virtue of its body of formative forces. It also did without higher forces which are expressed as capabilities of the soul and spirit. Up until the middle ages, one described this characteristic of minerals by saying: they have become "selfless". For this reason, one looked at the crystals with reverence. One had the feeling that these minerals had become entirely earthly. They had given up all higher qualities: life, soul and spirit, as well as light and warmth of their own.

For just this reason they have made possible an important — even decisive — step forward in evolution. By creating their own (mineral) kingdom, they have helped other beings — especially man — to a higher stage of evolution. We have already spoken of how the highest member of man's organization, his Ego, could incarnate because of the minerals; this has blazed a new path in world evolution.

The plant, which learned to take root in the earth, could then say: "I owe my present, higher form of existence to this lower kingdom." Man himself ought to look into the world and say to himself: "I, too, have reached this evolutionary stage — and can reach it daily anew — only because lower forms, who do without it, exist beneath me."

We already mentioned that there lived in this conception an older wisdom which we can again enliven by means of new knowledge. The poet, Christian Morgenstern, gave artistic expression to such a view in his poem "The Washing of the Feet."[10]

In looking at human nutrition, we come to the insight that the mastery of the mineral world represents a decisively important step toward allowing the Ego-organization to take part in it. The mineral challenges us every day to call forth this highest power in order for us to take part in earth evolution. At the same time, however, it challenges us to overcome the earthly forces and to learn how to rule them. Rudolf Steiner's statement regarding medicaments taken from the mineral world is applicable here: "It does honor to man to say that he also takes part in this raging battle, fought in the terrestrial environment, against the mineralization of the earth."[11]

We here meet some ideas presented from another point of view in *The Dynamics of Nutrition*. Even sugar, to the extent that it is mineralized, belongs to the mineral kingdom. In the previously mentioned medical lectures, Rudolf Steiner speaks of how it is necessary that man fight against the hardening forces within him. On the one hand, man needs these forces in order to be an earthly being, since they are formative forces — e.g. of the skeleton and brain — and also awaken the consciousness. On the other hand, they would make him sclerotic if he could not impress on them the stamp of his own individuality.

In this way, the threefold human organization is brought into the process of becoming human. The "becoming mineral" of man, which is the same as the tendency to become sclerotic, is concentrated in the head, but fills out the entire man from here. This "germ of mineralization of the whole man" must be constantly combatted. On the one hand, this ability comes from the opposite tendency of the metabolic pole. In contrast to the "salt process" of the human head, ancient medicine characterized this pole as the "sulfur process". On the other hand, however, a constant process of overcoming the "sclerotic" element must proceed from the nerve-sense pole itself. Just here, the actual element of human formation — the Ego-organization — is at work. We shall see later how this is at work in, for example, the lead process in man.

In this connection, Rudolf Steiner pointed to an important fact which can lead to an understanding of the activity of minerals in plant foods. It is known that various minerals can be found in all plants as so-called trace elements. Today, these are considered to be in living organisms in quantities of less than .005% micron. Their distribution in the plant — and in man — is so thin that one may speak here of a homeopathic process. Biochemical research therefore finds it difficult to determine the necessity for these trace elements. "Thus, it is unknown today — or at least not conclusively demonstrated — whether or not they fulfill a physiological function in the organism."[3] Rudolf Steiner, however, emphasized an entirely different aspect of the subject. To begin with, he developed an understanding of the efficacy of minerals as remedies and spoke specifically of a counter-process called forth by homeopathic potentization, i.e. the fine distribution of the mineral substance. This happens in order "to support everything which must be supported in the battle of man against the mineralizing tendency, against generally becoming sclerotic." In the plant, the mineral is freed from its condensed form and from the gravitational tendencies of the earth. It is raised by the plant toward an upward tendency and a process of lightness. It is thereby dispersed, homeopathically potentized and driven into a fine distribution. Thus it is "precisely in the mineral kingdom that those forces are laid bare which are opposed to the activity of the external mineral kingdom." With trace elements, especially, we support the forces which call us to the battle against mineralization. In other words: through the trace elements contained in our food (e.g. the precious metals in whole grains), we

213

appeal in a definite way to the region from whence the minerals came, the region of cosmic forces.

Modern spiritual research has emphasized with particular clarity the origin of minerals in the cosmic forces. The ancient mystery knowledge — as taught, for example, by Pythagoras — appeared in a less defined form in a personality like Paracelsus, who learned to understand the "language of metals" within the earth. According to Rudolf Steiner, this language, "which can only be perceived with spiritual hearing . . . recounts the memories of the earth, the things which the earth has gone through in the phases of Saturn, Sun, Moon, etc."[7] — that is, in its cosmic development. This is true not only of the coarser minerals like iron, magnesium, calcium, potassium, and sodium, but also for those mineral substances "which, to crude outer observation, appear not to play any role in the human organism." For these are not only confined to the weight of the depths of the earth, but they are also found "in a super-homeopathic concentration all over the earth's environment", in the atmosphere.

At this point, Rudolf Steiner specifically mentions lead as an example. Lead penetrates us not only through the air we breathe, but also "through food, where it appears in an infinitely minute concentration."

Here we have the bridge to the mineral content of our plant food, and from here we can gain new insight into its significance for man. By means of its mineral content, plant food makes a great contribution toward overcoming the necessary "process of becoming sclerotic" in man; it calls upon man's Ego-organization to make effective the original cosmic forces of the minerals with the help of the minerals themselves. Here again we come to the connection between the earthly and cosmic nutrition of man, as discussed in detail in *The Dynamics of Nutrition*. And we are also led back to Steiner's words, already quoted: "It does honor to man to say that he also takes part in this raging battle, fought in the terrestrial environment, against the mineralization of the earth."[1] For our considerations here, this is primarily true of the role played by table salt. Keeping in mind what we said about trace elements, we can say that man here participates, in his own being, in this "overcoming" [de-salting] process, a process in which the plant has eliminated one step since it has already incorporated the mineral into its own growth.

214

"What, then, does this Ego-organization have a special relationship to? This Ego-organization has a special relationship to the mineral in man. When you take in something mineral — e.g. by putting salt on your tongue — it is the Ego-organization which sets to work on this mineral. The salt moves on; it goes through all sorts of changes, goes through the intestines and further: but your salt is never abandoned by your Ego-organization."[12]

And what dissolves the salt on the tongue? The warmth which comes to it in the mouth. The saliva in which the salt dissolves is almost at the temperature of blood. The Ego-organization lives in this vital warmth. The warmth is the instrument of the Ego-organization whereby, during every moment of our lives, it holds the balance between hardening and sclerosis on the one hand and dissolution and inflammation on the other. Only in this way can we be truly human, not only in body but also in soul and spirit. And the mineral is the means whereby the Ego accomplishes this regulation. It needs the opposing force of the earthbound mineral in order to constantly practice overcoming it. But the Ego would not be able to do this if the mineral itself did not have a connection to the cosmos. This mineral has expelled the cosmic entities of light, warmth and life out of itself, but it is not resting; it is in constant motion between the earth and the cosmos, renewing itself and becoming younger in constant contact with the "world Ego" and the "womb of the world." This is the power of the Phoenix, as it appears in mythology; it is peculiar to the mineral and to the human Ego, which can therefore be seen as related.

We can thus understand that the Ego — because it takes in minerals — not only has to dissolve them in the digestive tract, but also has to permeate them with warmth, even to raise them up to the level of warmth itself. "When you eat a grain of table salt, this salt must be taken up by your own individual warmth. Everything mineral must be transformed into warmth-ether."[13] Otherwise, a person becomes ill. Only with this transformation can we say that the mineral has actually been taken up by the human organization. It can then take part in the various organic functions and can be condensed again, into the skeleton or an iron crystal in a red blood corpuscle.

Even those minerals which we take in with plant foods — the iron in spinach, the silicon and also flourine in grain, the calcium in milk, etc. — must take the path through warmth. This path is made easier and more accesible, however, when the plant has already taken the mineral a few steps further and has enlivened the mineral. If we had to take all the minerals we need directly from the inorganic world, the strength of our Ego would soon be exhausted. The edible plants help us to accomplish this important process toward becoming human because they take on part of our task. Thus, inorganic minerals — except table salt — serve primarily as medicaments. As such, they can be brought within our power to overcome them by means of potentization. When taken as food, the plant "potentizes" the minerals for us. Today, for example, by means of spectral analysis, all precious metals — i.e. not only iron but also gold, silver, etc. — have been found in grain. Thus wholegrain bread stimulates the human Ego-forces relative to the highest, most noble minerals which are to be found between the earth and the cosmos. Minerals thus provide the most extensive stimulation of the highest human activity — that of the Ego-organization.

Perhaps this is why insight into and knowledge of "mineral metabolism" could first be spoken of by modern spiritual research. In fact, it was only afterwards that modern natural science — unaware of the pioneering work of Rudolf Steiner — became aware of the role of minerals in human nutrition.

The Most Important Minerals in Human Nutrition

We have already named the primary minerals in human nutrition. Above all, there are eight with a special connection to protein: sodium, potassium, calcium, magnesium, iron, phosphorus, sulfur and chlorine. In addition there are the important trace elements: silicon, copper, lead and flourine. In this chapter we shall deal with all those which have not been dealt with already, or which have been discussed only in a limited way.

Many important functions related to the entire human organism are connected to the activity of minerals. Potassium and sodium are the indispensible substances which regulate the "water economy" and also the balance of acids and bases. Calcium is a key to the entire inner metabolism. Silicon appears as a ruling element in another way, and we may also speak of iron, a central element for man, in conjunction with copper. I have already described the special role of phoshorus in *The Dynamics of Nutrition,* and spiritual-scientific research has shed the light of knowledge upon magnesium and flourine. We have looked into the significance of sulfur in connection with protein. The problem of table salt was discussed — in my earlier book, as well as in the previous section of this chapter. The extent to which the entire mineral metabolism takes a significant part in warmth regulation was also dealt with in *The Dynamics of Nutrition.*

Water — The Indispensible Bodily Fluid

In the course of our studies, we have already clearly seen that — with the exception of table salt, where we accomplish the "pushing back of the earthly formative process" as soon as we dissolve salt in the mouth — mineral substances in our food appear in connection with living protein processes or are dissolved in the cellular fluid or in the extracellular "tissue fluids". Here not only the "homeopathic process," but also the fluid element as such, plays an essential role. In this regard, all bodily fluids are "mineral water," related to the water in the mineral springs of the earth. We are here led to the *significance and nature of the element of water* as such, and we shall have to deal with this subject. K. Lang also begins his discussion of minerals with a description of the functions of water. Recent research has had especially important results in this field, results which help to clarify both the potential and the limits of modern scientific methods. Before entering into this subject, however, let us try to approach the watery element from another direction.

As late as 1863, M.J. Schleiden characterized water as follows: "Since ancient times, the word water referred less to the chemical substance than to the state of fluidity ... without water, no life, no organism, would be conceivable. Can it be otherwise regarding the great organism which we call the earth?"[14] Schleiden was a botanist, still living in the shadow of the epoch of Goethe. In his book, *The Plant and its Life,* he attempted — in the manner of Goethe, whose "classical objectivity and flexibility of perception" he praises — to develop an "aesthetic of the plant worlds." He admits that "we in no way as yet have this teaching", i.e. the description of "the plant world as an hieroglyph

217

of the eternal" whereby "in the earthly form we look for and find indications of a super-earthly existence."

Schleiden — along with Schwann — is credited with discovering the cellular structure of plants. Schwann said clearly that the basis of cell formation is the blastema — a fluid formation out of which the actual cell is hardened. Schleiden expressed it more abstractly with the term "archetypal cell."

Rudolf Steiner pointed out that, around the middle of the 19th century, the basis of the plant was thought to be a "fluid element" out of which, "by means of a differentiation, the cells arose."[11] The cell was depicted as an organism "originating from a fluid being with the power of differentiation." In such views, there lived the remnants of an insight which saw the Archaeus — in the sense of Paracelsus — as "the basis for the activity of the organism's fluids." Today we speak of the etheric organism "which is essentially comprised of forces which work out from the cosmic periphery."

Goethe still worked out of such apprehensions when he put the words of the Greek philosopher Thales into the mouth of his Faust:[15]

Alles ist aus dem Wasser entsprungen
Alles wird von dem Wasser erhalten!
Ozean, goenn' uns dein ewiges Walten . . .
Du bist's, *der das* frischeste Leben erhaelt.

Everything arose from water,
Everything is contained in water!
Ocean, grant us your eternal power . . .
It is you who holds the freshest life.

Greek mythology depicts "Oceanos" as a divinity, a son of heaven and earth living in a state of constant change and indomindomitable fertility. One of his sons is Proteus, whose powers of change were depicted by Goethe in his "Classical Walpurgis Night" in *Faust*. The archetype of protein, the primeval protein atmosphere, appears as eternally forming and transforming. It is closely related to the origin of the mineral. He who still understands how to read the myth in Goethe's work can come faintly to perceive the secret of the watery element: "And should the water unfold itself, so would it livingly form itself . . ."[16]

218

During the time that Schwann and Schleiden lived, this knowledge was increasingly lost. Water became an object of physical and chemical research, which defined anew its universal significance for all life-processes. The "inner-sea" in the organism was discovered, the sea "on whose shores all of our cells live" — "which in adults consists of about 15 liters of salt water, with a composition roughly analagous to that of sea water."[17] The American author George W. Gray[18] devoted a chapter in his book to "the sea in which we live". Not only every organ, but also every single one of the perhaps hundreds of trillions of living cells in our bodies, bathe in this life-fluid and depend on its uninterrupted flow and on the consistency of its composition. Rudolf Steiner often pointed to this important fact, but he went beyond the conclusions of modern physiology. As Steiner described it, we have this phenomenon of sitting, with our solid mineral body, in a bath of our own bodily fluids. Thus, the force of buoyancy is active here, as it is outside of our bodies. This is the so-called Archimedian principle, which states that a body in a liquid becomes lighter by the weight of the liquid it displaces. In reality we live in opposition to gravity. "In fact, we don't live in that which physics makes of us, but rather in that which is overcome in physics,"[11] said Rudolf Steiner. This applies to the entire physical body, as well as to each of its individual organs. "Every blood corpuscle swims, devoid of weight." Rudolf Steiner, of course, illuminated these facts from a spiritual-scientific viewpoint.

We can observe that the principle working against this physical gravity is not centrifugal, but is rather a centripetal, etheric, formative force. "In the face of genuine knowledge, it is childish to believe that, in everything at play here — the ocean, the water in rivers, rising mist, falling raindrops, cloud formations — there is only that which physicists and chemists know about water. This is childish in the face of real knowledge. For at work in everything out there — in the powerful drops of the watery world, constantly rising as mist, forming clouds, descending as rain and fog, and everything else which water does on earth (water exerts a tremendous activity in the formation of geological structures) — in all this there work etheric streams . . ." This is especially significant for the brain. For "the brain swims in the cerebral fluid. Its weight is thus reduced from about 1500 g to only about 20 g . . . The etheric thus has a tremendous opportunity to work there . . .

219

The sum of the etheric forces which lift us from the earth can develop favorably in the cerebral fluid."[19] Moreover, the cerebral fluid is itself a "mineral water". That is to say, the typical mineral substances are dissolved in it, and thus raised into the sphere of etheric activity.

If we want to view the "fluid man" in his reality, we must see our body of formative forces active in and through him. This activity is at work in its movements, flow and circulation. It is also characteristic of these etheric formative forces that they live in rhythmic movements.

In order to form a correct picture of the activity of fluids in man, we must bear in mind that every organ and every tissue is filled with fluid. Even the hardest, most mineral formation — the enamel of the teeth — is 2.7% water. The skeleton is 44% water, the muscles 79% and brain 90%.[20] In fact, the human body is mostly organized liquids. Various minerals are dissolved throughout this fluid. For example, the muscles and the brain yield the following mineral spectra (related to their total substance, including the solid parts):

	Na	K	Ca	Mg	P	S
Muscles	0.072	0.360	0.007	0.023	0.220	0.250
Brain	0.17	0.33	0.012	0.016	0.38	0.13

One should consider that these figures relate to the organs of adults. Among children — as well as among fetuses — the relations are different, reflecting their much higher fluid content (e.g. a five-month fetus is about 91% water).

The rhythmical motion in this "fluid man" relates primarily to the so-called extra-cellular fluid, such as tissue fluid, brain fluid, etc. However, both the fluid within cells and that within particular organs are not at rest, but rather engaged in constant exchanges. For example, the liver is estimated to be 79% liquid, and constantly takes in and gives out fluids. The liver never remains substantially the same. It takes part in, and is indeed especially connected to, the total water economy of the organism, the dynamics of which have often been the object of physiological research.

Since the work of Claude Bernard, one has spoken of the "inner milieu" of this fluid organism, which displays an "unbelievable intensity of exchange . . . Every second, billions of water molecules and dissolved substances penetrate the walls of the capillaries and the membranes which surround each of our cells."[17] However, this interplay takes place according to strictly regulated laws. The aim of these laws is to keep the composition of the mineral portion of our "inner environment" constant. This is the necessary pre requisite for its functions, both for the activity of the "etheric streams" and for the "taking hold" by higher forces which serve to ensoul and enspirit the organism. "If this composition deviates even a little from the norm, the activity of all cells is seriously handicapped." The practical consequences for our nutrition are stated by J. Hamburger: "For example, the inner environment contains 200 mg potassium per liter. Too much or too little of this calcium is life-threatening, for the functioning of the heart muscles is then immediately affected. Now, the daily change in the type and amount of food eaten leads to a highly variable intake of potassium. Our bodily cells themselves, which contain more potassium than their surroundings, can, according to conditions, put out either very small or very large amounts of potassium. Every day, and in every person, the same potassium concentration remains stable, thereby acting as an effective regulatory system which avoids fluctuations. This regulatory system works so perfectly that it "leaves the observer amazed," for it apparently possesses "an infinitely more powerful, subtle, rigorous and efficacious organization than any other concentration of living beings."

What is at work in this grand and unsurpassable organization, this "regulatory system"? Here we come to the activity of the formative forces — the "etheric body" — the dynamics of which have been presented to us. In the words of Rudolf Steiner: "The essence of the organism is in its activity, not in its substances. The organization is not a relationship of matter, but rather an activity."[21] A substance which is not active must be excreted or else it has a pathological effect. An old saying here takes on new meaning: we eat ourselves sick, and digest ourselves to health.

In the example above, put forth by Hamburger, we have the idea that even the plant, which serves as our food, presents a living play of forces, expressed within a definite spectrum of mineral concentrations. Potassium, for example, is found primarily in plants. There are plants both rich and poor in potassium; the two extremes are represented by potatoes, over-rich in potassium, and rice, which is very low in potassium. We shall see later how this subject of potassium content presents a practical nutritional problem. First we must make clear what demands are put on the organization of formative forces — which regulates the constancy of the "inner environment" — by our eating these foods. We shall look at how not only too strenuous demands but also too little stimulation can arise from our daily food.

This regulation is expressed primarily in the so-called base and acid equilibrium, for potassium is one of the most important substances working in the alkaline realm. In recent years, this subject has often come under discussion, although not always in an appropriate way; the extended view offered by spiritual science is especially needed here.

Spiritual-Scientific Aspects

We have already mentioned the work of Snively and Sweeney.[22] Like all modern authors, they are quite generous in the dates they give for the evolution of man. Nonetheless, they point out that the salty fluid which surrounds our bodily cells is indeed an "ancient liquid." This amazing requirement for the development of the life-organization has been "preserved so well through time that in modern man both its composition and concentration are the same as when, in prehistoric times, life first appeared on dry land." "Sea water of a geological area in the far past is the phylogenetic ancestor of human extracellular fluid."

The authors also come to another interesting conclusion: "The exchange of water and dissolved substance with the surrounding fluids is an unceasing process of tremendous dimensions. This exchange is based on heretofore unknown physical or chemical processes. It is of no use to speculate about the nature of these ghost-pumps which begin their work months before we are born and continue it without pause until we die."

Could any clearer statement be made that in this case physical-chemical ideas fail, that the forces at work here are not physiochemical? The authors make an admirable admission: "Our knowledge of the composition of the basically different types of

222

bodily cells is, at best, sketchy . . . In fact, the working of these cells remains, as before, veiled in a mysterious darkness."

In this book, as well as in *The Dynamics of Nutrition,* we have often referred to the results of spiritual-scientific research into the evolution of the earth and of man. Rudolf Steiner describes how, in the earth's past, the human being was of much finer nature, consisting originally of an accumulation of warmth-air, progressing during the next stage of evolution to a form of watery substances which was condensed from the wider surroundings. The substances at that time were much finer than they are now. "Man swam around, so to speak, in an atmosphere filled up and permeated by thick water. He was a kind of water being — similar to those animals today which can hardly be discerned from the water."[23] His form was not fixed but constantly metamorphosing. He lived as a still unhardened being in an atmosphere "containing all the substances which today have become hard or liquid . . . all the metals and minerals."[24]

When, in a later evolutionary period, this "water-earth" solidified, man kept a remnant of it in the form of his bodily fluids. As we have seen, this remnant is still a true image of its origin, and it dominates the solid parts of the body. "Now, as the earth solidifies, it gradually becomes possible for the 'water man' to solidify his form and to take on a solid skeletal system." This was the time when the form of the earth itself "condensed more and more . . . and gradually the solid mineral core arose."[24] This phase, which represented an inwardization of the human being, was not only one in which man separated from his environment, but also the point at which he experienced the dawning of his individual existence. He could then encompass his own individual warmth by means of the power of the Ego which was bestowed on him. This made possible the rudiments of blood and of blood circulation, the "sea in which we live."

Only at this point can we say that matter actually reached the end of its process of development. The mineral form, as we know it today, was then complete. The matter which then appeared had, like the mineral we described at the beginning of this chapter, separated itself from its origin and became "selfless".

However, in another way, the mineral has remained connected to its higher origin. "The etheric body of the mineral surrounds and encases it from all sides." It can appear to us like an

223

echo of the mineral's evolution that even today it dissolves in the watery element, the bearer of the activity of the etheric forces.

We also find the higher members connected to the mineral element, although not in the physical world and therefore not accessible to physical observation. "When you observe a mineral clairvoyantly," however, "the following occurs: you see the physical body surrounded by the radiant light-figure of the etheric body; then you see the rays which separate more and more as they go into outer space . . . to the point where these rays unite; at that point you come to a place where, from all sides of the universe, the Egos of the minerals radiate towards us."[23]

It is only the physical body of the minerals that is here on earth. Their higher members are in the spiritual worlds, and we shall never understand the activity of the minerals until we take this other side of their existence into consideration. Their relationship to man — which is our first interest here — can only be understood if we bear in mind that, "in a certain sense, the situation of the minerals here on earth is exactly opposite to that of man. Man has his Ego within him, enclosed in his skin. Every person is a center for himself, a human center." This statement suggests the complete polarity — and therefore the affinity — between the minerals and the human Ego, which I have often tried to make clear; it also helps us to understand how, when we eat, "something spiritual flows into man."[23] In this way we can perhaps begin to sense why minerals in particular have such profound significance for human nutrition, and why they permeate all of our actual foodstuffs, thereby becoming our daily food.

We need to consider all of this before we turn again to that "process of tremendous dimensions" which reaches its peak in the acid base regulation of the organism.

The Human Fluid-Organism

According to modern calculations the fluids in the human body can be broken down as follows: the average adult human body is 45% by weight cellular fluid (i.e. fluids within cells). 15% moves freely as "extracellular fluid," consisting of both plasma and other fluids. The latter are primarily tissue fluids, but include cerebral/spinal fluid as well. Among the minerals dissolved in these fluids are five so-called alkaline-forming elements: sodium,

224

potassium, calcium, magnesium and iron. There are also three so-called acid-forming elements(phosphorus, sulfur and chlorine.)

Today, these dissolved substances are referred to as electrolytes, as they hold electrical charges in certain environments. One speaks of cationic electrolytes (cations) with a positive charge, and anions or negatively charged electrolytes. These properties, which are so important to the modern physical-chemical mode of analysis, have no essential significance for our presentation here.

All of these minerals are found in all the bodily fluids. Sodium, however, is found primarily in the extracellular fluids, and potassium primarily in the organs and cells.

All eight of these mineral substances are found in living protein. Protein is thus in a kind of equilibrium — it is amphoteric, i.e. it can appear either as a base or acid.

Phosphorus, sulfur and chlorine combine readily with the five metals to form so-called salts. Among these, sodium chloride (table salt) plays a special role, as we have already mentioned.

It is clear that table salt plays the most important role in the bodily fluids. It must always be present as a 0.9% solution in order for life to exist. In contrast, sea water has a 3% concentration of table salt, which is much higher. In man, we are dealing with a "fresh water stream" comparable, in its relationship to sea water, to the rivers and lakes of the earth. Rudolf Steiner made some important remarks concerning this relationship in one of his lectures to workers. Salt, and especially table salt, penetrates the solid earth from the ocean. At the same time, these salts bring the actual earth forces to the ground. So-called fresh water has a more cosmic orientation. In springs, especially, minerals are found in homeopathic concentrations. They thus exercise their curative power, as we can see with regard to the various curative mineral waters. "When you go by a spring and the wonderful, pure water pours forth . . . . that also refreshes the entire earth. The earth is there opened, as through eyes and sense organs, to cosmic space." Rudolf Steiner also spoke of the healing effect of water in his first medical course, in 1920.[11] For our present considerations, it is significant to realize that the bodily fluids, which today appear as "fresh water," have a two fold activity. On the one hand, we need their salty element, so that we may become earthly beings. Salt forms and preserves our bones and muscles.

225

It bestows earthly power upon us. On the other hand, the fresh-water character of our organism mediates the other pole of our nature, which is cosmically oriented, consisting of "both reproductive and spiritual forces, as well as those forces which bestow common sense."

In this connection, Rudolf Steiner brings forth an instructive example. "If milk contains too little salt, [the child] will get rickets." On the other hand: if a person gets too much salt he becomes too much of an "ocean," i.e. he becomes too salty, too earthbound and heavy. It thus follows that "there must always be a balance in man between salt intake and the intake of substances contained in the other foodstuffs."[25] This statement points to a new aspect of salt consumption. We have already spoken of the dangers of overconsumption.

Rudolf Steiner continues by pointing to plant foods and their two poles: the salt pole in the root and the phosphorus pole in the flower. The latter — of course in homeopathic concentration — appears in the flower pole and represents the cosmic light-forces which are necessary to enkindle the power of human thinking. "No thoughts without phosphorus," as Moleschott put it.

As we become aware of these relationships, the value of root and flower/fruit foods — and also of table salt — can again become clear to us. "So, we can say: for those organs in our human bodies which to a certain extent contain the fresh-water stream, we need light. For the muscles and bone, for that which should be salty, we need salt and the solid ingredients of our food. And between the two, there must be the proper balance."

It is important to note here that table salt is found not only in the blood and bodily fluids, but also in the various connective tissue substances such as fibers, cartilage and tendons, as well as in the skin. Diseased joints, cartilage muscles and connective tissue are, as a rule, overloaded with table salt. They thus have a tendency to hold water and to become inflamed. We have already mentioned kidney damage and the circulatory and heart diseases — so prevalent today — which result from too much table salt. All too often we see this destructive cycle: overconsumption of table salt — kidney damage — thirst — liver damage. A lacto-vegetarian diet can prevent and work against this vicious cycle.

The Sphere of Activity of Potassium

Along with sodium — and its salt form, as sodium chloride — potassium plays a large role in human mineral metabolism. In contrast to sodium, we find it primarily in the cell fluids, the organs, the muscles, the liver, the brain and the heart. Potassium has thus been called the "leading actor in cellular activity." We observe it in cell activity working in conjunction with protein; it is necessary for the organic processes of growth and regeneration. "When new tissue is to be formed, along with protein there must also be sufficient quantities of potassium in the diet."[22] Here we can point to the wealth of potassium in vegetables and fruits, thus seeing their significance for human nutrition — especially as regards the compounds of protein and potassium — in a new light.

Whereas sodium appears in the all-important "sea salt", potassium plays a special role in the solid earth and is thus important for plant fertilization. Potassium is the most important mediator between the mineral kingdom and plant roots. (F. Julius)

In spite of its indispensibility in the nutrition of man and animals, sodium is unimportant to the plant — although it does contain NaCl. In potassium, however, we find a quality which belongs especially to the plant element. This points to the fact that, by means of potassium, it is primarily the etheric formative forces which are at work. Sodium, on the other hand, stands in the service of the higher forces, of the soul-spiritual organization. Moreover, table salt (NaCl) is the only salt which man and the animals can assimilate in its pure mineral form. In contrast, a corresponding potassium salt acts as a poison, i.e. man cannot overcome potassium as he can sodium. The difference between the plant and the human/animal organization thus becomes clear. Of course, we must take other factors into consideration here. Although potassium is indispensible for plant life, it nonetheless poses a great riddle to researchers, both regarding its being taken in from the ground and its activity within the plant.

It has been known for some time now that the intake of so-called nutrients from the ground is by no means a passive absorption on the part of the plant — just as we also cannot speak of passive absorption in human beings. Here again, the physical-chemical processes are not the major factor. Rather, the intake of such substances takes place "only with the active cooperation of the living substance."[26] As one would expect, this confirms that here, too, the metabolic processes represent the direct activity of the etheric formative forces. An awareness gleaned from spiritual research applies to the plant as well as to man: "The organism is an activity, not an aggregation of substances."

It is interesting that plant nutrition is based upon imbalances which are, indeed, an expression of this activity. The plant cannot take any substance from the ground unless the root has at its disposal the oxygen necessary for breathing. This applies even to the intake of water. Such plant activities call forth "imbalances"—i.e. a chemical-energy tension. Hence, A. Frey-Wyssling can say: "Life consists of the constant disturbance of balance and the constant maintenance of imbalances." In spite of all the research in this field, natural-scientific methods have proven inadequate here: "How the plant alters the balance in the ground or nutrient solution to its benefit remains a mystery," according to Frey-Wyssling.

One significant fact, however, has been disclosed. It has clearly been shown that, even for plants, a pure, isolated solution of potassium, magnesium, calcium or the like is useless — indeed, even poisonous. By simply mixing two salts together, however, such a solution is no longer poisonous. For the living organism, it is always a question of the composition of the substances, not of the elements as such. The law applies to plants as well as to animals and man. Though isolated substances have a poisonous, destructive effect on the life system, in "balanced solutions" they become starting points for the development of life forces. In this regard, sea water, spring water, plant saps and human bodily fluids are all "balanced solutions," a fact which points us to the evolutionary principle that all living things have proceeded from the same creative source.

It should be mentioned here that these facts are especially important for plant fertilization. Turning again to Frey-Wyssling[26]: "The best fertilizer is animal manure." It contains significant quantities of nitrogen, phosphorus and potash. It is itself an organic composition of substances necessary to stimulate and develop the life forces of the plant.

These phenomena are also of great significance for human

nutrition, but we shall never grasp them in a realistic way without the extended research methods developed through spiritual science. The insights contained in Rudolf Steiner's agricultural lectures[5], for example, have shown themselves to be indispensable for our understanding of this subject.

Regarding our theme — water and minerals — we are pointed, in the second agricultural lecture, to the fact that these substances experience a kind of deadening in the ground. "In the earth, they become even more dead than they are outside." But for this very reason, mineral substances become "capable of being exposed to the most distant cosmic forces." This emancipation from the earth forces is strongest in the northern latitudes during the middle of winter. It brings forth "the greatest crystal-forming force." In this way, these minerals come under the influence of cosmic forces — the forces of their true origin and their spiritual home.

The Problem of Potassium Fertilization

In order for plants to thrive, to be filled with nutritional quality, this opening of the mineral in the ground to the cosmos, this interplay between earth and cosmos, must be promoted and activated; hence, the proper fertilizer is necessary. That is to say, the soil must be so enlivened that it is capable of "allowing to radiate in, out of the cosmic periphery, what the plants need." The introduction of mineral fertilizer is not necessary here. Rather, "it is a question of adding living forces to the fertilizer." For "even if we gradually built up a soil which was rich in this or that substance, it would not help the plant growth, unless — through fertilization — we could give to the plant the capacity to take what is in the soil into its own body." Here, too, the primary thing is the "dynamics." Even modern research points to this fact.

The plant is able to bring forth an interplay between inorganic forces and living protein. It builds up a protein which furthers the presence of the previously mentioned minerals, including potassium or potassium salts. This potassium content must be "worked on in such a way, in the interaction between earth and plant, that within the organic process it relates in the proper way to that which makes up the actual body — the protein — of the plant." This can be done with the help of the process described

229

in Steiner's agricultural lectures, where we learn that yarrow, with its "very homeopathic sulfur content, can be combined with potassium in an ideal way."[5]

Modern plant physiology reports that potassium is related to protein formation in the plant. A potassium deficiency disrupts the synthesis of protein. "With an adequate supply of potassium, the entire protein metabolism is disrupted."[27] Moreover, potassium has been related to an increase in the plant's assimilatory capacity as well as an increase in cellulose formation. The latter especially affects the ability of the grains to stand upright. It also affects the cellulose hulls of the seeds and their penetration by trace elements. The activity of potassium is related to the enzyme activity of the plant. This fact, in turn, is related to potassium's connection to the protein metabolism.

It is characteristic of potassium's activity, which is directed toward the life processes of protein, that there is more potassium in young leaves than in old. Grain, at the time when the ears are formed, has four to five times more potassium than when it is ripe. Calcium, on the other hand, is especially plentiful in older leaves.

Two potassium "specialists" in the plant world which are significant for human nutrition still need to be mentioned. They are the potato and the birch tree. We might ask what these two plants — so different from each other — have in common with regard to the potassium process?

Potassium Specialists in the Plant World: Potato, Rice and Birch

Let us first look at the potato. We mentioned it briefly in *The Dynamics of Nutrition,* pointing out that it is difficult to digest and that its starch structure is a great burden for the activity of the brain. In addition, its extremely high potassium content is well-known. Potassium makes up about 3/5 of the total ash content which Schneider reports to be 667 mg/% K_2O, as compared to tomatoes (297 mg/%), green lettuce (218 mg/%), celery (321 mg/%), and cauliflower (32.8 mg/%).

All these values are less than half of that of potatoes. The potassium content of fruits is generally lower still (e.g., apples have about 137 mg%). In contrast, whole grains have a higher

230

potassium content, e.g. 530 mg% in rye, and 502 mg% in wheat.[28] Processing lowers these values, however, so that wholegrain "crisp bread" has only 436 mg%, and "Steinmetz" yeast bread 275 mg%. The potassium content of rice is especially low. At 150 mg%, unpolished rice has approximately the same content as cow's milk (155 mg%).

Bunge was the first to compare the extremely low potassium content of rice to the high content of potatoes. In the second volume of his book on human physiology,[29] he dealt with the problem of potassium in human nutrition in great detail (as discussed in Chapter 8 of *The Dynamics of Nutrition,* with regard to table salt). Bunge clearly saw the dangers facing mankind from an overconsumption of table salt. He also spoke of rice: "It contains six times less potassium than the European grains (wheat, rye and barley), ten to twenty times less than the legumes, and twenty to thirty times less than potatoes." Even if these analyses are not precise, they correctly point out a tendency of rice, with regard to its potassium content, to have an antagonistic relationship towards the potato.

Potassium and sodium have a polar relationship in the cell and tissue fluids of the organism. Thus, a high intake of potassium necessitates a high intake of sodium, so a diet rich in potatoes usually results in a high table salt consumption. The German *Salzkartoffel* bears witness to this fact, as do other extremely popular (and equally unrecommended) potato products, such as french fries and potato chips, both made with lots of salt. With a diet including cereals, 1-2 g of NaCl daily is enough. With the daily consumption of potatoes, table salt consumption increases significantly — often going far beyond the physiological requirement (.5-5 g). This is especially true when potatoes are served as a side dish with meat (often oversalted). The overconsumption here can, according to Bunge, be as high as 20-30 g daily.

Rice, on the other hand, needs only very little salt. It is thus especially suited to a low-salt diet. Among the rice-eating peoples of the far east there is a conspicuously small desire for salt; hence the development of earthly forces is hindered. At the same time, the high phosphorus content of rice provides a basis for the development of spiritual forces.

The potato, on the other hand, comes from the west and has an opposite "signature". When man eats potatoes, he tends to

231

over-consume salt and thus becomes too earthly — too much bound to the earth, even in his thinking. Perhaps now we can understand why Rudolf Steiner connected the high potato consumption of the 19th century with the materialistic way of thinking of that time. Just as rice unburdens the brain metabolism, so potatoes impose an extra burden on it: "And materialism — which is produced in the frontal part of the brain — has come precisely because eating potatoes has become widespread in recent times."[29]

Brown rice not only has importance in our diet but becomes an equal member of the spectrum of seven grains. Its great advantages are its easy digestibility (especially for a small child's diet or for gastro-intestinal problems) and its ability to unburden the kidneys and circulatory system. These advantages were recognized by Bunge and have since been confirmed in many ways. The relatively low potassium content of whole-grain rice is important here for its water-reducing and "unburdening" properties.

Stimulated by Bunge, Bircher-Benner also did research in this area. He confirmed the benefits of "reducing table salt consumption in cases of acute and chronic kidney problems" and of eliminating table salt "for certain heart and vascular diseases."[30]

Bircher-Benner fully confirmed the results of Bunge's research and applied them practically. These results are again being considered by the medical world. The American Heart Association has come to the conclusion that, with regard to arteriosclerosis, high blood pressure and heart problems, "almost all cases of these diseases are essentially kidney-related." Moreover, more than half of the population of The United States dies from kidney-related problems (i.e. arteriosclerosis, hypertony and heart disease). As E.K. Dahl points out, one essential cause of kidney problems is the over-consumption of table salt. He puts the need for salt at 0.5g daily. Its consumption should not exceed 5g for healthy people and 2g for those disposed to high blood pressure.

In his book on nutrition for sick people,[31] A. Welsch reports that "sodium is largely responsible for the development and persistence of neurogenic hypertension and at times even of real hypertension. The positive results from over forty years of therapy with low salt diets also corroborate these findings. The research of Dahl and his colleagues stresses the significance of

232

table salt. It shows an unequivocal correlation between the incidence of hypertension in a population group and their average salt consumption."

Hence we can see that Bunge's conclusions have been fully confirmed by modern medicine and dietetics. His early research was aptly described by his student, Aberhalden, who said that he "was way ahead of his time." This comment also applies to Bunge's indications for a rice diet, which has since become accepted for cases of kidney disorders and hypertension. According to Kempner, the rice diet "has had amazing success. In many patients, blood pressure returned to normal, the size of the heart decreased and in some cases there were strong changes in the backs of the eyes and in the EKG results."[31]

An entirely different sphere of influence of potassium is opened to us by yet another plant, whose specialization regarding potassium and the protein process was first discovered by Rudolf Steiner. In his first medical course (1920)[11] and later, in speaking to physicians, Steiner pointed to the white birch (*Betula alba*) and to the extraordinary way it deals with these two processes, in the leaves on the one hand, and in the bark on the other hand. "The birch comes into existence in that the processes which take place with the formation of living protein are carried further into the leaves than is usually the case . . ." For this reason, the leaves (e.g. steeped as a tea) can stimulate the desalting process. And the bark, when processed into a medication, can work against the hardening tendencies of gout and rheumatism.

Birch-leaf tea, birch elixir and birch bitters are effective remedies for the widespread "salt tendencies" of the organism. Rudolf Steiner here again proved to be the originator of a new dietary cure, the effects of which are only beginning to be tested today.

In this connection, we should mention two authors in particular. In the second volume of his book on medicinal plants (*Heilpflanzenkunde, 1962*)[32], W. Pelikan gives an impressive description of the "healing virtures" of the white birch. He also mentions the beneficial effect of brich in the diet, along with a low salt diet. As a botanist, G. Grohmann has made a persuasive plant portrait of the birch. Through this outline, he has come to the same conclusions regarding the effects of birch.[33]

233

The Calcium Processes as the Masters of the Metabolism:
Calcium at Work in the Kingdoms of Nature

Along with potassium and sodium, calcium is the third important mineral which plays a leading role in human metabolism. We
shall thus take a look at this universally present substance.

Calcium, in the form of salts, is quantitatively the most plentiful mineral in the human body. These salts make up about 1.5-2%
of the bodily weight, and more than 99% of them are in the teeth
and bones. It is by means of calcium that man is most subjected to
earthly heaviness. The calcium in man is most active in the mineral world. Nevertheless, we shall see that the less than 1% calcium in the bodily fluids is, in its dynamic functions, more essential and more dominant than the 99% which — even in outer
appearence — rests in a solid and concentrated form in the skeleton. Between the strong solidification and the constant movement
of calcium in the organism there is an unceasing interplay.

In keeping with its dominant capacity for forming deposits,
calcium also appears within the earth as a plentiful, rock-forming
element. It is the fifth most plentiful element within the earth, and
its salt-like compounds are quite common in nature. We find it
there in two forms, similar to those found in the human skeleton.
As calcium carbonate, it forms the basis of our chalk mountains.
In the stalagtites and stalagmites of caves, as well as in pearls
and coral, we can recognize its formative processes. The many
fossils of animal forms lead us to its origin. On the other hand,
calcium phosphate appears, as apatite, in the archetypal image
of calcium. Calcium goes from the rock into the water. As is the
case with most salts, there is more in sea water (30-40%) than in
fresh water. The calcium concentration in the latter varies, but
the water in Berne, Switzerland, which is considered "hard" because of its high calcium content, has about 7 mg%.

Along with its being common in the earth, we find calcium
widespread within the plant world. Calcium carbonate is in the
leaf framework, calcium phosphate in the heartwood. Calcium
itself is especially concentrated in the bark of trees, most notably
in the oak.

In addition to this more static function, calcium has a dynamic function which makes it indispensible to the plant. No
plant grows without calcium, which plays a prominant role in the

234

entire liquid metabolism of the plant. Here too — although in a way different from the way it functions among the ensouled organisms — it plays a role in the regulation of acids and bases.

Nonetheless the true nature of calcium first reveals itself in the animal world, and this fact can lead us to its essence and origin. One could say that in the animal world calcium is in its true element. The phenomena associated with this fact can only be touched upon, but they appear both in morphology and physiology. In the former, calcium's inexhaustible formative power is revealed. This appears in many sea animals: the oysters with their centrifugal shell-formation, coral with its centripetal calcium deposits and the crabs, which alternately display both types of calcium deposits. In the skeletons of the vertebrates, the inexhaustible formative power of calcium serves to express the soul-nature of the individual species. If you compare the skeleton of a bird with that of a carnivore or a cow, you can see how the form is a direct expression of the drives and desires which the particular species has internalized. The same holds true of the human skeleton, which, in its form, is a wonderful expression of man's soul-spiritual nature.

In a previously mentioned lecture cycle,[7] Rudolf Steiner describes the developmental process of the animals in its connection with calcium. We are also led back to the primal protein atmosphere of Lemuria, in which animals actually "consisted of curdled protein. They had the consistency, say, of gelatin, or even that of present-day cartilage." Liquid calcium then flowed into these forms, a process we see repeated today in the formation of oyster shells, or even of the human skeleton. "This calcium had a special attraction to this gelatin, to this cartilage. It penetrated it and was impregnated by it . . . Thus, there gradually arose the animals with calcium in their bones."

Of course, these animals were altogether different from those on earth today. The atmosphere at that time had not yet progressed to present-day atmospheric air and ocean water, a metamorphosis which, according to Rudolf Steiner, took place later, during Atlantean times. The most important thing for us to consider here is the property of calcium, which makes it a bearer of soul qualities. Calcium is a medium for the soul world, allowing it to incarnate and live in the most diverse forms, both externally and internally. The soul element is as if frozen in the skeleton, and made liquid, mobile and dynamic in the blood and other bodily fluids. Calcium also lives within man, but here it is taken hold of by an even higher principle, which gives each person his individual form and leads him to his individual soul qualities.

Calcium Activity in Man

We have already mentioned the one percent of calcium which is dissolved in the human fluid organism. From a dynamic point of view, this calcium is extremely significant for all bodily functions. It is so versatile that we can here only touch upon a few aspects important for human nutrition.

In the book *Fundamentals of Therapy*[21], Rudolf Steiner and Ita Wegman describe the activity of calcium in the human fluid-organism, at first with regard to protein. "The formation of the organism is a transformation of protein, which works together with mineral forces. Such forces are found, for example, in calcium." This describes one side of the working of calcium, manifest in the formation of the skeleton which is based upon a constant building up and dissolution of its form. "A mere protein activity has to be transformed into an activity in which formative forces are at work which are called forth in calcium by the Ego-organization. This must take place in the formation of blood." Blood formation — in the broadest sense of the word — which begins in the bone marrow, points to the other side calcium's activity: the actual calcium process.

We might think, here, of the ability of blood to clot. Through the clotting process, man is prevented, by means of calcium, from "spilling out" and losing himself in the environment. He thus maintains his individual existence and can rest on his own foundation.

The "calming effect" of calcium can be seen in another important area. The sensitivity and ability to recover of the entire musculature — including the heart and the involuntary intestinal musculature — are dependent upon the calcium content of the blood. Thus both tetanic and non-tetanic cramps in the skeletal muscles can be relieved by an injection of calcium. This fact points to an interplay with the central nervous system. It is interesting that calcium has a dual function with the nerve cells. It can

236

neither "suppress over-sensitivity nor raise under-sensitivity back to the norm."[34] This phenomenon clearly shows the great extent to which calcium is the bearer of soul forces and plays a role in these processes. Calcium not only seals up the vessels (e.g. in bloodclotting) but it also suppresses the nerve-sense life to a human level. Over-sensitivity and over-excitability can be caused by a calcium deficiency. "A calcium deficiency is thus also of fundamental significance with regard to the soul life and nerves . . ."[6] The regulatory activity of calcium reaches as far as the acid/base equilibrium. Bersin writes: "If, within the tissue fluids, the acid level is pushed too far to the alkaline side, then the concentration of Ca+ (free calcium) drops to the point where over-sensitivity and muscle cramps appear. This, in turn, leads to heavy production of carbonic and lactic acids, by means of which the Ca+ concentration rises and the over-sensitivity is overcome."

In his agricultural course,[5] Rudolf Steiner spoke of this basic characteristic, saying that "calcium has a wonderful relationship to the human world of desires." Regarding its regulating and ordering qualities, he said: "Calcium creates order whenever the etheric body works too strongly, so that the astral cannot approach some part of the organism. It suppresses the etheric body, leaving the way free for the working of the astral body. This is the case with all calcium." A calcium process is found in ossification in the formative process of the human head, the "cold pole" of our being. This process suppresses the inflammatory processes. It causes allergic symptoms like nettle rash (*urticaria*) to die down.

Thus, we have before us the dual activity of calcium. On the one hand, it works toward the head-pole in the formation of the skeleton and the nerves. On the other hand, it is active in the blood and tissue fluids. Precisely in this quality can we see its regulating activity, which holds the balance between the realm of life and the soul realm.

Calcium is everywhere at work in the metabolism. It directs the enzyme activities, either promoting or suppressing them. It acts both as a partner and opponent of sodium and potassium, controlling the balance between base and acid. We thus describe not the "winter" calcium but, in effect, the "spring" (or "summer") calcium in man. One could also describe this "summer" calcium as nerve-sense and metabolic calcium. "Winter calcium is, so to speak, a self-satisfied being . . . As we move toward the spring, calcium has more desires. It then develops a kind of inner vitality."[35] Man bears the poles of winter and summer within himself, at the same time. Therefore, calcium unfolds this dual function within him.

On the metabolic side, it has an excretory effect, pushing out water and even detoxifying. Rudolf Steiner pointed to this calcium function by saying: "In the metabolic-limb man, it is at work, driving out the fluids."[36] On the other hand, calcium can become too solid in the sclerotic deposits, in stone formations and in the calcifying tendency as a whole.

Our central concern here is the leading role played by calcium in nutrition through all the above-mentioned functions. It can only fulfill its tasks when — through daily nutrition — the organism has sufficient calcium substance and force at its disposal. In general, we need about one gram of calcium daily to provide the necessary stimulation for our inner organic activity. How can we find this in our daily food?

The Calcium Process in Nutrition and Metabolism

We have already mentioned some foods rich in calcium, especially milk and milk products. However, many vegetables — like various cabbages and spinach — are also high in calcium, as are many fruits and cereals. A lacto-vegetarian diet would provide us with sufficient calcium. In contrast, meat, sausages and eggs are low in calcium. The most harmful effect today is produced by refined food products: refined factory sugar, refined flour, white pasta, bread and baked goods, etc. Our nutrition thus makes it difficult for us to get enough calcium. There is another equally important question: are we able to utilize in our metabolism the calcium available in our food? It is known that even the absorption of calcium in the intestines is an active process with many determining factors. Lactose promotes this absorption; above all, the hormone of the parathyroid gland has a stimulating effect.[37]

The regulation of the calcium metabolism in the organism appears to stand at the center of the human "calcium economy." There are about 300 mg of calcium in the blood plasma itself and calcium accomplishes its tasks in the entire organism from this starting point. On the one hand, calcium streams from the blood

238

into the bones. The latter are living tissue in a constant state of being built up and broken down and are in need of constant renewal. The break-down process of the bones frees calcium into the blood again. The bone tissue is thus a kind of calcium reserve which can be used in the regulation of the calcium metabolism. Of course, pathological conditions also occur here.

On the other hand, used calcium is taken by the blood to the kidneys and intestines to be excreted. According to modern research, when the skeleton is in a state of equilibrium, about 400 mg of calcium go into the bones each day, and the same amount flows back into the blood. About 200 mg are excreted through the intestines. The kidneys filter about 10,000 mg of calcium, but only excrete c. 1-3% of it. This process is controlled by the parathyroid glands. In addition is the quantitatively small, but qualitatively highly significant, amount of calcium which is necessary for the cellular fluid.

Even this brief overview reveals a tremendously subtle, all-pervasive, active regulation of the entire calcium metabolism. This activity is connected to the living organism, and to call it "automation" — as is often done today — is simply primitive. We can come much closer to this mystery by considering what has already been said about the calcium process as the bearer of the astral forces in the human organism. By means of calcium, we are in a position to incorporate all the processes of our etheric and physical organisms in the most varied ways, so that they are permeated by the soul. Every instant, we create our skeleton anew by means of calcium, in such a way that we can take hold of it with our individuality. At the same time, we also reconstitute the structure of our nerve organism anew every moment. Without this re-creation, the nerves would be unable to fulfill their function in a healthy manner. Bersin says clearly that "perhaps this explains the psychological disturbances which accompany a calcium deficiency."[34] By means of calcium, we constantly give directives to our metabolism, not only for the "utilization" of the calcium itself, but also for the placement of the entire metabolism in the service of ensouling the organism. This makes it an instrument of the "astral" organization, or one's own inner experience. Thus on the one hand, calcium must "calm" us, "suppressing" and perhaps even "sealing out" what storms in from the outer world. On the other hand, it must at the same time direct the entire metabolism. It promotes the digestion of protein, brings forth an optimal sugar synthesis, and stimulates the digestion of fats. It enters into the muscular metabolism, making the muscles capable of giving expression to the human form and movement. Is not calcium the "leading player in the metabolic processes?"[2] "Calcium creates order," as Rudolf Steiner said. But this "order" is the result of tremendous processes still beyond the grasp of our present faculties of comprehension. We can approach an understanding of it only by concentrating on the dynamics of calcium. The methods of spiritual science offer us indispensible help toward this end. Without it, we stand transfixed before a "wonderful mechanism", as it is called, which is perhaps of some significance, but which is by no means fully understandable.

Grasping this dynamic is, of course, no small task, as even a superficial look at the disturbances or dysfunction in the human calcium organism will confirm.

Disturbances in the Calcium Metabolism: Osteoporosis

Let us first look at the building up and breaking down of the bones. The preservation of the bones is dependent upon their activity; i.e. their use by the human soul-spiritual forces expressed in movement. One sees the same phenomenon in cripples and those who are bed-ridden, as well as among astronauts who are in a weightless environment: the breaking-down process becomes too strong, the bone begins to diminish, and *osteoporosis* can set in. We see clearly that ensouled movement — the struggle with and the overcoming of earthly gravity — is what maintains the equilibrium between the building up and breaking down of the bones. In addition, "hormonal regulation" by means of the parathyroid gland also plays an important role. Fleisch offers the following description: "If, for some reason, too little calcium is taken in, the calcium level in the blood tends to drop. This stimulates a gland — the parathyroid — to increase production of a hormone, parathormone. This hormone, in turn, stimulates the dissolution of the bones. The calcium released in this way brings the blood calcium level back to normal. In this way, a deficiency in the consumption of calcium is compensated for by an increased dissolution of the bones."[37] This sober formulation reveals the following: for the organism, the most important thing is to keep

240

the blood-calcium level constant. Only then can that force-organization take hold which is necessary for the ensoulment of the body. Even an illness — *osteoporosis* — is not too high a price to pay for this. However, this condition appears only when the limbs have not been moved sufficiently (i.e. have not been taken hold of by the soul) or when too little calcium is consumed. The latter occurs when there is either too little calcium in our food or when the available calcium is unable to fulfill its functions. Thus, on the one hand, we must take care to get enough calcium in our daily food, and on the other, we must consider how well it can be utilized.

Nutritional calcium can be "utilized" only when combined with the proper composition of other minerals — above all sodium, potassium and magnesium in the appropriate salt forms. Both too little and too much can upset the equilibrium. The organic basis of protein, carbohydrates and fats in which the calcium is embedded is equally important. In other words, the utilization of calcium depends upon the nutritional quality of the entire diet, thus posing a challenge to the inner forces of the organism which must be in a position to react properly. If not, "too much calcium is absorbed, and a slight increase in the blood calcium level leads to a decrease in parathormone production. That, in turn, means a decrease in parathormone production, which means a decrease in bone dissolution and a normalization of the blood calcium level," a regulation favoring the central function of the calcium in the blood: "Parathormone preserves the extremely important constancy of the blood calcium level ... it reacts to the slightest deviation." It is interesting that a new hormone has been recently discovered which is formed in the thyroid gland. Its effect is "antagonistic to that of parathormone."[37] Rudolf Steiner has already pointed to such a functional connection between the thyroid and parathyroid glands.[38]

As we have seen, *osteoporosis* arises from too strong a dissolution of the bones, while the remaining bone remains completely normal, i.e. the building up of the bone remains intact. This degeneration, which often occurs in old age, can also extend to the backbone. It can have various causes: deficient consumption or poor quality of calcium or dysfunctions in hormonal activity. The latter often appear in women during menopause, which shows the close relationship of the entire endocrine organism.

Rickets and Osteomalacia

We must also look at the other side, which takes us to the illness of rickets or *osteomalacia*, where the bones do not calcify enough. They remain, or become, soft, and tend to become deformed or — especially in old age — to fracture. Rudolf Steiner was able to shed some light on this complex process. He spoke of it often in his spiritual-scientific writings, but we shall confine ourselves here to a few indications specific to our theme of nutrition.

In an early lecture,[39] Rudolf Steiner stated a fundamental fact of the human form: it is dependent not only upon the hardening tendency in the bones and teeth, but also upon a softening tendency. The forces which at first use calcium to bring about hardening, formation and ensoulment "hold back something which has a softening tendency." We have seen that a rhythmical interplay of hardening and softening takes place in the human skeleton. Dissolution, breaking down and excretion are also essential to the human form, because the forces thus freed can be devoted to further evolution — to the development of higher soul-spiritual forces. If these forces become one-sidedly strong, however, the softening of the bones becomes pathological and we are faced with rickets (*osteomalacia*). "If man can master that which today appears unseasonably as rickets, even down in his bones, then he will be able to give himself his own form . . . he will then conquer the principle of hardening." This clearly means that the processes of calcification and decalcification are of a soul-spiritual origin. However, outside factors can also have their affects.

Rudolf Steiner approached this problem from another angle in a later lecture series,[40] where he also mentioned the polarity between ossification and its suppression. "In the human brain, we have a constant striving toward bone formation," but this formation of bone must be checked, so that "in the brain, we constantly have a nascent condition, the arising of rickets." This "suppressed development of rickets in the head," by means of which the head "can be the bearer of soul-spiritual processes," is made possible by the working of phosphorus in the brain. Here we have the basis for Steiner's phosphorus therapy for rickets. These indications also point to a process closely connected to phosphorus: light metabolism.

242

We have already seen that the absorption of calcium is also dependent upon the other substances in which it is embedded. Among these are the phosphates and magnesium, which are related to light metabolism. The role of vitamin D becomes clear here. It is often said today, in a simplistic way, that rickets is caused by a deficiency of vitamin D, the precursor of which — pro vitamin D — is produced in the organism itself. Only upon exposure to light in the skin — a kind of "phosphorizing" process — does it become an "anti-rickets" substance. Thus O. Wolff was correct when he wrote: "This vitamin itself is not a necessary building block of the organism. Rather by means of and through the organism it has a formative influence upon the body's calcification."[41] It is a well-known fact that therapy with vitamin D has done tremendous harm (cf. Vide-Stoss). Fleisch writes of an "overdose of vitamin D", whereby an increase of calcification takes place outside of the bones, e.g. in the kidneys and arteries. "These changes can be so serious that they result in death."

On the other hand, a dietary preparation conceived of by Rudolf Steiner (Calcon I and II)[42] which imitates and stimulates the calcium process has proven beneficial for both organic formation and nutrition. Regarding the nutritional aspect, however, we must repeat that the quality of the entire diet is of essential importance. The parent's commitment to bio-dynamic produce, a thoughtfully conceived and harmonious diet and proper medical treatment can counter the tendency to rickets even before the child's birth.

We must not overlook the great difficulties posed by modern conditions, however. Many factors have to be considered which hinder the proper incarnation of a new-born child. There is the poor quality of milk, including even mother's milk. Then we have the results of environmental pollution, which has reached such proportions that, as a result of smog, sunlight is reduced by about 8% on the earth. For many people, the light forces necessary for the small child reach the organism in a diminished form. In addition, modern hygienic and cosmetic measures often make the child's body less open to the inflow of cosmic forces. Finally, clothing — especially artificial fabrics which shut out even ultra-violet rays — can be a serious problem. One can see how many difficulties the new-born child encounters. In order to overcome these obstacles, tremendous insight and loving devotion on the

243

part of parents, physicians and all who care for children are necessary. One can see how much comes into play and finds expression in a phenomenon like rickets.

The feeding of infants and small children is a problem which requires altogether new guidelines. It should be clear that biodynamic food (which carries the *Demeter* trademark in Europe) is indispensible, and that food preparation must also take place in the right way. We should here mention the *Holle* foods for children, made by Holle KG, CH-4144 Arlesheim, Switzerland.

Calcium Metabolism and Phytin Activity

A question has recently come to the fore regarding the presence of phytin in cereals. Phytin is an organic substance found especially in the bran, the endosperm layers, and the germ. Thus, it is in all wholegrain flour. It is valuable as a phosphorus compound, but it can also form calcium salts which are insoluable and therefore difficult to digest, thereby diminishing the available calcium in food. In their classic work on flour and bread (1954), Neumann and Pelshenke wrote: "By means of fermentative splitting with phytase, as well as by means of calcium supplements, the metabolic disorders which could lead to rickets from a cereal diet can be overcome."[43] K. Lang wrote something similar in 1974[3]: "In short-term experiments, the phytin content of food did indeed prove to be a factor contributing to a decreased utilization of calcium . . . However, this phytin effect proved to be temporary and vanished after about three weeks . . ." "In general the cereals (except oats) contain a phytin-splitting enzyme (phytase)." It is significant that Lang also points to the limited value of animal experiments. "A reduction in the calcium content of the skeleton" was brought about "only under the extreme conditions of animal experiments. In human nutrition, it apparently plays practically no role." Regarding the intake of calcium, he states that "a number of small dosages given throughout the day are better absorbed than the same amount given all at once." Regarding the question of "whether phytic acid diminishes the calcium supply of man", he writes — in a more recent article — that "this danger has been overestimated."[44]

We mention these things only to show how complicated the calcium problem really is. We also hope to avoid a false evaluation of details which could cause us to lose our vision of the whole.

244

The Significance of "Brain Sand"

The problem of calcium in nutrition accompanies man throughout his entire life. As we mentioned in the chapter on milk, Rudolf Steiner said that "an overfeeding of calcium, by means of cow milk in childhood, can lead to the hardening of arteries in adulthood." In fact, we can observe a deposit of calcium in the arteries of older people, but this only becomes pathological when other conditions are present, e.g. the overconsumption of protein. The metabolism of fat and sugar also play a role here. We are thus faced with a very complex problem.

The same holds true for the formation of kidney stones, in which calcium metabolism plays an important role. In all cases — both over-calcification and pathological decalcification — there is, without a doubt, a disruption in the equilibrium of the processes of building up and breaking down in the organism.

The significance of this fact can be seen in one of Rudolf Steiner's lectures to workers,[45] where he turns to the problem of mineralization and of the need for man to work against these mineralizing forces in the living, formative process. Also "within the nerves mineral substances would be constantly created if we were not able to counter them." These mineral substances must first be formed in order for man to develop a normal intelligence, as can be seen, for example, in the phenomenon of "brain sand". This "brain sand" is well-known to anatomists and is described by Rauber-Kopsch, among others, as "yellow sand-like granules made up of calcium phosphate and carbonate and an organic base."[46] It is found in the pineal gland — a particularly significant organ in the history of human and animal evolution. Without going into details from a medical point of view, it is nonetheless important to look at Rudolf Steiner's statement on this subject. He said that within the brain, "sand is constantly deposited when you bring nutrients into your blood."[45] This "brain sand" is, as a crystal formation, "just as much subject to the forces of the cosmos" as the crystals in outer nature. Thus, we need this "brain sand" — it mediates the intelligence forces of the cosmos to us; for this reason, "without brain sand, we would be stupid", yet we must constantly dissolve it and build it anew. With every use of the brain — e.g. during a sense-perception — this "brain sand" arises. Yet the activity whereby we become conscious of this

245

sense-perception dissolves it again. "This dissolving of what comes into us is what brings about the fact that man can experience himself in such a way that he can say 'I'". "That is the most powerful dissolution of the brain sand; when we say 'I'". Our working against and offering resistance to the mineral forces within us enkindle our Ego-consciousness. In this process, however, we work against not only the earthly forces, but also against "the forces of the cosmos." This crystallizing and dissolving — building up and breaking down — is a general principle of our organism (the principle of formation and "unformation"), so that we can realize our individuality even on a physiological level. Everything which comes into mineral form — table salt, sugar, all the minerals in us, like iron, silicon,etc. — is subject to this law. All these substances put themselves at the service of the Ego-organization. "What we call our Ego-consciousness consists in this dissolving." However, we would dissolve too much if our food, with its minerals, did not work against this process, making possible the rhythmical development of new crystallization, new formation and new dissolution.

Nonetheless, the mineralization process reaches a kind of culmination, as part of the calcium process, in the formation of "brain sand" in the pineal gland. This amazing formation is made up of the same substances as our skeleton — calcium carbonate and phosphate — which is, ultimately, the entire calcium metabolism in man. And the proper crystallization and dissolution is closely connected to the development of our intelligence, our Ego-consciousness. In his *Occult Physiology*[47] Rudolf Steiner says that we incorporate in ourselves "the most dense process of becoming earthly" by means of calcium carbonate and phosphate. At the same time, we constantly oppose this with the "most active process", the warmth process which culminates in the blood and in the entire fluid organism. The warming process is dominant, and our individual soul-activity takes hold of it directly.

What we call the physical processes are merely the last result of what happens in the higher members — in the life-organization and soul-being. The pineal gland itself, in which the "brain sand" is found, is the condensed result of supersensible processes. "These streams become so dense that they take hold of the human bodily substance and form it" into such organs as the pineal

246

gland.

Here we can understand that a great deal of insight can be had into the interconnection between nutrition and consciousness, and between nutrition and feeble-mindedness.

The Acid/Base Equilibrium as the Interplay Between Bodily and Soul Forces

Equally significant is the process which is expressed in the regulation of the acid/base equilibrium in man. We can grasp this process in its full subtlety only if we can see it as the interplay between the bodily and soul forces. From a merely physiological or physical-chemical point of view, we cannot understand why the living organism expends so much effort in order to maintain this equilibrium at all times. The most we could say is that the balance preserves human health and that a strong deviation in either direction means sickness in man. A realistic orientation toward sickness and health is possible only with a consideration of the soul-spiritual element in man.

Let us begin by considering the physiological aspects of this subject to the extent that they aid our understanding of nutrition.

"Acidic" and "basic" are two chemical qualities which we find everywhere. When a mineral substance is dissolved, either an acid or a base can result. If they balance each other out, a salt results. Chemistry expresses this process in an abstract formula:

$$acid + base = salt \ and \ water.$$

Thus, we see that water — the fluid element — always takes part in this interplay. The measure of acidity (or alkalinity) today is even more abstract. One speaks of the so-called pH, which signifies the "negative of the logarithm of the hydrogen-ion concentration" in a liquid. Clearly this phenomenon of pH takes into account only one aspect of the totality of nature and man—namely the ability of these substances to develop electrical charges when dissolved in water. These substances are therefore also called electrolytes.

When Rudolf Steiner spoke of the formation of acids and bases, he did so in reference to man. For example, he once said to a class in the Waldorf School: "So, you have all seen these experiments. But now think of what is going on in your body. If you

247

move your limbs, an acid is always formed. But if you sit still, and only exert yourself mentally, something alkaline arises in your brain."[48] Speaking to physicians, he said: "It is a question of understanding these processes as they relate to the development of the earth and the development of man. Then, one finds that alkali support those effects in man which begin in the mouth and are continued in the digestion, from the front to back. All other processes which go from front to back are also related to them. Alkali are related to the direction from front to back, acids to the opposite direction. Only when one looks upon the contrast between the human 'front' and 'back' can one come to the actual polarity between acids and bases. Salt relates to this by directing itself toward the earth, standing vertically upon both opposites. All processes which proceed from above downwards have something salty in them."[11]

These statements show us that Rudolf Steiner's approach to such problems was, indeed, dynamic. It also was one which considered man at the center. In both instances, we are referred to phenomena we can learn to observe.

It is well-known to modern physiology that an active muscle forms lactic acid, which is then broken down during its "recovery phase". The formation of acids is an expression of the activity of the human will. On the other hand, the resting head — typical of everything resting or passive (from one point of view) — is characterized by alkali. Tension and relaxation appear here as a polarity. With alkali, we inwardize our being, we remain within ourselves; with acids, we externalize our being and become active and aggressive. Even litmus paper (produced from a plant) shows us this polarity: it turns red in acids and blue in bases.

These characteristics bring us closer to an understanding of the polarity but they are by no means exhaustive. For example, human skin is acidic. This "acid coat" that we constantly form and replenish is an important bastion against outer influences like bacteria, again showing the active nature of acids. The same is true of stomach acid; it aggressively breaks down our food, which still has an external character. Here we can also look at the relationship of acids to the soul life. We may speak, for example, of a person "souring" to something — or even being a "sourpuss". Such people can be especially sensitive, even oversensitive and easily injured, yet they can tend to be rigid. This leads us to see the activity of the astral in acidity. (cf. *The Dynamics of Nutrition,* Chapter 3).

The alkaline element, on the other hand, has been seen here as the "resting element". It is also the element of plant life. The leaves of plants generally have an affinity to the basic element. They are a great reservoir of base-forming elements such as potassium and calcium. Within man, they correspond to the formation of the liver, while the gall bladder expresses the astral element. We find, therefore, that the alkali first appear as an expression of the life forces. It is interesting to note here that the plant develops acidic forces in the formation of blossom, fruit and seed. The acids in fruit (including many berries) as well as the formation of acid in grain are typical indications of an element which leads the plant beyond its life-organization and touches upon the astral world.

Within man, the basic element in the liver and brain serves as a foundation for the taking hold of the forces of individuality. This also applies to the alkaline small intestines, where the strongest Ego-impulses enter into the digestion. (cf. *The Dynamics of Nutrition,* Chapter 3).

These facts are also of significance for human blood, which is slightly — but nonetheless clearly — alkaline. This alkaline tinge apparently serves as a basis for the working of the Ego within this central fluid. That man holds on with such power to the stability of this reaction that he must and can re-establish it constantly if he wants to remain healthy may be seen as an expression of a definite relationship among the members of man's being. The following diagram, based on the pH spectrum of blood plasma,[22] shows us that modern physiology is also interested in these matters.

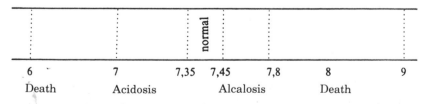

6	7	7,35	7,45	7,8	8	9
Death	Acidosis		Alcalosis		Death	

We see here that the basis necessary for a healthy working together of the members of man's being lies in the slim margin between pH 7.35 and 7.45. Should the pH sink below this, the symptoms of acidosis — an acidification of the blood — appear. The reaction cannot go below pH 7 without coming into a realm no longer compatible with human life. By the same token, a critical point of alkalosis in the blood is reached at pH 7.8, which also brings man to the threshold of death. These processes — which are directly related to nutrition — have rightly been given special attention, although a number of false conclusions have been reached.

Basically, we can say that the human organism exerts all its forces in order to maintain the proper reaction in the blood — as we can see, for example in the so-called "alkaline reserve" which one calls upon to combat an acidification of the blood. Apparently the danger of acidosis plays a greater role than the danger of alkalosis. The "buffering capacity" of the blood and other bodily fluids results from a complicated chemical system which is primarily related to alkaline bicarbonate. The greatest factor determining the pH of the blood is the relationship of carbonic acid to bicarbonate. A deficit of the latter leads to acidosis; a surplus leads to alkalosis.

Regulation takes place at the same time in the "outer court" of the blood, in the tissue fluids which function as a "watchman", thus sparing the blood as long as possible from a change of reaction. As a result, man is protected against acid or alkaline elements in his food directly affecting the blood. In other words: the blood itself, as the central workplace of the members of man's being, is protected as long as possible from the effects of an imbalanced diet or improper life style. However, this takes place at the expense of all the other activities and organic functions. The blood itself becomes acidic or alkaline only in extreme situations — e.g. in a diabetic coma, or in the alkalosis following the lack of carbonic acid.

However, two other physiological possibilities are open to the organism for this regulation — the kidney functions and respiration — so that the blood is protected in three ways from over-acidity or over-alkalinity.

Nonetheless, the dangers here are both complex and severe. As long as man followed his healthy nutritional instincts, he was for the most part protected. In our times, these dangers have increased. One can well imagine that an overburdening of this three-fold regulatory system soon leads to a pathological weakening of the kidneys, the respiration, and the skin, and from there to the functioning of all other organs. The "metabolic slag" accumulates, and various ill-boding symptoms appear.

Experience shows us that the danger of acidosis is greater than that of alkalosis, since the blood must remain in the alkaline realm. Thus, special attention must be paid to this aspect of nutrition. We have already seen that the mineral content of the blood plays a decisive role here. However, the determining factor in man is not so much the actual composition of food as the process or activity it calls forth within man.

In this regard, a diet based on animal foods — with poultry, fish, meat, sausages, and even eggs — is "acidifying" in that it furthers the acidic element. Fruits and seeds are also acidic. What effect do they have within the body? Fruits and fruit juices are neutralized by the organism and can then even have an alkalizing effect. They stimulate this process of regulation. And what about cereals? This question has lead to a number of studies.

B. Thomas[49] gave some exact indications when, in 1964, he wrote that "dough made from flour with bran in it is more strongly buffered, and thereby prevents a quick displacement of the pH toward the acidic." This buffering effect of wholegrain flours is the result of their high phytin content — especially its phosphorus component — which we previously mentioned.

The most important acidic fermentation products in bread are lactic and acetic acids. Along with them are buteric, citric and other acids. Even formic acid plays a role worth noting. According to Thomas, the lactic acid content is "far below the level which can be considered as disadvantageous to the health". On the other hand, the acetic acid content "is only slightly below the level where a reaction takes place."

Before speaking of the acidifying effect of bread — especially wholegrain bread — on the tissue fluids, however, we must keep in mind that man needs acidic food within certain limits. One may speak of the unfavorable effect of cereals only when they are the sole food eaten over a long period of time. If they are taken in combination with vegetables, however, there is no such unfavorable effect. The legumes are an exception here, and their acidifying power is considerable. Among the berries, cranberries with their high benzoate content should be mentioned. In addition, hazelnuts and walnuts — both high in phosphorus — also stimulate the formation of acids. Milk, on the other hand, promotes the forming of alkali.

The diet of our modern civilization — rich in meat products, refined flour and animal fat — all too often overtaxes the organism with regard to the acid/base equilibrium. Psychological burdens often add to the problem. Then, as E.A. Schmid[6] so graphically put it, "the organism is soon forced to store the harmful decomposition products somewhere in the body — at first temporarily — e.g. in the muscles, joints, cartilage, nerves." The kidneys, liver and spleen are chronically overburdened. The result of these tendencies toward acidification and mineral deposits in the organism can be seen in a number of illnesses. We then find not only gastric and intestinal disorders and stone formation, but also what Paracelsus called the "Tartar diseases" — gout, rheumatism, and arthritis. Schmid also points out quite rightly that many forms of so-called nervousness, migraines and psychoneurological disorders originate in the same manner.

Actually, Bircher-Benner had already observed and described this condition. He directed attention especially to the "acid poisoning" resulting from an overconsumption of animal protein. The resulting acids — especially uric acid — provide the "putrid morass" in which many unfortunate chronic diseases thrive, e.g. rheumatism, arteriosclerosis, gout, diabetes, and multiple sclerosis. These dangers have increased since the lifetime of Bircher-Benner.

There are other problems associated with this area of study. We have spoken of lactic and formic acids, and have pointed to the necessity of the sour-acidic element for our human life. But what about the processes of acidification and their significance for our health? Let us look at this question.

The Significance of Lactic Acid: Sauerkraut as a special dietary food

Though he didn't mention it by name, Rudolf Steiner was referring to lactic acid when he spoke of the acid formed in the active muscle. This insight takes us from the formation of acid as a soul activity to the physiology of acids. Lactic acid — like acetic acid — is a human physiological product. This holds true at least for "dextrorotary" lactic acid found in human tissue. The majority of this muscular lactic acid is converted back to glycogen in a few minutes. The muscle is thus de-acidified and becomes alkaline, a fact substantiated by F. Eichholtz[50] who writes that "the fate of lactic acid and other organic acids is different from that of inorganic acids. The latter are formed in the body after eating meat, eggs, cheese, etc. and include sulfuric and phosphoric acids." These "raging acids then take the corresponding base out of the bones or tissues." But the other acids leave their bases free so that "a flood of organic acids of this type has practically no meaning for the acid/base equilibrium." These acids build no salts which could form as metabolic precipitates. Their effect is thus to allow an alkaline excess.

Lactic acid has an important physiological property which comes into play in the "acid coat" of the skin: its disinfectant effect. It stops the growth of bacteria and works against putrefaction. Lactic acid is therefore a natural protection of the body against infection, thus providing the basis for one of the healthful effects of sour milk products (e.g. yogurt) as well as for sauerkraut. At the same time, lactic acid acts as a preservative of protein, fat and carbohydrates. As a result, such fermented products can be preserved, although freezing partially breaks down the ferments. The consumption of sauerkraut has thus been called "ferment therapy". The value of pickled vegetables also depends upon the same factors. Foods pickled with lactic acid are easier to digest and they stimulate the digestion. For ill persons with chronic constipation, sauerkraut is a medicinal food. Products with lactic acid have a laxative effect and also protect the intestinal flora. Sauerkraut, especially, is high in calcium, potassium and magnesium and is thus antagonistic to sodium. It is therefore a diuretic and works against inflammation. It is thus a good food for those with arthritis and kidney or heart diseases — though it should be made without table salt. It also supports the detoxifying function of the liver. These few indications point to the great significance of lactic acid — and the entire fermenting process — for and within man.

The formic acid process proceeds in a different but no less significant way, both in nature and man. The spiritual research of Rudolf Steiner has shed a new light on it.

Two More Indispensible Acids: Oxalic and Formic Acid

Formic acid is also indispensible for the organism of man and animal. As its name shows (*formica* is latin for "ant"; formic acid

253

is formed as a poison by ants for their defense), it has an active, aggressive character. In the higher animals and in man it is closely related to oxalic acid, which also plays an important role in the plant world.

Oxalic acid "is formed in all growing [plant] tissues and is excreted as calcium oxalate in the new permanent tissue."[26] Oxalic acid is also found in human beings and animals. Modern research has discovered that dysfunctions of the oxalate metabolism often result not only in the formation of oxalate stones in the kidneys but also in oxalate deposits in various tissues. In this case, the transition from oxalic to formic acid appears to be disrupted.[51]

Rudolf Steiner's discussion of this subject goes much further and opens a broader perspective. As we said, oxalic acid is found in both plant and animal. "In reality, oxalic acid is found in all vegetation, even if only in homeopathic doses." Insects transform it into formic acid. "And, in fact, we constantly breath in formic acid — even if in tiny doses — from the atmosphere."

Rudolf Steiner, in one of his lectures[7], asks what this process means to man. The fact that man transforms oxalic acid into formic acid was already known to the medieval alchemists, although they did not see it as merely a chemical transformation but as a human, formative process. They said to themselves, "there, in the digestive tract, we are dealing primarily with processes which are under the influence of oxalic acid." In the breathing organism, however, oxalic acid is transformed into formic acid by means of glycerin. The result is carbon dioxide, which is then exhaled.

This process can be realistically described as follows: "If man did not develop oxalic acid in his digestive tract, he would not be able to live; i.e. his etheric body would have no foundation in his organism. If, on the other hand, he could not convert oxalic acid into formic acid, then his astral body would have no foundation in his organism." It becomes once more apparent, in this case, that the most important thing is the activity of the organism, the *dynamics*. In his lectures on bees (1923),[52] Steiner put it concisely: "We have formic acid as the basis for soul and spirit."

This process is important for the entire dynamics of nutrition. "Life consists of work and not of matter. This is the most important point — people should know that life does not consist of con-

254

suming cabbage and beets, but rather, of what the body must do when cabbage or beet substance enters into it."

Nonetheless, it is important that these substances stimulate the necessary activities. "What you eat during your life is always transformed" — to a certain extent — "into formic acid." And when you get sick and do not have enough formic acid in you, that is very bad for your body, which then "forms too much uric acid, which leads to arthritis or rheumatism."

It is thus important that we take in oxalic acid in the right way with our food. As we noted, it is found in the young, vital tissue of all plants. Recent research has shown that the oxalic content of fruit and vegetables is usually above 10 mg/100 g fresh substance.[44] It is much higher in spinach (60-200 mg/100 g) and in beets, a fact which may be related to their stimulation of the process of cellular respiration. There is still more oxalic acid in sorrel, celery and rhubarb leaves. In fact, the latter can have so much oxalic acid that one may not be able to overcome it. This inability can further the formation of oxalate stones as well as kidney diseases in general. So we see that "as much as we need the stimulation which comes from the oxalic acid in plant foods, when consumed in large quantities, it is no longer a harmless nutrient."[44]

We can also see here that the acidification of the organism is connected to an ensouling gesture. Oxalic acid is a weak acid which is formed in the generally alkaline regions of the plant — i.e. in the etheric realm. Formic acid, a typical animal "venom" or poison, is stronger. When raised up in the human organism, it serves as a basis for the development of soul and spirit. If this process cannot be controlled, it leads to illness.

We have tried to give an overview of the most important and interesting aspects of the acid/base regulation. There now remains the task of characterizing a few more mineral substances as they work in man. Let us begin with silicon.

Silicon as Foundation for the Ego-Organization

Silicon is present in all the kingdoms of nature and in man. It is the second most common (chemical) element in the earth's crust. Who has not admired a quartz crystal in which silicon most purely reveals its formative power and transparency?

In the organic world, silicon appears not only as formed, but also as formable. In water, it forms the most varied colloids, hence playing a special role in human connective tissue.

Silicic acid is a weak acid found in all plants. It appears in a special way in cereals, and this has implications for our nutrition.

Today, silicon has been discovered in almost all human organs and tissues. Its concentration in the blood — both in plasma and in red corpuscles — is given at 1 mg/ml. The human body contains about one gram of silicon[3]. Berson mentions the following values: human epidermis, 106 mcg SiO_2/g, nails 56, hair 90, tendons 28, and muscles 18 mcg SiO_2/g. Adults excrete about 10 mg. of silicic acid daily in their urine.

Although these indications might justify speaking of a silicon metabolism, K. Lang writes of this trace element that "in physiological concentrations, simple silicic acid is a harmless substance. In spite of its alien character and constant presence, it does not cause any harm in the organism."[3]

This statement clearly reveals the helplessness of the analytic method. It also explains why silicon is today considered insignificant for human nutrition. Rudolf Steiner was the first to investigate and describe the working of silicic acid in both agriculture and medicine. Studies in both fields yield important results for human nutrition.

We shall limit ourselves here to a short discussion, since the subject has been treated extensively elsewhere.[53 54 55] We have also mentioned the role of silicon in Chapter 10 of *The Dynamics of Nutrition* and shall take this as our starting point.

The activity of silicon in man becomes comprehensible when we consider its mineral nature. Accordingly, silicic acid works "through the metabolism into those parts of the human organism where the living becomes lifeless."[21] We thus find it in the skin, nails, hair, etc. It is also in the sense organs and nerves, as well as in the tendons, connective tissue and muscles. It always has a formative effect, and it stands in the service of those forces individualizing man. "It forms the physical basis of the Ego-organization. The latter needs the silicic acid process in the organism, right up to the point where the process of formation comes up against the outer and inner [unconscious] world."

Silicon is always active as a process, even where, as in the nerve-sense pole, it can be materially recognized. In the metabolism, it unfolds a dynamic activity. Furthermore, it provides us with an example of how an acid can be put in the service of a higher force — the Ego.

Steiner described the task of silicon quite precisely in a way which can help us to understand its significance for human nutrition. He writes: "Silicic acid has a two fold task. Within the body, it sets the limit for the processes of mere growth, nutrition, etc. Outwardly, it shuts off the body from the external, natural processes, so that the organism is not consigned to merely continuing these processes, but can, rather, develop its own."[21] The function of silicon is thus both inwardizing and individualizing.

What does this mean for our nutrition? In *The Dynamics of Nutrition* we saw that, in the processes of nutrition, man must hold back the natural forces. He must learn to resist them and to use the ingested substance to build up an organism in his own image and in accord with his own individuality. This extremely important process is facilitated by a substance which we can eat with our daily food. Silicic acid is given to us in whole grains and wholegrain products. Although all grains — especially barley and millet — contain this indispensible substance, even Kollath doesn't mention this fact in his book,[28] in the tables of trace elements in grain. He merely mentions that silicon is found, along with many other elements, in the skin of fruit. Thomas[49] also mentions silicon only as part of the ingredients of wheat, without elaborating further.

With regard to nutrition, therefore, the silicic acid process is virtually unknown. And even though its importance for the skin, hair, etc. has been recognized, its true nature has yet to be grasped.

Silicic acid resists the nature forces in the digestion, thus calling forth the activity of the individual Ego-forces. Inwardly, it acts in accordance with its second task. It not only helps to put substances in the service of nutrition and growth, but it also helps make them open to processes of consciousness. Rudolf Steiner again put this precisely: "One can speak of a special silicic acid organism, as a member of the entire organism. The sensitivity of the organs to one another — a basis for healthy life processes — rests on this. In addition, it is the basis for the proper relationship of the organs to the working of soul and spirit within, and the proper sealing out of the nature forces coming from with-

257

out."[21] Mere life is suppressed, pushed back, and put into the service of a higher power — a power which not only sculpts and forms the organism, but which also forms consciousness. Silicon thus stimulates a central, human, formative process. By means of whole grains, milk (which also contains silicon), and plant foods in general, it can unfold its unique activity within the human body.

Flourine and Magnesium

We can continue by saying a few words about another trace element, often spoken of today, which has not been adequately dealt with in its relation to nutrition. This element is flourine. Rudolf Steiner was able to provide us with a knowledge of the essentials of it, even though flourine was hardly spoken of at the time.

In the first medical course[11] (given in 1920) Steiner mentions the connection between flourine and the teeth, as well as the sources of flourine in our food. Its relationship to magnesium is also touched upon. "Dissolved as they are in the human organism, flourine and magnesium play an especially prominent role in the growth of the child up to the change of teeth. The solidifying and hardening which in this case occurs in the human organism is an extended interplay of the forces of magnesium and flourine. The forces of flourine work in man like a sculptor. The magnesium forces have a radiating effect, but flourine holds back this radiation." These two substances work dynamically with each other, and both the flourine and magnesium processes are to be found throughout the entire human being. Even the teeth are formed out of the entire human formative process, and they constantly interact with it, even after they appear to be complete. In his important work on *The Degeneration of Culture and the Decay of Teeth*[56] (1962), A. Roos points to this problem and shows the relationship to our deficient food quality.

Today, we have definite information about the relationship between flourine and magnesium in the formation of the teeth. H.J. Schmidt writes that "in healthy dentine, there is a balance between flourine and magnesium,"[57] and that both substances must be present in the proper relationship for the formation of the teeth. This also holds true for calcium, which is necessary for forming teeth. Schmidt also mentions silicon — whose forces we

258

have already examined — in discussing the process of teeth formation.

In speaking of the importance of flourine with regard to nutrition, Rudolf Steiner said that it is important, "by means of a proper diet, to have an adequate intake of flourine and magnesium." At a later date, he explained that "it is not necessary to introduce fluorine in the diet, since the fluorine process is in the plants." There then follows a decisive statement: "It is only a question of the organism being so organized that it masters the extraordinarily complex process which is connected to the intake of fluorine." In practice, this means that the problem is not solved by taking in isolated fluorine, for example in drinking water or fluorine tablets. If the fluorine is to be effective, it must be taken in as part of a diet of such quality that it bears the fluorine processes within it and stimulates these processes within the human organism.

H.J. Schmidt points to an interesting study by Pazurek which relates the decreased incidence of tooth decay in school children to an increase in their consumption of whole grain rye bread. "Rye — as opposed to wheat — contains fluorine. So, in eating this wholegrain bread, the children have at their disposal all the minerals — including the decisive fluorine — which are necessary for the function of healthy teeth." Barley and millet are also rich in fluorine. Kollath gives the following values for fluorine: barley, 20-480 mg/100 g; millet 20-90; rice 67-80. A diet of wholegrains is guaranteed to stimulate the fluorine process — in conjunction with all other necessary minerals — for the formation of teeth. G. Bredemann gives a long list of foods which contain fluorine.[58]

There is another important point here. In the final lecture of his first medical course,[11] Rudolf Steiner spoke of the process of tooth formation. He pointed out its mineralizing tendency, which proceeds from within outwards. There is a movement within man which runs in the opposite direction — from outside inwards, and from front to back. This is the peristaltic movement of the intestines. These polaric movements are functionally related to each other, and "this movement of the intestines is inwardly connected to the utilization of fluorine in the human organism." To regulate this process, it may be necessary for a physician to "give the digestion something to calm it." This is done in order to correspondingly calm the movement of the intestines when a decay of the teeth is observed.

This sketchy outline — to which we shall add a few words about magnesium — shows us how comprehensive a view is necessary in order to do justice to reality.

Magnesium appears in the chlorophyll of green plants, thus revealing its relationship to the radiant force of the sunlight. When burned, its flame is even brighter than sunlight.

Its role in man is twofold. On the one hand — like calcium — it is found in the bones and teeth, and there we have the "radiating effect" which was described earlier. Its other activity is in the metabolism. It is "involved in practically all reactions of the intermediate metabolism in which a phosphorylated substrate plays a role." Magnesium thus combines with another "light-bearing substance," phosphorus, and takes part in all its vital functions, which are related to almost every active enzyme process. Its presence in the brain is also significant, and it is found especially in the nutritive substance of the grey cerebral cortex. It is also active in the lateral muscles, thus playing an essential role in the heart's activity. Finally, it has been found at the reproductive pole, in male semen. These facts are sufficient to show that magnesium is indispensible for man. The daily requirement is estimated to be 100-120 mg for adults.

Magnesium comes to us through fresh, green vegetables and salads. Wholegrain products (especially barley and rye) and milk are also important sources of magnesium. Fruit also has magnesium, so we can be assured of an adequate supply with a lacto-vegetarian diet.

Phosphorus Processes

Even modern nutritional science is aware of the tremendous significance of phosphorus for the entire metabolism. It is characteristic that most phosphorus is found in the skeleton (530 g), with a bit in the muscles (58.5 g) and only 4.6 g in the brain, in spite of its prominent role in the latter organ.

Understandably, the phosphorus metabolism is most intense in the bones, where a typical crystal (calcium phosphate) is constantly being formed and dissolved. This interplay is regulated by the parathyroid gland, which controls not only the calcium, but also the phosphorus level of the blood.

260

The role of phosphorus in the inner metabolism of carbohydrates has also been recognized, a fact which, quantitatively, applies primarily to muscle activity. However, it also has a very special relationship to the metabolism of the central nervous system from a qualitative point of view. This brings us to where we left off in Chapter 10 of *The Dynamics of Nutrition.*

We have quoted Rudolf Steiner's statement: "Phosphorus is beneficial when it is taken in with food in the right way." And we mentioned grain — especially rice — as well as hazelnuts as being especially high in phosphorus. Milk can be added to this list, as well as a lacto-vegetarian diet in general. If the food is of high quality, it can offer an adequate supply of phosphorus.

Meat and eggs are also rich in phosphorus, but these foods work in an altogether different way and contribute to the danger of an acidification of the organism. As phosphoric acid, phosphorus works toward the acid side of the pH balance.

The Key Position of Iron

The last mineral we shall look at is iron. Quantitatively, it is only a trace element, but it nonetheless occupies a key position in human metabolism. Today it is one of the best-researched mineral substances. In addition, we have Rudolf Steiner's spiritual research to thank for much of our understanding of this metal. As with silicon, there are important, anthroposophically oriented studies on iron,[59] but we shall confine ourselves to a narrow outline.

Even in ancient times, it was known that iron is necessary for human life. Thousands of years before the discovery of iron in blood ash (1713), its dietary and medicinal effects were known and applied. It was not until the 20th century, however, that a comprehensive study of iron metabolism was made. This resulted in new insight into the importance of iron for human nutrition. At the same time, Rudolf Steiner, using the methods of modern spiritual research, explained the functions of iron and offered new insights into its dietary and therapeutic applications. Meanwhile, nutritional science was also studying this subject, stimulated by the work of physiologist G. von Bunge at the turn of the century.

Iron Activity Within Man

The central activity of iron certainly takes place within the blood. It there mediates the respiration — the absorption of oxygen and the excretion of carbon dioxide. Even a relatively slight iron deficiency causes symptoms of illness. In a similar way, iron mediates the "inner respiration" — the exchange of oxygen between the blood and the organs and tissues. We must therefore speak realistically of an iron "phantom" which permeates not only the blood (both red corpuscles and plasma) but also every cell of the body in a constant, rhythmic movement.

Rudolf Steiner pointed out that iron constantly protects the blood from dissolution — i.e. it brings about a constant healing activity. By means of the crystallizing capacity of metabolic iron, the red blood corpuscle can fulfill its actual function: to connect man to the outer world, while at the same time protecting him from outer influences.

A simple fact points to the enormous intensity of the blood processes. Out of a total of roughly 25 trillion erythrocytes, some 208 billion perish every day and must be produced anew. Iron is crystallized in every one of these blood corpuscles. This stream of production and decay does not occur uniformly. Rather, it follows a 24-hour rhythm with a daily high and low point. This daily rhythm is similar to the daily rhythm in which 25,920 breaths are taken, corresponding to the number of years the sun takes to go through the entire zodiac.

Thus, by means of iron, man partakes of the life of the cosmos and at the same time impresses his earthly life with his own individuality. "The physical-sense world meets another world — one which requires the activity of supersensible systems of forces — more directly in our blood than in any other substance,"[47] explained Rudolf Steiner.

Even the process outside of the blood — in the muscles and bodily cells — serves the mediation between human and extrahuman forces. Iron battles the food we eat, especially the protein, breaking it down and destroying it so that its foreign nature — a constant source of illness — is overcome. In the human interior as well, iron serves to regulate the protein forces. It harmonizes the life processes borne by protein with the formative forces necessary for the development of consciousness. Its true home is in the

262

rhythmic system, and its activity is always one of mediation. Without iron, man could, perhaps, attain to life, but he would remain at the level of the plants. Iron makes it possible for him to incorporate his soul-spiritual aspect into his life-body. By means of iron, man's Ego incarnates in the world: it becomes a participant in earthly events.

The Significance of Nutritional Iron

This brings us to the central role of iron in the human being. The fact that we take in iron in our daily food points to its importance as a nutrient. As we see the dynamics of iron in man, we can also come to understand its significance in the soil and plant-formation processes. Rudolf Steiner once showed how plants — e.g. wild strawberries — are able to draw up traces of iron out of the soil. "The root of the strawberry is quite powerful, and it draws in traces of iron from afar."[60] Wild strawberries are thus used as a special dietary food to stimulate the blood processes.

Grains are also an important source of iron for man. Prof. A. Fleisch[61] points out that wholegrain bread has seven times more iron than bread from refined flour, and that this fact alone makes it more valuable. Barley, oats and rye are richest in iron, and wheat contains relatively less. Fleisch also writes that "during the war, the scientific management of nutrition greatly reduced the proportion of refined products, and thereby increased the amount of whole foods available." As a result, the health of the Swiss population during the war remained sound — indeed, it even improved. (Transl. Note: During the Second World War, the refinement of grain and the feeding of grain to animals were largely prohibited in order to insure the self-sufficiency of Switzerland). Especially significant was the "clear increase in hemoglobin — the red blood particles — among the 700 people tested during their conversion to a diet high in dark bread and vegetables." The average increase was 27.3% among the children and 19.3% among adults.

In 1964, B. Thomas of Berlin published a "comprehensive presentation of the bread question."[49] Regarding the iron content of grain, he presents the following analysis of grain as it is milled to make white flour, using data available up to 1962.

Wheat flour: at 60% Milling: 25.4 mg% Fe
                at 70% Milling: 44.1 mg% Fe
                at 80% Milling: 50.0 mg% Fe
                at 90% Milling: 69.0 mg% Fe

The corresponding figures for rye are 48.1, 61.1, 74.0, 87.0 mg% Fe. There is thus a clear increase in iron as the milling occurs. Thomas cited further studies of the utilization of iron with regard to how much it has been milled. According to these studies, cracked wheat bread offers twice as much iron as white bread. Experiments with animals showed that this iron "is more effectively used for growth and for the formation of hemoglobin." "The regeneration of hemoglobin in anemic rats was effectively 30% greater when they were fed wholegrain bread than when they were fed an equivalent amount of iron in the form of ash mixed with endosperm flour."

Further Activities of Iron in Man

Although the amount of iron in the human body as determined by modern research appears rather modest, quantitatively seen, it is one of the more important minerals in the body. It comes to about 5.85 grams in an adult and is distributed roughly as follows:

Hemoglobin Iron		3.25 g
Myoglobin Iron		0.6 g
Cell Haemin	circa	1 g
Plasma Iron		3—4 mg
Deposit Iron	circa	1 g

These figures are not especially valuable, but they do show us that iron is most concentrated in the blood, although it is found throughout the entire human organism. The constant renewal of red corpuscles points to the extraordinary activity and intensity of the iron metabolism.

In this regard, the liver—and especially the reticulo-endothelial system, a tissue structure especially potent in formative forces — plays a major role. It takes in the iron from the decayed red blood corpuscles and transfers it to the hemoglobin. This takes place in a daily rhythm. In the morning, during the "assimilatory

264

phase", the liver cells take in the iron. Then, in the evening, during the "secretionary phase," this iron is given over to the blood-forming areas of the bone marrow. There is thus a higher iron content in the blood serum during the morning, and a correspondingly lower concentration during the evening. It has been surmised by some that this rhythm of day and night — the great importance of which we dealt with in Chapter 5 of *The Dynamics of Nutrition* — is "directed" from a higher place. For example, one researcher says that it is "beyond a doubt that above all cosmic and other stimuli from without are in this way transmitted to the appropriate organs."[62]

This is the rhythm which Rudolf Steiner so often pointed to — the 24-hour rhythm, during which time a person breathes about 25,920 times, corresponding to the number of years needed for the sun (at the vernal equinox) to go through the entire zodiac. "You there have a rhythm in the world process which is expressed on a large scale, which is expressed in the life of the individual and which is expressed in the breathing process of a single day."[11]

It has since been discovered that this rhythm is also found in the daily building up and breaking down of human blood. Here we can see that iron itself is led over from the death processes of the decaying erythrocytes to a rebirth in the red blood corpuscles being built up with the help of the cosmic rhythmic process. Iron goes through a daily process of death and rebirth, and the director — the motive force — of this process is the human Ego itself. Indeed, Rudolf Steiner spoke of this 24-hour rhythm as the "Ego rhythm," i.e. the Ego uses this rhythm to work in the body.

What does the iron receive when it is subjected to the world of cosmic forces by means of rhythm? This is the previously mentioned "cardinal question of medicine." Indeed, the blood is constantly healed by iron. Rudolf Steiner expressed it as follows: "If we look at the blood, we look at something which — in man, because of his human constitution — tends always towards illness. Blood is simply ill by its very nature . . . The blood process is such that nature herself must constantly bring healing — nature, by means of a mineral, iron, must constantly heal the blood."[11]

This allows us to understand the recently discovered fact that there is no functional difference between young and old erythrocytes. "A 110-day-old erythrocyte is just as capable as one five days old. In contrast to the human being as a whole, the red blood corpuscles work fully until their deaths."[63] They are constantly rejuvenated and healed by means of iron, filled with cosmic formative forces.

Healing Forces Through Iron

The healing process of iron in the blood presents an arche-typal picture of the working of iron in general. We can also look at another point, presented by Rudolf Steiner and Ita Wegman in *The Fundamentals of Therapy*:[21] the nerve substance — because of its activity — undergoes a constant decay. It is known that the nerve substance, as well as red blood cells, is incapable of repro-ducing . However, the blood obtains its formative force by means of the iron activity in the erythrocytes, whereas the nerves do not have such an iron element. Nonetheless, modern research has shown that the nerve cells, especially in the so-called excited state, display a strong metabolism, expressed in a high phosphate activity. Even the energy involved in the central nervous system is relatively high, if we consider that this tissue does not do any perceptible work. For example, a person at rest uses c. 18% of his oxygen in his brain. This means that the brain requires one fifth of the body's oxygen, although at 1.6 kg it comprises less than one fortieth of the weight of a 70 kg person.

Rudolf Steiner pointed out that these nervous processes are not normal, but are, by nature, "illness processes which con-stantly permeate the organism."[11] Indeed, our organism would need a tremendous amount of oxygen if all organs had the same requirements as the brain. Our respiratory system could by no means handle this amount.

The tremendous oxygen requirement of the central nervous system shows us that a constant process of breaking down, of dying, must be compensated for. This regeneration process — i.e. external and cell respiration taken together — is dependent on the presence of iron. Iron is found not only in the hemoglobin, but also in the so-called hemic enzymes of all cells — including nerve cells. In other words, even the nerve cells require the activity of iron for their regeneration. Indeed, they need it in quite an intensive form. We here again have a process of healing which is constantly accomplished by means of iron. These iron-laden, hemic enzymes are in fact transformed blood components. Thus

266

we can say that, to the extent that this iron blood-element reaches into the nerve tissue, the healing activity of the blood extends into the illness-producing processes of the nervous system. "Illness-producing processes take place in the nerve processes. They go to the point where they are healed by the blood processes which constantly work against this."[21] This healing process is the working of iron.

The Radiant Iron Activity in the Human Organism

Iron does not only work on the upper part of man from the blood. Its activity also reaches into the metabolic processes of the lower part. In his lectures on *Occult Physiology*[47], Rudolf Steiner described how the blood process is extended into the bile process — a "dull life process" in which iron plays a special role. Bile, in turn, struggles against the incoming foodstuffs — especially the fats — in order to overcome their foreign quality. Thus, another illness-producing tendency is healed, this time from the metabolic pole. For if the foodstuffs were not overcome and divested of their foreign character by being broken down and destroyed, then their effects would extend to the interior of man. And this would cause illness.

In his first medical course[11], Steiner spoke of a "radiant iron activity" which permeates man from above and counters the stagnating protein activity. These two poles must constantly balance each other out. We need not confine our thinking here to the meeting of iron with nutritional protein: that takes place on the coarsest and lowest level. Steiner pointed out that original protein is formed by the human metabolism for the various organs. This protein stands opposed to the iron radiation, holding it back and balancing it out. "This battle is constantly taking place in the organism."[11]

Consider the peculiar fact that there is no iron in the human organism which is not connected to some protein. Is this not an image of such a polarity? These iron-protein compounds fill the entire body. Everywhere, and at all times, they must balance the tension among themselves and effect a process of healing, for protein alone would have a pathological effect within man.

During the third phase of life, between the ages of fourteen and twenty-one, it is especially important for one to find the "right balance between iron and protein." Otherwise "those

267

symptoms appear which are manifest as anemia." Protein alone cannot produce blood. "Without iron, the blood would dissolve completely."[64]

What is the actual spiritual nature of iron? What forces make use of this substance, penetrating the entire human being right into each cell? A key to answering this question can be found in Rudolf Steiner's *Occult Physiology*. He says that there is something in the red blood corpuscles which "is at the point where it makes the transition to lifelessness." Physical-chemical processes play into our blood, and "they are necessary in order for our Ego to participate in the physical world." This points to iron — an inorganic, mineral, even crystalline element — in the erythrocytes. Without iron, the blood decomposes; a deficiency (or an excess) of iron makes it ill. Metallic iron incorporates a death-element into the flowing life-forces of the blood. This makes the red blood corpuscles both sensitive and yet resistant. With protein alone, we would live, but we would *only* live, we would only fulfill vegetative functions. By means of iron, we are led right down onto the earth. Our Ego experiences the resistance of the solid earthly element in metallic iron. Thus it can develop consciousness and participate in the physical world. Rudolf Steiner's discovery here paves the way for a true understanding of the working of iron in man.

Let us now sum up: Iron permeates the entire organism. It appears in its most concentrated and mineralized form in the blood. It is always combined with protein. This iron-protein structure appears in various forms, mediating between the dull life processes and the consciousness-awakening death processes. It mediates between sleeping and waking. Its true "home" is thus in the rhythmic organism. It joins forces with the circulatory system. There, in the human blood, it first exercises its healing function — i.e. by adding the necessary mineral component to the protein there. Protein alone, as the bearer of the life function, is buoyant. The red blood corpuscles swim in the blood. By means of iron, they receive the necessary weight and earthly heaviness. This is the physiological basis for the ensoulment of our bodies; we can develop feelings in our human bodies in that we find the balance between sleeping and waking, between unconscious life conditions and consciousness-waking death forces. Since the life forces belong to the etheric body and consciousness formation to the astral body, we can understand Rudolf Steiner when he says: "In the addition to and subtraction from the iron content, we have an important regulator of the activity of blood circulation, i.e. of the interplay between the etheric and astral organisms of man."[64]

Iron in the Course of Human Life

Since iron mediates between the forces of life and consciousness, could it be that the iron content of the child's organism — which proceeds from the dominance of vegetative forces, to the development of consciousness, to the ensoulment of the body at puberty — is an expression of this fact? Recent research has come up with some interesting results in this connection. It was determined that "the iron content per kg of body weight drops down to very low values during the first years of life." In fact, "a clear iron deficiency" sets in, and the erythrocytes become hypochromic and microcytic. Even serum iron drops about 60-80%. This process continues, essentially, until the sixth year of life, although the serum iron returns to normal at about the third year. "Up to the thirteenth year, the absolute and relative amounts of iron continously increase."[62]

What can this tell us? During the first seven-year period, the child's organism grows considerably. The protein forces dominate. The milk diet of the infant contains little iron. The life of sleep and the vegetative forces are primarily engaged. At three years, a turning point occurs. The serum iron — but not the hemoglobin iron — increases. The Ego experiences its first stage of incarnation — not in the erythrocytes, in the iron crystals, but in a fluid medium, in the etheric body. At this point, said Rudolf Steiner, there is "the greatest chance for the person to get ill. The healing iron impulse is too weak with regard to the protein pole."[65]

Between the ages of eleven and thirteen, the child's weight increases about 25%, but his iron content, about 35%. Iron is victorious over protein. The person proceeds to "earthly maturity." The hemoglobin iron rises to its normal adult level. The child in puberty can now ensoul his body. His Ego can become "a participant in the physical world." The increased iron in the organism provides more of a chance to overcome illness. "When the second teeth come in, the inner predisposition to sickness ends . . . During his second life-period, man is actually healthiest in his inner

269

being." Only then does he have the capacity to develop the mediating power of iron in both directions — toward the consciousness and the life sides. For only then are both of these poles physiologically mature. This opens up a new possibility for, and danger of, illness.

Iron in Nutrition and in Diets

From the above-mentioned facts, we can see the central role played by iron in the course of a person's life, especially during childhood. Such knowledge points to the care we must take in feeding children with regard to the quality and quantity of iron (and protein as well) that they receive.

The ideal composition of iron and protein can be sought in nature, as we have seen in the case of grain and hazelnuts. In addition, almonds (4 mg%) and walnuts (3 mg%) are also rich in iron.

The iron content of nettle varies from place to place. It is remarkable for its versatility in cooking — the young leaves can be used in soup or as a vegetable, salad or seasoning. Also rich in iron are celery, radishes, apples, cherries, plums, peaches, apricots and strawberries. G.A. Schmid[6] has pointed out that ferrous (Fe^3) compounds predominate in raw, green leaves, and this makes for greater absorption through digestion.

The preparation of food also plays a central role in our relation to this vital metal. For example, the washing, cutting and peeling of vegetables can bring forth a loss of iron. This loss is dependent on time, temperature and the surface area of the food. Heating, sterilizing and drying, however, do not cause an appreciable loss of iron. Dried fruits and vegetables thus retain their iron content. In contrast, juicing and pulverizing bring on high losses of iron. For example, apples can lose up to 90% of their iron when they are made into apple sauce.[66] These facts must be considered when judging the amount of iron in one's diet.

It is often said that animal foods — meat, liver, even caviar and oysters — are high in iron. In this connection, however, we must consider the profound difference between plant and animal foods. (cf. *The Dynamics of Nutrition,* Chapter 9)

The high incidence of iron deficiency today is a symptom of the poor quality of our food in general. In West Germany, "10-12%

of the population are deficient in iron," as is "every other woman of child-bearing age." Iron deficiency is thus rightly called the most common mineral deficiency.[67] The situation is similar in other countries. Mount[68] gives similar figures for England and the U.S.A., especially for mothers and young girls.

The importance of the iron problem in nutrition is thus clear. The preparation "Fragador" is of use in assuring a proper intake and utilization of iron. It contains, among other things, iron in plant form (*Fragaria vesca, Anisum, Urtica dioica*), mineral iron (*Vivianit*) and iron-rich wheat germ. Furthermore, it stimulates the body's own iron metabolism. (It is available from Weleda, Inc., Spring Valley, New York, 10977).

Let us now turn toward the one remaining realm of substances we need to consider: that of the so-called vitamins.

References

The World of Minerals—

1. R. Tigerstedt, *Lehrbuch der Physiologie des Menschen,* Vol. I, Leipzig 1897.
2. G. v.Bunge, *Physiologie des Menschen,* 1901.
3. K. Lang, *Biochemie der Ernährung,* Darmstadt 1974.
4. H. D. Cremer, *Mineralien als Nahrungsbestandteile,* Basel 1953.
5. Rudolf Steiner, *Geisteswissenschaftliche Grundlagen zum Gedeihen der Landwirtschaft,* Dornach 1979 (GA 327). English translation, *Agriculture,* London 1977.
6. G. A. Schmid, *Sinnvolle Ernährung-Gesundes Leben,* Zürich 1933.
7. Rudolf Steiner, *Mysteriengestaltungen,* Dornach 1974 (GA 232). English translation, *Mystery Knowledge and Mystery Centers,* London 1973.
8. Rudolf Steiner, *Makrokosmos und Mikrokosmos,* Dornach 1962 (GA 119). English translation, *Macrocosm and Microcosm,* London 1968. Reference is here made to the fifth lecture.
9. Rudolf Steiner, *Theosophie,* Dornach 1978 (GA 9). English translation, *Theosophy,* New York 1971.
10. Christian Morgenstern, "Wir fanden einen Pfad," Munich, 1921.
11. Rudolf Steiner, *Geisteswissenschaft und Medizin,* Dornach 1976 (GA 312). English translation, *Spiritual Science and Medicine,* London 1975.
12. Rudolf Steiner, *Die Weltgeschichte in anthroposophischer Beleuchtung und als Grundlage der Erkenntnis des Menschengeistes,* Dornach 1980 (GA 233). English translation, *World History in the Light of Anthroposophy,* London 1977.

13. Rudolf Steiner, *Der Mensch als Zusammenklang des schaffenden, bildenden und gestaltenden Weltenwortes*, Dornach 1978 (GA 230). English translation, *Man as Symphony of the Creative Word*, London 1979.
14. M.J. Schleiden, *Die Pflanze und ihr Leben*, Leipzig 1864.
15. J.W. Goethe, *Faust*, Part 2, "Klassische Walpurgisnacht".
16. J.W. Goethe, "Sprüche in Versen".
17. J. Hamburger, *Macht und Ohnmacht der Medizin*, Munich 1973.
18. George W. Grey, *Auf Vorposten der Medizin*, Zürich 1944.
19. Rudolf Steiner, *Anthroposophie. Eine Zusammenfassung nach einundzwanzig Jahren*, Dornach 1981 (GA 234). English translation, *Anthroposophy, An Introduction*, Spring Valley 1961.
20. Documenta Geigy, "Wissenschaftliche Tabellen," Basel 1955.
21. Rudolf Steiner/Ita Wegman, *Grundlegendes für eine Erweiterung der Heilkunst nach geisteswissenschaftlichen Erkenntnissen* Dornach 1977 (GA 27). English translation, *Fundamentals of Therapy*, London 1967.
22. Snively/Sweeney, *Elektrolyt - und Wasserhaushalt*, München-Berlin 1958.
23. Rudolf Steiner, *Welt, Erde und Mensch*, Dornach 1974 (GA 105). English translation, *Universe, Earth and Man,* London 1955.
24. Rudolf Steiner, *Aegyptische Mythen und Mysterien*, Dornach 1978 (GA 106). English translation, *Egyptian Myths and Mysteries*, New York 1971.
25. Rudolf Steiner, Lecture given in Dornach, 9 February 1924, under the title "Der Flüssigkeitskreislauf der Erde im Verhältnis zum Weltall," published in *Natur und Mensch in geisteswissenschaftlicher Bertrachtung*, Dornach 1967 (GA 352).
26. A. Frey-Wyssling, *Stoffwechsel der Pflanzen*, Zürich 1949.
27. Konrad Mengel, *Ernährung und Stoffwechsel der Pflanze*, Jena 1965.
28. W. Kollath, *Getreide und Mensch*, Homburg 1964.
29. Rudolf Steiner, Lecture given in Dornach, 23 January 1924, under the title "Von der Ernährung," published in *Natur und Mensch in geisteswissenschaftlicher Betrachtung*, Dornach 1967 (GA 352).
30. M. Bircher-Benner, *Ernährungskrankheiten*, Part 2, 1942.
31. A. Welsch, *Krankenernährung*, Stuttgart 1965.
32. W. Pelikan, *Heilpflanzenkunde*, Vol. II, Dornach 1962.
33. G. Grohmann, in "Wesentliches und Weisendes zu den Heilmitteln der Weleda," Arlesheim 1961.
34. Bersin, *Biochemie der Mineral - und Spurenelemente*, Frankfurt/M. 1963.
35. Rudolf Steiner, *Das Miterleben des Jahreslaufes in vier kosmischen Imaginationen*, Dornach 1980 (GA 229). English translation, *The Four Seasons and the Archangels*, London 1968.
36. Rudolf Steiner, Lecture given in Den Haag, 15 November 1923.

37. H. Fleisch/U. Tröhler, "Kalzium bei Gesunden und Kranken," in *Schriftenreihe der Schweiz. Vereinigung für Ernährung*, Heft 18, Bern 1972.

38. Rudolf Steiner, Lecture given in Dornach, 2 December 1922, under the title "Ueber die Schilddrüse und die Hormone," published in *Ueber Gesundheit und Krankheit. Grundlagen einer geisteswissenschaftlichen Sinneslehre*, Dornach 1967 (GA 348).

39. Rudolf Steiner, Lecture given in Berlin, 21 October 1907.

40. Rudolf Steiner, *Physiologisch - Therapeutisches auf Grundlage der Geisteswissenschaft*, Dornach 1975 (GA 314). Reference is here made to a lecture given 9 October 1920.

41. O. Wolff, in "Wesentliches und Weisendes zu den Heilmitteln der Weleda," Arlesheim 1961.

42. Rudolf Steiner, Lecture given in Dornach, 17 February 1923, under the title "Vom Leben der Erde in Vergangenheit und Zukunft. Ueber Heilkräfte in der menschlichen Natur," published in *Vom Leben des Menschen und der Erde. Ueber das Wesen des Christentums*, Dornach 1980 (GA 349).

43. Neumann/Pelshenke, *Brotgetreide und Brot*, Berlin 1954.

44. K. Lang, in *Ernährungs-Umschau*, 8/1976, Frankfurt/M.

45. Rudolf Steiner, Lecture given in Dornach, 9 August 1922, published in *Die Erkenntnis des Menschenwesens nach Leib, Seele und Geist. Ueber frühe Erdzustände*, Dornach 1976 (GA 347).

46. Rauber-Kopsch, *Lehrbuch der Anatomie*, Vol. III, Leipzig 1940.

47. Rudolf Steiner, *Eine okkulte Physiologie*, Dornach 1978 (GA 128). English translation, *An Occult Physiology*, London 1951.

48. F. H. Julius, *Grundlagen einer phänomenologischen Chemie*, Part II, Stuttgart 1965.

49. B. Thomas, *Die Nähr - und Ballaststoffe der Getreidemehle in ihrer Bedeutung für die Brotnahrung*, Stuttgart 1964.

50. F. Eichholtz, *Die biologische Milchsäure*, Bad Soden.

51. H. Mennert/H. Förster, *Stoffwechselkrankheiten*, Stuttgart, 1975.

52. Rudolf Steiner, "Ueber das Wesen der Bienen", nine lectures published in GA 351. English translation, *Nine Lectures on Bees*, Spring Valley 1975.

53. "Heilmittel für typische Krankheiten", 2. Folge, Dornach 1960.

54. G. Schmidt/U. Renzenbrink, *Das Getreide als menschengemässe Nahrung*, Vol. I, Dornach 1957.

55. H. Knauer, *Erdenantlitz und Erdenstoffe*, Dornach 1961.

56. A. Roos, *Kulturzerfall und Zahnverderbnis*, Bern 1962.

57. H.J. Schmidt, *Karies-Prophylaxe durch Fluor - Therapie*, Heidelberg 1951.

58. G. Bredemann, *Biochemie und Physiologie des Fluors*, Berlin 1951.

59. "Heilmittel für typische Krankheiten," 4. Folge, Dornach 1962.

60. Rudolf Steiner, Lecture given in Dornach, 9 September 1924.

61. A. Fleisch, *Ernähren wir uns richtig?*, Stuttgart 1961.
62. W. Keiderling, u.a., *Eisenstoffwechsel*, Stuttgart 1959.
63. P.G. Frick, "Der Erythrozyt als Beispiel biologischer Zweck-mässigkeit," in *Schweiz. Med. Wochenschrift*, Heft 91, page 1245 ff, 1961.
64. Rudolf Steiner, Lecture given in Dornach, 24 October 1923, under the title "Ueber die Natur der Kometen," published in *Mensch und Welt. Das Wirken des Geistes in der Natur. Ueber das Wesen der Bienen*, Dornach 1978 (GA 351). The lecture has not been published in English.
65. Rudolf Steiner, "Anthroposophische Grundlagen für die Arznei-kunst," published in *Physiologisch - Therapeutisches auf Grundlage der Geisteswissenschaft*, Dornach 1975 (GA 314).
66. *Ernährungs - Umschau*, 4/1976, Frankfurt/M.
67. "Eisenmangel - häufiger als vermutet," in *Ernährungs -Umschau*, 9/1976, Frankfurt/M.
68. J. L. Mount, *Food and Health of Western Man*, London 1975.

The publication dates mentioned refer to the latest editions available in German and English.

Chapter VI

The So-Called Vitamins: The Necessity of Correcting Our Current Viewpoint

The Question

The observant reader will have noticed how little we have mentioned a topic of considerable interest today: that of the so-called vitamins.

Whole libraries could be filled with the literature on this subject. Yet many researchers, even today, insist that much in this field is still unclear, and that totally unexpected results may come from future research. For example, Henry Sebrell of Columbia University writes: "Although we know a lot about vitamins, it is clear that we are still at the beginning of understanding how they actually work."[1] And K. Lang[2] wrote in 1974: "The understanding of the biochemical effect of vitamins is at present insufficient... We have only an inadequate idea about the human requirements for vitamins."

In spite of such clear indications, however, there is no other field of nutrition which has even approached vitamin research in public interest, with the result that many "dilettante" views have been widespread.

How did this come about? What are these so-called vitamins in the opinions of those who have researched them? How has this research developed? What help can a spiritual-scientific method of consideration offer in coming to grips with this problem?

The History of Vitamin Research

It does not come as a surprise that vitamin research began only during the end of the last century, under rather peculiar

275

circumstances. At that time the classical nutrients had been discovered and characterized in a primitive way. Proteins, carbohydrates and fats were recognized as "energy carriers," and their "caloric values" were determined. A *terra incognita* — described in the last chapter — was entered into, as various minerals were discovered to be both necessary and yet devoid of caloric value. At the same time, substances were discovered which would take on the name of "hormones". "It was discovered that a whole series of endocrine glands — pineal, mucus, thyroid, adrenal etc. — produce one or more hormones which influence the function or development of other parts of the body. These substances appeared to be catalysts, and were extremely potent."[3] Thus writes R. Shyrock, who also notes the astonishing fact that adrenaline, isolated from the adrenal glands, is still effective in a dilution of 1:300,000,000. Regarding the similarly potent thyroid, he writes: "This tiny pinch of substance determines either complete idiocy or normal mental capacities."

These discoveries paved the way for a search for similar "subtle" substances in nutrition. Lunau is credited as being the first researcher in this field. His experiments with milk in 1881 attracted much attention and gave his research its initial direction. Lunau was a student of G.v. Bunge who, as we have seen, did much research on milk.

Bunge refused to recognize new, special substances called "vitamins." For most researchers, however, it was only natural that they should adhere to the notion of matter — even if "subtle" — and thus proceed in their original direction.

From the beginning, vitamin research recognized dynamic effects; tremendous effects were induced with tiny amounts of substance and, along with enzymes and hormones, "vitamins" were classified as catalysts. Moreover, mineral research had to learn to deal with "traces" of substance. Although the facts themselves brought scientists to the verge of a dynamic approach, materialistic thinking — the materialistic mode of consideration — still prevailed.

When Funk coined the word "vitamin" in 1911, the path to a proper consideration of these substances was already blocked. He succumbed to a double error. First, these substances are not chemical "amines," as he thought. Second, and more important, he confused the material bearer of certain forces with the forces

276

themselves, not seeing that the former are merely the expression of the latter. The whole of vitamin research thus went down a one-sided path.

Methodological Viewpoints

In Chapter I, we spoke of Rudolf Steiner's answer to the research which was formally established by Drummond in 1920. It is worthwhile for us to look again at Steiner's lecture to physicians (January 3, 1924)[4], where he tried to show young doctors and medical students what prerequisites are necessary for grasping the actual functions of the human organism. "Thus, I can't know anything about the significance of an organ by merely observing it alone, as is common today. I must consider it in relation to the whole organism . . . To begin with, we need a viewpoint of man entirely different from that which comes from chemistry and merely investigates chemical affinities and forces." He then goes on to speak of milk research. "What have these people done? They have said: milk not only has these components which we know, but also another substance, vitamins. They had to posit another, extremely subtle substance — the vitamin. They invented this substance."

One should not jump to the erroneous conclusion that Rudolf Steiner refused to recognize the so-called vitamin substances which were then isolated. Rather, he questioned the method involved: that of killing, isolating and chemically analyzing living organs to obtain substances which were then said to be responsible for various organic activities. In reality, these substances were, at most, the remnants of an interplay between organic activities and their material carriers. It is similar to taking apart a watch and spreading the parts out before oneself. But "the watch is what the thought of the watch-maker has made it. And, when looking at milk and its components, the thought of the 'watch-maker' is that earthly qualities are contained in the components, the qualities which the individual parts derive from the earth." For, by means of analysis, these components are torn out of their living connections — out of the original quality of formative forces from which they were created and remained active.

In this regard, Wilhelm Pelikan said that "all of these substances are denatured — i.e. spoiled — some more quickly, others more slowly . . . Upon being denatured, they approach a condition which the modern chemist can grasp, formulate and synthesize."[5]

Vitamins also decay and become ineffective as soon as they are removed from the subtle framework of the living organism. Actually, they are "directive functions of the life-processes which are joined to the element of formative forces — the etheric body."[5]

These formative forces constitute the etheric organization of every plant and can continue to be effective when a foodstuff is prepared (e.g. cleaned, cooked, etc.), but not when the individual components are removed and used as ingredients. The forces belong to a world which is opposite to the physical, earthly world — a world which is centripetal rather then centrifugal. Thus, the chemistry of living things is different from the chemistry of earthly things. Rudolf Steiner coined the term "antichemistry" to describe it. And it is here that we find the true nutritive forces. This brings us back to a discussion of the dynamics of substance.

"One must have the resolve to do more than just accept the existence of these things. It's not a question of something hidden being discovered. Such things — like vitamins — they are inventions, by means of which people simply state what is already there. A whole new way of looking at these things must take hold."[4]

Still, vitamin research was pursued in the old, inadequate way until, after more than fifty years of remarkable work, the final conclusion was "that we still are just beginning to understand how they [vitamins] really work."

It had to come about that conscientious researchers learned to recognize the limits of their methods and to confess a certain uncertainty, e.g. regarding the "effective mechanism" as well as the "minimum requirements" of certain substances. As early as 1963, W. Kraut wrote: "In scientific discussion, one must be aware of the uncertainty regarding vitamins: the variations in their presence in food stuffs and, even more importantly, the still greater variations in the requirements of different people, and in the same individual under different circumstances."[6] K. Lang, in 1974, wrote that "our orientation regarding the requirements for vitamins among human beings is, in the strict sense of the word, inadequate . . . for the vitamin requirements are not static quantities, but are, rather, variable."[3] Yet, in spite of this, all too many "experts" act as if they could give exact "vitamin"

278

requirements — especially to the general public.

K. Muenzel, writing in the *Vitamin Compendium Roche, 1968*[1], made a significant contribution in this regard. He deals with the problem of how such substances are synthesized and combined into so-called "multiple vitamins." He discovered that even in the synthetic vitamins, the individual components can react with each other. "The chemical interactions, especially among the water-soluble vitamins and their functional groups, lead more or less quickly to changes in the molecules, and thus to a loss of the particular vitamin effect. This disadvantageous interaction occurs not only among the vitamins, but also between the vitamins and other substances . . ." such as dyes, sweeteners, and stablizers.

As a result, in spite of a reasonably high "practical stability," the "efficacy of the active ingredients [in synthetic vitamins] invariably diminishes." For this reason, an excess of active ingredients — usually 10% to 60% — is added, in addition to various artificial stabilizers. Because of the sensitivity of many vitamins, a guarantee of stability is possible only if an excess is added."

This shows us that the public is faced with impenetrable factors in buying these preparations, since a scientific control of their efficacy in human beings is quite impossible. More important, we also see that even with the greatest technical mastery, these substances can be subjected to chemical and physical laws only with tremendous exertion, because these laws are essentially foreign to them. In spite of the large expenditures for tests on rats and human beings — which occur under quite artificial conditions — it is easy to see how many illusions are connected with the modern vitamin industry.

There also remains the important question of multiple vitamins. It is said that "the chemical interactions" among the various vitamins decrease their efficacy, and that these "vitamins" must be artificially isolated from one another. The question thus arises: how does nature herself do it, where everything is in a constant state of interaction, and every grain of cereal, every vegetable, is a sort of "multiple vitamin"? Are the substances isolated in living beings, or do they work in a way different from their artificial imitations? Or could it be that their activity is altogether different from anything that can be explained by chemical models? Could it be that a whole different play of forces

279

is at work in living beings than we find in the whole ABC of vitamins produced from the test tube — a play of forces which cannot be grasped by such a method? In any event, Rudolf Steiner's statement appears all the more justified: "An entirely different way of looking at things must take hold . . ."

It is well-known that a qualitatively and quantitatively adequate diet presents no problem regarding a "vitamin deficiency." G.A. Schmid is certainly right when he says, "With a careful — even if not very plentiful — diet of naturally nutritious and mostly fresh food, a person's vitamin requirements are easily met."[7] We would put it differently. There is no question of vitamins. The real question is: how do we obtain the necessary forces through our nutrition?

It is "the reaction within us against the foodstuffs, which we actually experience as that which stimulates us and supports our life."[8]

New Insights

Recently, modern research itself has left the old path and come to some new conceptions of vitamins. In light of the problems with multiple vitamins, researchers are beginning to realize that these substances can only be seen in the living interplay of a dynamic whole. For the most part, they are effective merely by their material presence — as so-called catalysts, mediators, stimulators and "directors" of various processes, often involving many other links in a complicated chain.

The *Vitamin Compendium, Roche, 1970* is useful here. Regarding vitamins, these "agents necessary for life," we read that they "mediate the processes of building up and breaking down without themselves being used as building material . . . In contrast to nutrients — which are the building blocks and storage material of the organism — vitamins function as catalysts . . . Research into these biochemical processes is in full swing . . ."[9]

A basic insight begins to emerge here. In the final analysis, the whole complexity of functions of enzymes, hormones, vitamins and trace elements (which were historically researched at the same time) belongs to *one* realm of a higher order. Thus, even the material extracts are intricately interrelated, and all are expressions of higher forces and activities. It is still a long way to this insight, however, and questionable whether modern researchers will dare take such a big step.

The fact that the production of so-called vitamins is connected to a person's receiving an adequate amount of sunlight could lead one to see cosmic influences at work here. We spoke of this matter in connection with calcium and so-called vitamin D. The situation with so-called vitamin A is similar.

All this, however, should not keep us from seeing that modern vitamin research is a strong expression of materialism, and that modern humanity is subjected to this senseless "vitamin hullabaloo" because it has become incapable of applying a "different mode of consideration." Vitamins have thus become an expression of our western civilization. A pharmacist in the USA once expressed this by saying, "When a customer asks me for a vitamin preparation, then I know that he has succumbed to western materialism. If he asks for a soya product, then his world view, as a rule, comes from eastern occultism." This complex issue will form the basis for our last chapter.

First, let us take a practical example from modern vitamin research and try to show how Rudolf Steiner employed this "other mode of consideration." This example takes us to the ubiquitous so-called vitamin C — ascorbic acid — and the disease known as the scourge of the sea, scurvy.

The Other Mode of Consideration

The disease called "scurvy" appears to have been known in Greece. Pliny gives an exact description of it in his *Historia Naturalis* (70 A.D.). Especially interesting is the mention made, in a tenth century Norwegian saga, of the disease "skyrbjugr." It is assumed that this is related to the German word "Schorbuk" or "Scharbock", from the fifteenth century, which can be traced back to the Latin "scorbutus." In 1531, J. Echt published his work *De Scorbuto,* and in 1663, Moellenbrock published a compendium of medicinal herbs, wherein spoonwort is described as a remedy for scurvy. Spoonwort — called scurvy grass, or *Cochlearia* in Latin — is an old remedy for scurvy.

This points us to something significant. The medieval doctors and practitioners obviously knew about the inner connection between this plant and scurvy, and they were able to heal the disease as a result.

Such knowledge grew out of instinctive forces. In our time, light has been shed on this subject from two sides. In his first medical course (1920)[10], Rudolf Steiner pointed to spoonwort, but without referring to traditional lore. He described its effects as the result of modern spiritual-scientific research. His point of departure was a description of the protein process in man and plants and its opposite, the salt process, as expressed in the potassium and sodium salts. From there, he went on to a desription of *Cochlearia officinalis* — scurvy grass. "This plant is also interesting to study; it contains sulfur-like and sulfurous oils." This points to a property, typical of the cruciferous plants, which makes them suited as medicinal herbs (e.g. watercress, horse radish, shepherd's purse). But the main thing is that these sulfurous oils work on the plant's protein, causing an acceleration in protein formation, because sulfur fires up the metabolism and stimulates the formative forces: "Sulfur, introduced as a medicine, makes the phsyical activities of the organism more suitable to the working of the etheric . . ."[11]

Scurvy grass grows especially well along the sea shore. It there becomes a salty plant, bringing forth the counter-process of sulfur, a kind of holding back of the protein process. These two tendencies — the "sluggish protein process" and the "accelerated protein process" — bring about a balance in *Cochlearia* "by means of an amazing natural instinct." The reason for its medicinal properties is to be found here: "There is a constant working together of the sluggish principle of inertia and the principle of acceleration in the growth of scurvy grass. This makes spoonwort (because of its inner relationship to the disease) especially suitable in cases of, say, scurvy. For the process at work in scurvy is remarkably similar to the process I have just described."

This statement by Rudolf Steiner points us to the true nature both of the disease, scurvy and of the healing process by means of *Cochlearia*. Perhaps it also opens a door to the question of so-called vitamin C.

What are the symptoms of scurvy? Weakness, exhaustion, decreased productivity, sometimes stunted growth, and in the acute stages, hemorrhaging in the entire body, as an expression of the impaired mesenchyma function.

The mesenchyma — as K. Lang notes — plays a key role in both scurvy and in the normal functions of so-called vitamin C.

282

It is a connective tissue which appears during the early embryonic stages and forms the first intercellular fluid. Dr. Stark[12] described it as follows: "The mesenchyma tissue with its intercellular fluid has a special significance in the young germ with regard to the movement and exchange of matter. It eases the especially intensive metabolic processes of the upbuilding period... The mesenchymal cells are capable of amoeba-like movement..." It is universal in character: from it proceed many differentiated tissues such as cartilage, bone and dentine on the one hand, vascular, intestinal and skeletal muscles on the other hand, as well as lymphosytes and red blood corpuscles. The mesenchyma thus has a tremendous formative capability. It is the site of an inexhaustible formative-force activity which lasts all during life. At the same time, it is a sphere of action of protein, as we have described in a previous chapter.

With scurvy, these formative forces are diminished and hindered, a result of what Rudolf Steiner — in speaking of scurvy grass — described as the sluggish "inertial principle" of the salt pole, as opposed to the "acceleration principle" of the sulfur pole. This sluggishness of the formative forces results from a one-sided diet: a deficiency of fresh fruit, vegetables and plant formative-forces in general. The descriptions of scurvy epidemics on ships, etc. make this clear. When Winkelmann[13], for example, described the south pole exploration of Amundsen, he mentioned that "as many fruits and vegetables as at all possible were taken." Lemons and oranges have been known for centuries as "anti-scurvy foods." They prevented scurvy — i.e. they stimulated the formative-force activity of the mesenchyma so that it could develop adequately even under various pressures. Thus, the balance between the salt pole — the hardening forces of form — and the sulfur pole — the dissolving forces of fire — could remain intact. Scurvy grass produces this balance by its very nature, and is thus an effective remedy for scurvy.

Folk medicine also describes *Cochlearia* as effective against bleeding gums and bloody noses, as a stimulant of liver and kidneys, and as "an excellent remedy against scurvy."[14]

And modern chemistry has also made an interesting discovery: scurvy grass, like many cruciferous plants, is an important and rich source of vitamin C.

In his work on medicinal plants, Wilhelm Pelikan writes that "the salt processes, rising up through the root, want to express the 'radiating' earthly forces. But the sulfur forces 'hold together the organizing forces of the protein substance', i.e. they support the activity of the formative-force organization . . . (and) accelerate the life rhythm . . ."[15] As Rudolf Steiner said, the activities in the organism are made "more acceptable to the entering of the etheric formative process." Thus we may assume that the formative process — which can be isolated from scurvy grass in the form of "vitamin C" — is related to this balance between inertial and accelerated protein formation. In the final analysis, all production of this "ascorbic acid" in living beings is the result of a living etheric interplay and is truly significant only when such formative activity is at work.

We might ask: what was known in 1920 about vitamin C? This was the year that the name "vitamin C" was introduced, although Funk, in 1912, had already spoken of an "antiscurvy vitamin." It was not chemically isolated until 1933, after which date it could be chemically synthesized. Vitamin C was discovered in the organism as "ascorbic acid" which becomes oxalic acid — a substance formed in the growing tissues of all plants — which Rudolf Steiner described as the foundation for etheric activity.

Ascorbic acid is thus understandably very sensitive. It is found primarily in plants, especially in buckthorn, rosehips, and sulfur-rich vegetables like cabbages and cress. And it is not surprising that the above-mentioned dietary aid — "Fragador" — contains *Cochlearia*.

By using the example of scurvy grass, we hoped to show how, in past times, instinctive insight penetrated the processes in the plant and thus came to a real understanding of nutrition and medicines. This old knowledge has been lost. It was replaced by a chemical-analytical natural science, whose child is modern vitamin research. The latter — in spite of its many successes — had no alternative but to remain at the most elementary stage as regards reality because it has been one-sidedly fixated on dead substance. In contrast, the spiritual research of Rudolf Steiner renewed the old insights through the forces of consciousness, combining these insights with the attitude of natural science. The result can be seen in a most persuasive way if we are aware of these considerations; they bear witness to the "entirely different mode of consideration" which must take hold, especially regarding the so-called vitamins.

Above all, we come to realize that we are called to free ourselves from "vitamin thinking" — to overcome it, and to replace it with a dynamic method which allows us to see into the reality of nutrition.

In a lecture to workers[16] in 1923, Rudolf Steiner spoke of the oxalic-formic acid process. Is it mere coincidence that he there spoke of the milk experiments of Bunge's pupils which seem to have resulted in a "new scientific discovery in the modern style — the vitamin?" He then goes on to speak of scurvy — "a very ugly disease." Patients could not be healed by the individual, isolated components of milk. "They weren't cured by any of it — not by any of the components." But when the components are together (in specially prepared milk), they can, indeed cure scurvy. The individual components cannot heal — only the whole can heal. Why? Because the "whole" is "within the etheric body." And if we separate it and analyze the parts, what remains? — The vitamin.

We see here that Rudolf Steiner's perceptions were up-to-date with the other research of his time. We also see that he used this "other mode of consideration" and sought to bring it to his audience. In this light, then, do we really need to go into the widespread synthetically prepared vitamins? These pseudo-substances may be called "vitamins" and their effects may be described, but they no longer have much connection to the living forces in nature and in man.

References
The so-called Vitamins —

1. *Vitamine 1967-1968,* Roche, Basel 1968.
2. K. Lang, *Biochemie der Ernährung,* Darmstadt 1974.
3. R. Shryock, *Entwicklung der modernen Medizin,* Stuttgart 1947.
4. Rudolf Steiner, Lecture given in Dornach, 3 January 1924, published in *Meditative Betrachtungen und Anleitungen zur Vertiefung der Heilkunst,* Dornach 1967 (GA 316).
5. W. Pelikan, "Von den Vitaminen," in *Der Sanddorn* Arlesheim 1964.

6. W. Kraut, *Vitamine*, 1963.
7. E.A. Schmid, *Sinnvolle Ernährung-gesundes Leben*, Zürich 1953.
8. Rudolf Steiner, Lecture given in Dornach, 6 January 1922, under the title "Die körperliche Erziehung im besonderen," published in *Die gesunde Entwicklung des Leiblich-Physischen als Grundlage der freien Entfaltung des Seelisch-Geistigen*, Dornach 1978 (GA 303). English translation, *Lectures to Teachers*, London 1948.
9. *Vitamin-Kompendium*, Hoffmann-La Roche, Basel 1970.
10. Rudolf Steiner, *Geisteswissenschaft und Medizin*, Dornach 1976 (GA 312). English translation, *Spiritual Science and Medicine*, London 1975.
11. Rudolf Steiner/Ita Wegman, *Grundlegendes für eine Erweiterung der Heilkunst nach geisteswissenschaftlichen Erkenntnissen*, Dornach 1977 (GA 27). English translation, *Fundamentals of Therapy*, London 1967.
12. D. Stark, *Embryologie*, Stuttgart 1955.
13. Winkelmann, *Die Vitamine*, Basel 1951.
14. Dinand, *Taschenbuch der Heilpflanzen*, Esslingen 1929.
15. W. Pelikan, *Heilpflanzenkunde*, Band 1, Dornach 1958.
16. Rudolf Steiner, "Ueber das Wesen der Bienen," a series of nine lectures published in *Mensch und Welt. Das Wirken des Geistes in der Natur. Ueber das Wesen der Bienen.*, Dornach 1978 (GA 351). English translation, *Nine Lectures on Bees*, Spring Valley 1975.

The publication dates mentioned refer to the latest editions available in German and English.

Chapter VII

Nutrition in the East and West:
The Hygienic Task of the Middle

Our Knowledge of Nutrition:
Inherited Traditions and New Beliefs

Our present-day nutrition has grown out of the occidental cultures throughout thousands of years. The foods spoken of in this book for the most part stem from this inheritance of post-Atlantean times. The breeding of the seven grains, the cultivation of our various fruits from wild fruit, the cultivation of olive trees, sugar cane, honey — in a word, everything which forms the basis of our nutrition — stand as a mighty and plentiful inheritance from the past. Without this, our present nutrition would be inconceivable.

The broad spectrum of our present nutrition bears unmistakable signs of influence from the eastern as well as from the western cultures. Rice came from the east; corn from the west. Sugar cane was brought by Alexander the Great from India, and potatoes were brought to Europe by the explorers of the western hemisphere at the dawn of the new age. Many vegetables — to say nothing of herbs and spices — came to us from ancient cultures. And let us not forget the domestic animals — milk cows, sheep, goats, etc. — which have come to us.

This rich inheritance flowed together and formed the foundation of western nutritional culture up to the threshold of the twentieth century. But, during the last third of the nineteenth century, there occurred a profound change: the emergence of technical thinking, which grew rapidly as the result of natural-scientific research. Thus, true materialism became firmly established, molding western man and heavily influencing his nutrition. Only what the "five senses" and the intellect could grasp was seen to be of any value, and the knowledge grasped in this way was raised to the status of a new, infallible authority. What can be grasped through the senses and calculating thinking has actually become the new idol of our century, and unlimited recognition of this idol has been demanded of everyone. Such thinking became the basis of all modern schooling, which every small child has to take up. Thus, in place of the old, faded, spiritual idea of God, a new authority was set up, one which exercised an even greater influence on man, compelling him to submit unconditionally to a new infallible dogma based on statistics and computation.

"The experience gathered through natural science has the great advantage of being tested and obtained by everyone. Not only that, but it also makes the claim — based on its methodological procedure — of being *the only certain experience,* and of being the knowledge before which every experience must prove its legitimacy."[1] Thus did H.G. Gadamer describe the task of "a new anthropology." He limits the concept of objective "experience" to what can be experienced through the senses, thus agreeing with Kant.

In its time, this sort of thinking was progressive; it brought a new, comprehensive world-view to the continuing shadow of tradition, speculation and subjectivity. One of the consequences for human nutrition can be expressed in the saying:"Man is what he eats." A new belief came to the old tradition.

"Concentration on Things of This World"

The above-mentioned saying, though over a hundred years old, can still be heard today. During the 1840's, the German philosopher Ludwig Feuerbach, describing his materialistic world-view, predicted the end of philosophy. He coined the saying which — like his whole philosophy — found both passionate approval and disapproval among his contemporaries. Researchers like Moleschott and Buechner not only saw it as a new insight into the relationship between man and nature. "Concentration on this world" was demanded by Feuerbach in his writings. "Only a sense-perceptible being is a true and real being." Above all,

288

Feuerbach fought against traditional theology, though he also took issue with the philosophy of Hegel. He accepted the thesis — both new and justified at that time — of "making man the object of philosophy" and, indeed, its "sole, universal and highest object."[2] Because he rejected any separation of body and spirit or mind, he came to such one-sided conclusions as are reflected in the above sentence. Nonetheless, he performed a service in directing attention to man's actual experience instead of getting lost in metaphysical speculation. He thus presented the logical philosophical consequence to a development which had long since been made in natural science. Rudolf Steiner speaks about Feuerbach, in this connection, in his *Riddles of Philosophy.*[2]

Feuerbach's "radical world view" exercised tremendous influence on Ludwig Buechner, whose book, *Force and Matter,* moved in triumph through the educated world at that time. Beuchner was a physician, and he saw Feuerbach's philosophical orientation toward man as a duty for medical thinking as well. He saw his own "raw materialism" confirmed in Feurbach's thinking. In working to increase the albeit one-sided results of natural science, Buechner helped spread the conviction that "without an understanding of the results of natural science and of the methods by which these results are obtained, no comprehensive world-view is possible today."[3] Thus did Rudolf Steiner speak of Buechner, in an essay published after his death in 1899. Steiner added, however, that the relationship between "matter and force," indisputably proven by experience, actually "finds its explanation through the phenomena of the spirit." Only then can one come "to an understanding of the relationship between the brain and the consciousness." Buechner considered it a fact "that matter contains not only physical, but also spiritual forces . . .," although there is "no spirit without matter" and "no matter without spirit." He thus described his world-view as "neither idealistic, spiritualistic nor materialistic, but rather as simply natural."

Thus, even before the turn of the century, we find points of departure which could have gone beyond the dogma of the one-sided and exclusive validity of sense experience. Although such insights have never been silenced, they have not, as yet, broken the bonds laid on them by natural science.

For example, P. Vogler writes: "One can affirm natural-scientific methods, as well as the knowledge gained by these methods, without expecting to find man as a totality in the individual scientific facts."[4] He thus discovered the boundaries of the scientific method but could not bring himself to consider another method. H.G. Gadamer is also aware of this threshold. He writes:[1] "It seems reasonable to me to imagine a perfect cybernetics, where the distinction between man and machine would really dissolve. Our knowledge of human beings, then, would reach its fulfillment if it were able to produce such 'machine men.' Here, we should take Steinbruch's warning to heart: that there are basically 'no insights from the fields of cybernetics and linquistics which point to any difference between what man *can* do, and what automata *cannot* do." Does this not point to the cleft between the science of the sense-perceptible and the reality of man? "Thus today, we see science itself coming into conflict with our consciousness of human worth." Not only the "horrible prospects" of modern genetic research and the "hideous picture" of the destructive force of atomic energy stand before his mind's eye. "More and more, the atom bomb is proving to be just one particular instance of the world-wide self-endangerment of human life on this planet which science has led to."[1] This is the result of Feuerbach's "concentration on 'this world'." We put the question: is nutritional science an exception to all this, or is it also leading to a similar abyss? This question appears appropriate today, and we shall try to answer it in the light of our subject.

Technical Thinking in Nutrition

There is no doubt about it: "technical thinking" has become the ruling principle of nutritional science. And western civilization has produced this thinking. The warmth technology (drying) of the last century was followed by the cold technology (refrigeration) of this. There arose "convenience foods" and technically processed foods of various types. In America, the output of frozen food has exceeded ten billion pounds annually, compared to 325 million pounds in 1939. Then there is the ever-growing — and increasingly unsurveyable — host of artificial additives: flavorings, colorings, vitamins, stabilizers and preservatives. The American *Dictionary of Nutrition* (1975)[5] tells us that "some 10,000 chemicals are used in America for these purposes." In his book on *The Food and Health of Western Man,*[6] J.L. Mount cites seven prophecies for the year 2,000 made by prominent individuals:

1) economic synthesis of amino acids and protein;
2) economic synthesis of sugar, fat and carbohydrates;
3) economic synthesis of all known vitamins and flavorings;
4) profitable extraction of protein from leaves and weeds, and the production of protein from micro-organisms;
5) all consumer goods provided in plastic and "stay-fresh" packages;
6) prepared meals available from automats;
7) food produced from a mixture of natural derivatives (e.g. leaf protein) and artificial products (e.g. synthetic fat).

This dramatic — or even apocalyptic — perspective is well on its way to being realized. Indeed, there is hardly a person in any civilized country who really understands what he eats.

In 1967 George Borgstrom wrote: "In order to deal with the biggest problem of our time, we first have to free ourselves from our technical thinking."[7] The analytic method— the basis of all technology — allows us only an "analytic mosaic," but "never a realistic picture" of the human being. "A total picture must be created, with regard to the nutritional requirements and physiological constitution of man as well as to the social fabric." Yet, no one can say how to create this total picture, because no one has dared attack the problem at its roots.

Even Borgstrom has little to say here. He simply notes that "by the end of the century, the total weight of artificial fertilizer used will be greater than the total weight of all the human beings on earth . . ." — unless the price of oil changes the calculation. Borgstrom does not even question what quality of food would then result.

Rudolf Steiner, however, addressed this matter in 1924, in a prophetic way. He spoke of fertilizer as "among the most interesting things." There are "really extraordinary mysteries" there. And the "materialistic farmer" who "thinks about these things somewhat" can "calculate about how many decades it will be in this century before agricultural products have degenerated so far that they can no longer be used for human nutrition." For "with the materialistic world conception, agriculture has come the furthest from rational principles."[8]

Anyone who looks at the development of nutrition since 1924 would have to agree that the same statement could be made about nutrition as well as agriculture.

The Eating Behavior of Western Man

Another point is also important in this regard. One often hears of the problem of mass food-consumption today. There is talk of the inner attitude of man toward eating or, to use a modern catch-phrase, of the behavioral psychology of nutrition. H. Glatzel,[9] for example, has made an earnest, if inadequate, attempt to address this problem. He begins by announcing that the concept of behavioral research comes from the field of zoology, and thus makes clear how one-sided this research is. Moreover, his image of the human being *vis a vis* nutrition is largely influenced by the materialism of the nineteenth and twentieth centuries. Thus, V. Pudel[10] is justified in complaining that "human nutrition is considered almost exclusively from a technological or physiological point of view." He then asserts that "unfortunately, civilized man — like the laboratory rat — has formed many eating habits . . . which are not in harmony with the needs of his body." Granted, the results he cites are based on experiments where people were treated more like laboratory rabbits than like human beings, but this very fact points to a significant aspect of the way man eats today. People today are unable to form sound judgments. For example, Pudel states: "To begin with, the physiological aspect is of no concern to the eater. The better a meal tastes the more favorably will he judge it — and he will adjust his behavior accordingly. Taste is a factor which can lead to human behavior which is contrary to biological requirements. Unhealthy foods are gladly eaten as long as they taste good."

We considered this problem in *The Dynamics of Nutrition* and will now look at it from another angle. It goes without saying that we need tasty food; we are instinctively led to it in order to attain those forces necessary for existence on earth. Hunger and thirst have, in themselves, an objective character. But it is a sign of an extensive loss of instinct that today they are overpowered by the subjective element. The objective nutritional needs are thus separated from the subjective desire for pleasure.

Pudel also points to another side of the problem, that of "nervous over-eating." He writes: "About 30% of the population —

292

most of them women — react to psychological tension, conflicts, overwork, frustration, fear, and even to boredom, with an increase in appetite."[10] Other people, though, react with a decreased appetite. We greatly see here how nutrition can be influenced by subjective impressions, a recognizable characteristic of modern western man.

Let us again cite Pudel: "Today we can prepare a meal for ourselves at any time and under any conditions. It is simply a question of money, and not one of adequate technology."[10] This fact is, in itself, not new. What is new is that it applies to practically everyone today, rather than to a privileged few. And this is an achievement of western civilization. "These situations, to put it harshly, corrupt our inner regulation of appetite and satisfaction. We are forced to deal with improper nutrition and over-eating."

The Socio-Economic Aspect of Nutrition

There is another vital element which needs to be considered. We have spoken of the rise of western technology which has profoundly changed our nutrition by increasingly removing man from his position as the measure of all things. Along with this technology have arisen socio-economic models which have achieved an awesome mastery within the last few decades. We thus come, from the mechanization of nutrition itself, to the principles of modern economics. They have led to tremendous concentrations of power — a kind of world rulership of nearly unsurveyable dimensions. These concentrations of power have been methodically formed into effective instruments for controlling the food supply of the entire world.

One example is the international wheat trade. It is handled by a few large American firms which hold a virtual world monopoly amongst themselves. There can be no doubt that this is used to serve certain political, social and economic goals. On one hand, the USA and Soviet Russia (i.e. west and east) work together here, perhaps toward certain hidden ends. On the other hand, the disparity between the rich and poor nations is used (*via* the so-called north-south dialogue) in order to secure for certain countries an "economic and political dominance" such as has never existed before. A report from the American CIA[11] says that "Washington would then practically have the power of life and death over the people in needy countries."

293

In reality, the methods used to control the food market are applied virtually undisguised in order to secure a monopoly for certain institutions. This is coupled with enormous speculation.

For example, special methods of advertising have been developed in order to alter people's life-habits in a certain direction. In Mexico, for example, such methods were used to reduce the percentage of breast-fed babies from 98% (in 1960) to 40% (in 1968). The supposedly superior value of high-technology baby formulas was impressed on the population by means of such advertising.[12]

Moreover, in spite of widespread, so-called "developmental assistance," it is doubtful that hunger has really been reduced in the world. The report of a U.S. Senate committee on "Nutrition and the International Situation" reads: "We do not distribute our food surpluses to those who need them most, but rather according to our foreign policy interests."[13] One could begin to doubt that there are any truly humanitarian impulses at work in this field.

Much of what we have touched upon here is called "the inheritance of colonialism", "neo-colonialism", "capitalist power grabbing" etc. It is then contrasted to "socialism in the economic, political and cultural-educational realm" which would supposedly represent the true interests of "the poor and oppressed." Let us guard ourselves from such over-simplified views. In reality, all of these views and methods are cast from the die of the same materialistic world view. So-called monopoly capitalism and socialism are thus merely two different systems or methods for achieving the same thing: the hindrance of true spiritual and cultural progress.

Spiritual-Scientific Considerations

Present-day nutritional behavior is a symptom of the current soul-spiritual situation of humanity in general. Man has left the protection of a realm of instincts previously in harmony with higher beings. He has thus fallen into a lack of direction, as he seeks increasingly to follow the animal side of his nature. One may speak of a "lack of purpose" in eating, but we need to go even beyond that concept to arrive at the essence of the situation. As we have shown, there is a well-founded pleasure in eating. In earlier times people enjoyed their generally nutritious food and thus experienced the unity of their subjective and objective nutritional needs. This was expressed in a grace, such as the following:

> The bread is not our food.
> What us in bread does feed
> Is God's eternal Word,
> Is spirit and life indeed.

Such prayers brought about an attitude in the soul, when people ate, of following not only their personal psychological needs but also their super-personal spiritual needs. To put it in spiritual-scientific terms: "Man has higher pleasures because, in addition to his three bodily members [his animal organization] he has a fourth, the Ego." However, the Ego can be subject to forces "which bring about desires which do not stem from the sense-world, yet can only be satisfied by the senses." To be sure, man's Ego wants and needs to "enjoy the spiritual in the sensory." But, to the extent that "the Ego has produced [these desires] for some purpose other than serving the spirit" — to the extent that the forces that we take in with our food are not of a spiritual nature which furthers our existence as human beings on the earth — eating becomes what modern behavioral research calls "purposeless." "The Ego is removed from the true spiritual reality of the world to the extent that its desires in the sense-world do not stem from the spirit."[14]

The reader will surely recognize Rudolf Steiner's reasoning here. The phrases above were taken from his basic work, *An Outline of Occult Science* (1909). He goes on to say: "A sensory pleasure which is an expression of the spirit signifies an ascent and development of the Ego. One that is not an expression of the spirit signifies a corresponding impoverishment and decline." This is the enormous danger which western civilization faces today.

Rudolf Steiner approached this question elsewhere: "Eating and drinking are done every day on impulse, from instinct. It really takes a very long time before someone who is evolving spiritually, so to speak, includes these things in his spiritual life ... For eating and drinking will only be included when we can understand why we need to rhythmically ingest physical substance in order to serve the progress of the entire world. Furthermore, we must understand the relationship of physical substance to the spiritual life, and the ways in which the metabolism is not only physical, but also spiritual because of its rhythms."[15] In this way "we get into the habit of not just letting eating be a physical

295

fact. We get into the habit of recognizing, for example, the role played by the spirit when a fruit ripens in the sun . . ."

These words point to a concrete task of modern man, that of finding a new hygienic impulse. Let us first consider how western materialism has resulted in this separation of the subjective needs of the soul and the objective needs of the spirit. This separation has resulted not only in a theoretical-intellectual dependence, but also in a physical dependence on matter. For "a person becomes a materialist when he is completely dependent on matter, when his soul is compelled to follow the needs dictated by life. That is a completely different materialism from the one which merely lives in thoughts and ideas."[15]

This materialism is especially entrenched in the west, where the highest ideals are the enjoyment of earthly possessions, material well-being and the mastery of matter and machines. It is expressed in nutrition in two ways: the technical processing and, when possible, the artificial synthesis of foods on the one hand, and the intensification of the pleasure in food by means of the clever manipulation of human instincts and the "sophisticated" packaging of food on the other hand. Ultimately, as we shall see in the next section, western man strives by those means for eternal existence on earth.

"Physical Immortality" Through Nutrition in the West

This striving towards immortality comes to expression in a peculiar way in Dr. Reymond Bernard's book, *Creation of the Superman*.[16] It has been very popular in America and may thus be viewed as symptomatic. This book announces "the immortality of the physical body on earth" as a goal to be striven for both through occult means and through nutrition. "Immortality can be achieved now, in the physical world." "One fifth of our brain cells are inactive as a result of poisoning by wrong nutrition." Bernard claims that, by rejuvenating our body through hygienic practices, we can overcome death — i.e. heal the diseases of old age. The "dead food" of the present is to be replaced by food which contains "the elixir of eternal youth."

What diet is to help bring this about? Bernard develops a vegetarian diet, albeit on an altogether different basis from the

296

one which we put forth. He condemns all meat because of the toxic effect which leads to death, aging and sickness in man. In addition, he condemns milk and especially milk products like curds, cheese and butter, recommending instead peanut butter, all other legumes for their protein content, and various seeds like sesame, sunflower and pumpkin.

He also has an interesting attitude toward bread. "Eating bread, like drinking alcohol, is a perverse habit," since both produce arteriosclerosis. Wholewheat bread especially promotes acidity in the blood, and Bernard contrasts it to raw sweet corn, which he considers to be the healthiest grain.

It is not surprising to see refined sugar eliminated from this diet, although it is noteworthy that table salt is also forbidden as a purely mineral substance which man cannot digest and which therefore has a hardening effect. On the other hand, "organic minerals" and "vitamins" are highly touted. Bernard also rejects all cooked food, since "cooked food is dead." This also applies to all preserved foods.

His "healthy diet" is then divided into seven steps which a person is to attain one at a time: the "bloodless, fleshless" diet, the vegetarian diet, the raw food diet, the raw fruit and nut diet and then the two "truly healthy" diets of raw fruits and vegetables and, finally of raw fruit alone.

Curiously, an eighth diet is added to these seven: the "cosmic ray diet." It is the nutrition of the superman who — no longer needing earthly food — has only cosmic rays as the source of his life and nutrition. "Only the cosmic ray diet makes physical immortality possible."

The errors, illusions and absurdities in this theory are obvious. Yet it is typical of the tendency in the west today to strive for an eternal life on earth, free from sickness, old age and the difficulties of normal life on earth.

The whole thing is surrounded by a certain idea of "eugenics" which strives to give the newborn child a brain which is capable of physical immortality.

Clearly we are dealing here with a theory drawing on ancient sources of occult wisdom, but it is full of misunderstandings, distortions, absurdities. Just think of our discussion of the importance of milk, the necessity of table salt for human thinking, or the animal-like quality of legumes. A raw food diet is important

297

as a therapy, yet even then it needs to be complemented by cooked foods in order to stimulate the inner "warmth man". Finally, the "cosmic ray diet" is a distorted allusion to the "cosmic nutrition" we spoke of in *The Dynamics of Nutrition.*

This nutritional concept is a symptom of the tendency in the west to promote an eternal physical existence. At the same time, however, it points to certain streams coming from the far east with increasing strength. The Masdasnan and Oshawa diets, Macrobiotics etc. appeal especially to young people yearning for a world-view which can free them from the oppressive weight of materialism.

Let us therefore turn to these movements, looking at some symptomatic examples which can reveal their general tendencies.

"Liberation from Earth Existence" Through Eastern Nutritional Practices

We here come to an opposite nutritional goal which consists in freeing one's self from "the four principles of earthly life" — birth, death, old age and sickness — by means of certain yoga techniques and their corresponding nutritional practices. The striving is to become free of these "earthly principles" until one lives exclusively in the spiritual world, since we do not belong to the "categories of past, present and future" but rather to eternity. One must therefore fully renounce materialism in order to attain the 3 H's: happy, holy and healthy. The person who treads this path will, in the end, achieve "Krishna Consciousness" and transform this life of birth, death, sickness and old age into an immortal life.[17]

Here we see a tendency opposite to that of the west. Earthly life with its burdens appears as a misfortune and a deception, keeping us from spiritual reality. Nutrition, therefore, should purify us and free us from these earthly burdens.

The macrobiotic system, on the other hand, does not pursue this end directly. Rather, it promises, by means of its diet, "health and eternal happiness, the art of longevity and rejuvenation," and unification with the "invisible treasure inherited from the ancestors: the All-one principle of freedom, health, happiness and world peace."[18]

The diet which is to realize these aims has "ten types of eating

298

and drinking", with the principles of yin and yang being of primary significance. Every food is either yin or yang, and it is a question of finding "a good balance" between them. Once you know how to evaluate a food, it is no longer difficult to eat "properly". Here again, almost all animal products — including butter, cheese and milk — are to be avoided. Animal protein is first to be reduced and then eliminated. At the seventh, highest level, there remain only cereals. "All animal protein is avoided for biological and physiological reasons. Thinking human beings are to be created . . . Only through thinking does one attain to understanding, health and happiness. Correct thinking is yin-yang thinking. Yin-yang thinking is the key to the kingdom of heaven."[18]

This teaching is doubtless based on deep insight into the essence of man and nature. It has, however, been frozen and reduced to dogma and is, in many respects, as little understood as the above-mentioned western diets. Above all, it no longer corresponds to the human constitution today — especially in western man.

Humanity today does not need rules, but knowledge and insight, not fixed traditions, but the development of new capacities, not an escapist "key to the kingdom of heaven", but the carrying of the spiritual into the earthly realm. The goal of eastern occult teaching (e.g. the Buddhist path of liberation) is the elimination of suffering and the "thirst which draws one into re-birth", and the attainment of nirvana. "Nirvana is the extinguishing of the individual, the liberating knowledge that there is no 'I' and no 'my'."[19]

A diet of rice is most appropriate to this end. It has been the standard grain in the far east for thousands of years and holds "first place" in the macrobiotic diet. All other food is merely preparation for the great goal of "satori, or the kingdom of heaven." One thus learns a sure path of eating one's way into heaven! Of course, the nature of this "heaven" is not clearly described. However, if it refers to a state of consciousness, one can be sure that it is not appropriate for our developmental epoch.

Eastern Teachings in the Light of Modern Spiritual Research

It is interesting to find "thinking" emphasized in works, such as Oshawa's, inspired from the east. This thinking is experienced as the spiritual in man, which at the same time reflects the spiritual in the universe. This spiritual element is yang, the heavenly, illumining, cosmic thinking, corresponding to the human head (i.e. to be found above), seen only through spiritual but never through physical means. It is an element through which "man feels himself to be a member of the entire universe."[20] In ancient times, as this thinking stood at the beginning of its development, yoga was a path to this "thinking", to this "grasping of the world in ideas." At that time, nutrition also served this goal. Rudolf Steiner emphasized the fact that "by means of rice, man is made into a thinker."[21] Since then, however, this thinking has become a general property of humanity. It has become individualized and abstract on its way to becoming the intellect. "What we find today on the street was then achieved through tremendous effort." Rudolf Steiner arrived at this insight through an exact spiritual study of the ancient eastern spiritual streams. He then had to say: "To expect a human soul today to live in Brahma, to expect that of a human soul living in the west today — that is an anachronism; it is sheer nonsense."[22] For "the man of the west today already has that which the man of the *Bhagavad Gita* sought. He has it in his concepts and ideas." Then "man had an altogether different spititual and soul constitution." It passively surrendered itself to an absorption in world-thinking. Today, however, we "must exert ourselves to be active" in order to fill our abstract concepts with spiritual content again.

Yoga made use of breathing in order that one might live in this world-thinking. "In his ascent to super-sensible vision, the oriental yogi wove together conscious breathing with conscious thinking." Modern day man can no longer do this. "He must, by means of meditation, raise thinking from a merely logical life to one of perception . . . The Oriental once experienced the world within himself, and he still retains an echo of this in his spiritual life. The man of the west is at the beginning of his experience. He is on the way to finding himself in the world. If a westerner were

300

to become a yogi, he would have to be a tremendous egotist. For nature has already given him the feeling of self which the easterner had only in a dreamlike way."[23] Thus Rudolf Steiner described the contrast between the way of the ancient east and that of modern times, an insight which also applies to nutrition. We can no longer blindly follow the ancient macrobiotic system as if in a dream. Rather, we must work to achieve a new conscious knowledge of man and food. And we must learn which foods serve the present-day spiritual development of man, and why they do so. For this end, conscious knowledge and freedom are necessary.

Let us again emphasize the fact that a lofty wisdom was certainly living in these ancient oriental teachings, and that it extended into the field of nutrition. What was valid in ancient times, however, is not necessarily so today. Rudolf Steiner provides some examples of this in his lectures on the *Bhagavad Gita*.[22] The ancient Indian called all plant food "soft, gentle food". To him, the average diet today would be "sharp and sour". Today "dark food" ("Tamas") is basically meat and meat products, but for the ancient Indian, who thought in a very different way, "Tamas food" was something which we would now not even consider as food — namely "what is rotten, foul and putrid."

The false overestimation of soybeans also belongs to this chapter. Oshawa, for example, recommends feeding even small children with "kokkoh" — a product of rice and soybeans — although he of course also recommends many foods still of value today. As we said, a spiritual theory of nutrition was once at the basis of such diets.

How can people of today not only achieve a sound judgment about the nutritional tendencies in the east and west, but also come to a new view of nutrition in harmony with the times and with the spiritual nature of man and the world? This question leads us to something of extreme importance: understanding the hygienic task of central Europe.

The Concept of Health in West and East

We must look at the concept of health in order to answer such questions. As we said in *The Dynamics of Nutrition*, every concept of health must come to terms with the problem of aging and dying.

301

The modern concept of health — as it has arisen under the influence of western civilization — is essentially determined by a materialistic view of the world. In 1755, an English physician said: "Health is the state of being whole and unharmed. Health is also the freedom from infirmity, pain and illness." He called health "a spiritual and moral well-being, a state of liberation, purity and goodness, or the grace of God," thus attempting to include man as a soul-spiritual being with man as a bodily being in the striving for health.

Modern concepts of health have grown much more abstract. They speak, for example, of a "state of complete physiological, mental and social well-being." Who could we then call healthy? A technologist in London, Prof. Thring, made an attempt to graphically portray "happiness." He found that, with increasing technology and its application, general "happiness" no longer increases. In fact, it begins to decline. "Instead of bad nutrition from shortages, we have bad nutrition from overconsumption and overweight," wrote M. Pyke, commenting on this issue in his book *Bread for Four Billion*.[24]

What is the basic attitude in the west toward health? Ivan Illich[25] writes: "Progress in medicine meant the constant striving to improve human health through ever new technology, to eliminate suffering and illness, and to increase the span of life." This is symptomatic of what we mentioned before: the striving to produce the "superman", to attain physical immortality, and to eliminate everything spiritual. What is here called "hygienics" is an attempt to eliminate sickness and suffering whether through medicines, drugs, innoculations or what have you. Man should no longer be subject to the possibility of sickness or pain, since these disturb his "happiness". Thus, the goal of all striving for health is the elimination of sickness, old age, suffering and death.

We met these "four principles of earthly life" in discussing the eastern concept of health, where their elimination was also proclaimed as an ideal: the overcoming of the bondage to the earth through the attainment of spiritual immortality — or, perhaps, "unborn-ness". Ultimately, nutrition should serve to free a person from having to incarnate again on the earth. Thus, there would no longer be any suffering, illness or death.

Now let us leave these two illusory concepts of health and try to find one in accordance with reality. We shall have unexpected

302

help on this path. For example, the Austrian poet Peter Rosegger[26] wrote a remarkable essay on this subject at the turn of the century, characterizing much that dominates our striving for health even today. "Many people have made it their life's task to live for their health. Never have there been so many health associations, health pamphlets, journals and books, as today . . . Health is the best! This is the first article of faith of those who, when they have health, really don't know how to use it." Rudolf Steiner also spoke of such a "health fever". "With how many means, and in how many ways, do most people today struggle for health?"[27] But what is health in reality?

Rosegger had already described how superficial and one-sided certain views of health can be in our time. In addition, the theories of nutrition arising from such views are often laden with human egotism. Above all, a realistic view of the human being is lacking — a view which can lead to a realistic nutrition. Unprejudiced observation should confirm a statement made by Rudolf Steiner in 1907: "Everything is health-bringing which causes a person to make himself a center of creativity and production."[28]

Here, the entire human personality is called upon in its spiritual, soul, and bodily nature; it is called to activity, productivity and the accomplishment of something positive.

Ivan Illich also calls upon such a force when he emphasizes the "mobilization of the forces of self-healing" instead of the "health-impairing removal of responsibility" and the "total care" which appear as tendencies in modern medicine.[25] Some examples may help to clarify these matters.

A Realistic Striving for Health

In the last few decades, western medicine has been increasingly occupied with the question of so-called immunity. For example, people are given inoculations to make them immune to certain diseases. A weak virus may be used, calling forth an immunological reaction in the body which then supposedly protects the person against the more serious form of the disease. The overcoming of these viruses, which act as "poison" within the person, give him resistance or immunity. These immunological forces are also at work in another way, as can be seen especially well in cases of transplants, e.g. of skin tissue. It then frequently happens

303

that the tissue is not accepted but rejected by the organism. The justified conclusion from this is "that every person is capable of differentiating foreign cells from his own,"[29] an insight which forms the basis of the concept of "immunological individuality." "These distinctive marks of our individuality are found in every one of our cells ... thus every one of the billions of cells in our body bears our reflection."[28] We are here faced with an extremely interesting phenomenon, which shows how our Ego-organization forms everything in us, right down into the physical body. Here again, resistance — the defensive reaction — is the central element. Since the basis for it is inherited, we may assume that man has gained this faculty in the course of his evolution. Among animals, this faculty applies only to species and not to individual animals within one species.

Along with these forces of resistance is "a system of surveillance and suppression." This "consists of a host of some 20 billion specialized cells which circulate ceaselessly throughout the organism, going into every last corner." These are the lymphocytes and other similar cells.

We see that the entire human organism grows strong in resisting elements in its environment — whether these are viruses, bacteria, allergenics, or other bearers of forces foreign to the body. These forces of resistance are developed at all times and in all places. We could even say that the entire external world is "poison" for man. Every other force, substance, being or person is a "poison" to him, which must be resisted and overcome. Yet, at the same time, this "poisoning" is a "de-poisoning", or, to put it in other words, a process of becoming sick and then healthy. Whether this "poison" comes directly or indirectly, as a substance or as a force, it is taken into the organism, digested, and overcome, and thus we are enriched, developed and strengthened. "What we have thus taken in from outer nature makes us strong and is of use to us," said Rudolf Steiner. He then added an important result of his research: "Spiritual science shows us that the entire human organism is built up — if you will — solely of things which were originally poison."[30] Our individuality in the realm of earthly corporeality is thus born from learning to overcome and differentiate ourselves from the environment. This is the process of poisoning and de-poisoning.

Steiner goes on to say: "We obtained the ability to eat the foods we do today, in that we learned to make ourselves immune to their harmful influences. We become all the more strong, to the extent that we incorporate substances into ourselves in this way. And we make ourselves weak with regard to nature when we reject her substances."[30]

This throws an important light on the fact, shown by modern research, that, although many of our food crops contain more or less "poisonous" substances, we have learned to overcome many of these substances and are strengthened each time we overcome or "detoxify" them. Thus, these substances are not basically "undesirable plant substances found in our natural foods," as K. Lang described them.[31] Rather, these various poisonous substances call forth the human Ego-nature. By giving us the possibility of getting sick, they also give us the ability to get well.

This brings us to an important insight which Rudolf Steiner put as follows: "Every possibility of becoming strong in the face of outer influences rests on the possibility of taking on illness — of becoming ill. Thus, *illness is the precondition of health.*"[30] He went on to say: "It is not possible to avoid sickness if one wants to have health."

This profound knowledge led Rudolf Steiner to the creation of a realistic concept of health which can be of tremendous significance for the whole field of nutrition as well. We must learn to interpret these words correctly, however, or they can lead to misunderstandings and error.

It is clear that only the possibility of becoming ill gives us the possibility of attaining health. Thus, at every moment, we are "healthy" in another way, just as every person has his own individual health. Health is just as individual as immunity, as the physiological individuality. Health is also a constantly-attained balance of all of man's forces and the members of his being — it is a unity. Health is a force which has been wrested from sickness, suffering and pain. Peter Rosegger's statement still rings true: "The happiest time is that of convalescence."[26]

The art of life and nutrition demands that we take in what furthers this convalescence: only as much "poison" as we can overcome, only those "poisons" which we are up to dealing with, only those "poisons" which further our lives today, rather than those which make us ill.

305

Seen in this light, the problem of food crops is "anthropo-centric". For — through the wisdom of nature or the artfulness of man — edible plants have been directed toward man. If we learn to cultivate and care for them, in a way appropriate to each species, then they will have a healing effect. They will be similarly healing if they are prepared, combined and eaten in the quantities which man is prepared for.

Of course there are undesirable substances which have come into our food as the residues of pesticides, fertilizers or environmental pollution, e.g. lead, mercury, and many others. Not only is man not up to these substances, but they also do not belong in his food, they are alien to his nature. They can only be used to a limited extent, and then only if properly extracted and prepared as medicines.

Practical Examples

Substances such as hemoglutin, which can be found in soybeans, led Pythagoras to the important saying: "Keep away from beans!" They are alien to the actual nature of plants. They have taken an animal-like quality, and we are not able to deal with them: they pose a hindering force within us when we eat them. Let us remember that the "artificial meat" developed in the west is made of soya precisely because it is similar to animal flesh. Here, the west has taken up something from the east, something which also belongs to the character of the western materialistic striving for health. Even a so-called vegetarian is thus able to have artificial meat from soybeans, prepared with chicken-breast flavor!

Among the "undesirable" substances in plants is one which is extremely poisonous, hydrocyanic acid. It is significant that about one thousand different plants, from some ninety families, are known to contain hydrocyanic acid. For example, the amygdalin found in bitter almonds has actually led to fatal poisonings. It is interesting to note that all rose-like plants bear some kind of hydrocyanic acid process, at least for a while. When the seed comes to the earth, however, the cyanide disappears; it is deadened — detoxified — by the earth forces. This leads us to ask if, perhaps, cyanide does not come from the earth at all. Natural science has long had an answer to this: every meteor contains cyanide, and it brings this tremendously potent poison down to the earth from the cosmos. Blackthorn — a rosaceous plant — has cyanic acid in its seeds, and thus "poisons" itself in a very subtle way. When we eat the fruit of plants which contain cyanide, our liver has to exercise a process of detoxification, a process of resisting the poison. If the liver cannot do this, it becomes ill. In the process of overcoming the poison, however, the liver actually becomes healthy. We also know that meteors contain cyanide in addition to the three metals, iron, cobalt and nickel. This discovery was made by Rudolf Steiner in 1906,[30] long before natural scientists came to it themselves. Moreover, spiritual science could determine the significance of this cyanide for the earth and man. Meteoric substance is actually a condensation of sun forces, as we have shown; its activity in man leads to a constant stimulation of the human will-forces through the liver.

Steiner spoke of these spiritual-scientific results in a lecture to workers in Dornach.[32] He said that we should turn our attention to the process of constant combination and dissolution of carbon and nitrogen (the components of cyanide). These substances are necessary, he said, because "in order for us even to live, there must be a constant poisoning within us, and also a constant de-poisoning." Here again, we see the basic theme: "Sickness is the necessary precondition of health." We also see the meterors (and comets as well) which bear this process to the earth as "the heroes of freedom in the universe. They contain that substance which, in the human being, is connected with free activity — with the activity of the will." Cyanide, in conjunction with iron, stimulates the will-forces in man.

We should also add that Steiner saw a great importance in almond milk and recommended adding one bitter almond to each ten or twelve almonds. This brings forth a controlled process of poisoning and de-poisoning — one which we can handle — and can thus strengthen our health and will-forces.

There are many other examples, such as oxalic acid, which is converted to formic acid in man (cf. chapter 5), another process of poisoning and de-poisoning. Here again, it is a question of the dosage. Unripe fruit, for example, contains more oxalic acid than we can overcome, and we thus instinctively avoid it.

Timely Nutritional Hygiene in Accordance with the Spirit

Such considerations give us insight into the true process of health, which is more comprehensive than one might at first imagine. Here again our thoughts meet those of Rosegger who, from a different point of view, and yet with a healthy human intellect, was able to approach the problem. "Precisely for self-development, for strengthening the will and character, for equanimity in viewing the world, for appreciating existence, occasional illness is better than constant health, which can lead only to superficial and self-seeking men."[26]

We come ever closer to a true striving for health in recognizing that "it is not possible to escape illness if one wishes to be healthy." "Human life is identical to a process of illness", as well as to "a process of health" which we gain in the struggle with the former.[33] This realistic striving for health is stimulated and supported by our daily nutrition. Today, however, we must increasingly develop a consciousness of what we are connecting ourselves to when we eat. Whether they come from the earth or from the cosmos, we must understand those forces which stimulate us to a de-poisoning, to an overcoming of illness: in a word, to becoming healthy. We need insight into how our food should be prepared, how much of it we should eat, and how it should be combined.

This would become a true "macrobiotics", a dynamic theory of nutrition based on a science expanded through spiritual science. Such a view, as we have striven to present in this book, can free us from all dogma of east and west: dogma which would enchant us either into trying to eliminate illness in order to have an eternal, "healthy" life on earth (the western dogma), or into attempting to escape the earth and illness, in order to attain eternal health (the eastern dogma).

Neither approach can further our ultimate goals as human beings on earth. Between the east and west there is a hygienic impulse of the center which longs to be established as a unifying force that can bridge the gulf in the right way. It can allow a true striving for health — in accordance with the times — to develop beyond everything that pertains merely to nation and race. Both east (working from the past) and west (working towards the future) have valuable contributions to make.

308

The lofty wisdom living in the ancient cultures of India, Persia, Egypt and Greece show us what man is capable of, spiritually. This spirituality was, however, born out of a dreamlike clairvoyance which had to disappear if man were to attain to freedom, independence and an individual spirituality; it developed into intellect and thinking, from which our modern natural and nutritional science proceeded, in its abstract, materialistic form. As a result, man as the "measure of things" was lost to us in the field of nutrition, replaced by the machine, calories, chemical synthesis and even by so-called vitamins. At the same time, the human will lost its guidance and is now increasingly threatened with being lost in the abyss of subhuman drives.

In this connection, Rudolf Steiner pointed to an important symptom which has become more pronounced since his time. In his lectures in Vienna on *The Tension Between East and West*[22], he spoke of a "very clear difference between the language of the European physiologists, and that of the American physiologists." The American physiologists would speak, for example, of the human brain in connection with the development of the will. They would then conclude that "if you want to know the individuality of a person, you must look to his will . . ."

This tendency appears to have developed in an important way since then. For instance, we spoke of the American physiologist, Roger Williams[34]. He was the first westerner to speak of the biochemical individuality of the human being, and even wrote a whole book on the subject. In this book he speaks of the human metabolic organization, which forms the basis for the will. In the chapter on "Individuality in Nutrition", he concludes that every human individual has his own nutritional needs and physiological requirements. Thus, the "wisdom of eating" is one of the fundamental "wisdoms of our bodies." Through it, we reestablish the biochemical individuality in us with every meal, creating the basis not only for unfolding our thinking, but for unfolding our willing as well.

The American neurologist, J.C. Eccles[35], comes to a similar conclusion from a different point of view. Coming from neurophysiology to the question of human self-consciousness, he concluded that "the doctrine of materialism" must be rejected, that "the uniqueness of my consciously experienced self goes back to the uniqueness of my genetic make up." Processes in the material world are "necessary, but not sufficient conditions for conscious experiences and for a conscious experience of myself." Thus, there is "no scientific basis for rejecting the possibility of an after-life." This refers neither to making the present physical body eternal, nor to retreating back to a body-free existence. Rather, we have here a statement which comes from an experience of the immortality of the human Ego-consciousness, as such. Eccles' book then comes to an interesting conclusion: "Fundamental problems, such as the role of the brain-mind liason during perception or free will, remain outside the realm of all imaginable research." But then he adds: "It appears as though these problems can only be solved at the expense of changing science in a way which is, as yet, hardly imaginable."

Here we have no *ignorabimus,* no unconquerable limit to knowledge, no materialistic narrowness. Rather, it is a fore-shadowing—and even a hope for—future research into the human individuality, right down into his biochemical individuality. Once again, the problem of free will is noted as the cardinal prob-lem of human, self-conscious existence, leading to the insight that "by studying the will, one must penetrate to the soul-spiritual element in man."[23] Thus did Rudolf Steiner speak of the human will as a mystery of the future which western materialism — in studying metabolism and nutrition — will bring to light. Steiner went on: "Thus, one might say that our own America is man's instinctive leaning towards the human will forces." It is the re-gion where the center can come to know the essential nature of the west, where "Europe and America can meet in agreement." And we begin to build a bridge to the ancient wisdom of the far east when we fill our own thinking — which has been rigidified as intellect — with a new vitality. This was begun by Goethe, continued by Hegel, Fichte, and Schelling, and developed by Rudolf Steiner as the fundamental method of modern spiritual science. Through it, we shall be able to found a genuine nutri-tional hygiene in accord with the times and with the spirit — an impulse which can stand as a center between east and west, and which will have, as its middle point, a new concept of health.

Oshawa has written of a "meeting between the far east and the far west, which could lead to a new civilization,"[18] but he is unable to build the bridge to such a meeting. Still, the path to this meeting is present today. It must be recognized and realized

310

through the impulse springing from the spiritual center. Such is the path that can lead out of the present catastrophic situation: a situation of hunger, improper nutrition and over-eating.

What we call "experience" is today still considered by many to come only from the physical senses and from the intellect. Through modern spiritual science, however, we see that experience can reach with certainty into the realm of the super-sensible, the realm beyond the physical senses. Such awareness must become a basis of the new nutritional hygiene, a new "dynamics of nutrition."

Today, we are called upon to grasp the key for overcoming the urgent problems of our time. In this vein, we cite a passage from a lecture by Rudolf Steiner[36] given under different external conditions, yet under the same inner circumstances we may find at present:

> The fact that humanity is in a more desperate situation today than it has been in the past is not due to physical causes. Rather, it is due to the spiritual attitude of man himself. If people are in grave danger today, it is because of a false application of the mind — because of false thinking. In order to overcome this dire situation, nothing else will work except to replace false thinking with true thinking . . .

We must come to terms, from many different angles, with this superstition: that if people can only have bread, and enough of it, then their thinking will also be improved.

This book represents a modest attempt to find a way out of the tremendous nutritional difficulties of our time. We adhere here to the insight that "because trouble is caused by the incorrect thinking of man, only correct thinking can alleviate man's troubles."

The materialistic "success thinking" of the modern west which has infiltrated the entire world is incapable of "correct" thinking. Equally incapable are the ancient spiritual treasures from the east, which are anachronistic today. Rather, such "correct" thinking must come out of the present-day spiritual life. Moreover, it must be capable of seeing that "everything external and physical can only be understood . . . when it is seen as an image of something super-sensible and spiritual."[37] It must see that, in the matter which we consume as our daily food, there is an infinite fullness of spiritual forces and effects. Only such cognitive capacities, and the strength for accepting responsi-

311

bility, can free man from the catastrophe which looms as a danger in the present-day nutritional situation.

The writers of the new report to the "Club of Rome" are therefore right in saying that "human society today stands before a task of heretofore unknown dimensions with regard to the problem of nutrition."[38] Our troubles will be overcome only if we can progress from insight into nutrition to daily nutritional practices which are in accord with the spirit.

References
Eastern and Western Nutrition—

1. H.G. Gadamer, "Aufgabe einer neuen Anthropologie," in *Neue Anthropologie*, Band 1, Stuttgart 1972.
2. Ludwig Feuerbach, *Rudolf Steiner: Die Rätsel der Philosophie*, 1901.
3. Rudolf Steiner, Essay on Ludwig Büchner, published in *Gesammelte Aufsätze zur Kultur-und-Zeitgeschichte 1887-1901*, Dornach 1966 (GA 31).
4. P. Vogler, "Disziplinärer Methodenkontext und Menschenbild," in *Neue Anthropologie*, Band 1, Stuttgart 1972.
5. Ashley/Duggal, *Dictionary of Nutrition*, New York 1976.
6. J.L. Mount, *The Food and Health of Western Man*, London 1975.
7. G. Borgström, *Der Hungrige Planet*, 1965.
8. Rudolf Steiner, Lecture given in Koberwitz, 16 June 1924, published in *Geisteswissenschaftliche Grundlagen zum Gedeihen der Landwirtschaft*, Dornach 1979 (GA 327). English translation, *Agriculture*, London 1977.
9. H. Glatzel, *Verhaltensphysiologie der Ernährung*, München 1973.
10. V. Pudel, "Wie erlebt der Esser seine Essensgeschichte?" in *Der massenverpflegte Mensch*, Knorr Caterplan Symposium, 1976.
11. *Weizen als Waffe*, Hamburg 1976.
12. R.H. Strahm, *Ueberentwicklung-Unterentwicklung*, Stein bei Nürnberg, 1975.
13. A.M. Holenstein/J. Power, *Hunger, Welternährung zwischen Hoffnung und Skandal*, Frankfurt/M. 1976.
14. Rudolf Steiner, *Geheimwissenschaft im Umriss*, Dornach 1977 (GA 13). English translation, *Occult Science-An Outline*, Spring Valley, 1972.
15. Rudolf Steiner, *Exkurse in das Gebiet des Markus-Evangeliums*, Dornach 1963 (GA 124). English translation, *Background to the Gospel of St. Mark*, London 1968. Reference is here made to the seventh lecture given in Berlin, 28 February 1911.

16. Reymond Bernard, *Creation of Superman*, Moketumne Hill, CA 1970.
17. *Easy Journey to Other Planets*, New York 1975.
18. G. Oshawa, *Zen Makrobiotik*, Hamburg 1971.
19. J. Wunderli, *Schritte nach innen,* Freiburg 1975.
20. Rudolf Steiner, *Die Naturwissenschaft und die weltgeschichtliche Entwicklung der Menschheit seit dem Altertum*, Dornach 1969 (GA 325) Reference is here made to the lecture given in Stuttgart, 22 May 1921.
21. Rudolf Steiner, Lecture given on nutrition in 1905. No other details given in the German text.
22. Rudolf Steiner, *Die okkulten Grundlagen der Bhagavad Gita,*

The publication dates mentioned refer to the latest editions available in German and English.

Typesetting — The Printer (William J. McLaughlin)
Book Production — Bookmaster — (H.L. Cartter)
Text Paper — 60# smooth opaque
Cover — 17 point Kivar 3, Linen Finish
Book Manufacturing — Thomson-Shore, Inc.